Infant and Toddler Mental Health

Models of Clinical Intervention With Infants and Their Families

Infant and Toddler Mental Health

Models of Clinical Intervention
With Infants and Their Families

Edited by

J. Martín Maldonado-Durán, M.D.

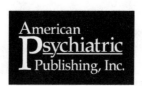

Washington, DC
London, England

Manufactured in Canada on acid-free paper
06 05 04 03 02   5 4 3 2 1
First Edition

American Psychiatric Publishing, Inc.
1400 K Street, N.W.
Washington, DC 20005
www.appi.org

Library of Congress Cataloging-in-Publication Data
Infant and toddler mental health : models of clinical intervention with infants and their families / edited by J. Martín Maldonado-Durán.—1st ed.
    p. ; cm.
  Includes bibliographical references and index.
  ISBN 1-58562-086-6 (alk. paper)
  1. Infants—Mental health. 2. Toddlers—Mental health. 3. Family psychotherapy. 4. Parent and child. 5. Mental illness. I. Maldonado-Durán, J. Martín.
  [DNLM: 1. Mental Health—Child. 2. Mental Health—Infant.
3. Family Therapy. 4. Mental Disorders—therapy—Child. 5. Mental Disorders—therapy—Infant. 6. Parent-Child Disorders—Infant.
WS 105.5.M3 I428 2002]
RJ502.5 .I465 2002
618.92′89—dc21
                                                    2002067892

British Library Cataloguing in Publication Data
A CIP record is available from the British Library.

Dedicated to Maria-Raquel, Maria-Ximena, and Ana-Marcela

Contents

I

Theoretical
Framework

II

Therapeutic Approaches to Relationships and Their Disturbances

III

Therapeutic Approaches to Psychophysiological Disturbances

IV
Illustrative Case Examples

Contributors

Kathryn E. Barnard, R.N., Ph.D.

Professor of Nursing and Adjunct Professor of Psychology; Affiliate, Center for Human Development and Disability, University of Washington, Seattle, Washington, U.S.A.

J. Armando Barriguete, M.D.

Staff Psychiatrist, Eating Disorders Clinic, Instituto Nacional de la Nutrición, México City, Mexico; Visiting Professor Paris XIII University, Paris, France; Professor and Director Euro-America Virtual University France-Mexico

Efrain Bleiberg, M.D.

Director, Child and Family Center, Menninger Clinic; Faculty, Karl Menninger School of Psychiatry and Mental Health Sciences, Topeka, Kansas, U.S.A.

Alice Eberhart-Wright, M.A.

Clinical Infant/Family Specialist, Region VII Head Start Quality Improvement Center, Community Development Institute, Raytown, Missouri, U.S.A.

Elizabeth Fivaz-Depeursinge, Ph.D., P.D., M.E.R.

Professor of Clinical Ethology and Co-Director, Center for Family Studies, University of Lausanne School of Medicine, Lausanne, Switzerland

Peter Fonagy, Ph.D., F.B.A.

Sigmund Freud Memorial Professor, University College, and Director of Research, Anna Freud Centre, London, U.K.; Director, Child and Family Center, Menninger Clinic, Topeka, Kansas, U.S.A.

J. Miguel Hoffmann, M.D.

Director, Center for Human Development, Buenos Aires, Argentina; Vice President, World Association for Infant Mental Health

Teresa Lartigue, Ph.D.

Researcher, Reproductive Health Center, National Institute of Perinatology; Researcher, National System for Investigators, National Council for Science and Technology; Child Psychoanalyst, Mexican Association for Psychoanalysis, Mexico City, Mexico

Serge Lebovici, M.D.

Professor Emeritus, University of Paris XIII Leonardo Da Vinci. Honorary Director, Infant Mental Health Service, Bobigny, CEDEX, Paris, France (deceased)

Alicia F. Lieberman, Ph.D.

Professor of Psychiatry, University of San Francisco; Senior Psychologist, Infant Parent Program, San Francisco General Hospital, San Francisco, California, U.S.A.

J. Martín Maldonado-Durán, M.D.

Family Service and Guidance Center, Topeka, Kansas; Investigator, Child and Family Center, Menninger Clinic, Topeka, Kansas; Adjunct Professor for Infant Psychopathology, Kansas State University, Manhattan; Clinical Professor, University of Kansas, Kansas City

Susan McDonough, M.S.W., Ph.D

Researcher, University of Michigan, Ann Arbor, Michigan, U.S.A.

Charles Millhuff, D.O.

Child and Adolescent Psychiatrist, Family Service and Guidance Center; Faculty, Karl Menninger School of Psychiatry and Mental Health Sciences, Topeka, Kansas, U.S.A.

Klaus Minde, M.D., F.R.C.P.C.

Former Chairman, Division of Child Psychiatry and Professor of Psychiatry and Pediatrics, McGill University; Director, Department of Psychiatry, Montreal Children's Hospital, Montreal, Canada

Richard J. Pines, D.O.

Medical Director of Child and Adolescent Psychiatry, St. Alphonsus Regional Medical Center, Boise, Idaho, U.S.A.

J. Luis Salinas, M.D.

Psychiatrist and Family Therapist, Instituto Nacional de la Nutrición, Mexico City, Mexico; Guest Professor, University of Paris XIII, Paris, France

J. Manuel Sauceda-Garcia, M.D.

Child and Adolescent Psychiatrist and Senior Advisor for Research, Hospital Juan N. Navarro (Child Psychiatric Hospital), Mexico City; Member, National Academy of Medicine, Mexico

Kristen Sligar, R.N., M.S.N.

Investigator, University of Washington, Seattle, Washington, U.S.A.

JoAnne Solchany, R.N., Ph.D.

Investigator, University of Washington, Seattle, Washington, U.S.A.

Lucile Ware, M.D.

Researcher, Child and Family Center, The Menninger Clinic; Child and Adolescent Psychiatrist and Psychoanalyst, Topeka, Kansas, U.S.A.

Hisako Watanabe, M.D., Ph.D.

Director of Infant, Child and Adolescent Mental Health Unit; Assistant Professor, Department of Pediatrics, School of Medicine, Keio University, Japan

Preface

The field of infant and toddler mental health is a rapidly expanding area of endeavor. One is tempted to say that this work is still in its infancy. There are several excellent resources that describe infant behavioral and emotional difficulties and other psychosocial challenges affecting young children (e.g., Lieberman et al. 1997; Zeanah 2000). Yet there is a dearth of literature that presents specific methods for assessing and treating infants and young children, particularly in the context of the family in which they live. It is an unfortunate reality that in many cases children do not literally "live" with their family. Clinicians are all too familiar with neglected, abused, or abandoned children. Nevertheless, even these children cannot be understood and treated outside the human or family environment in which they were born.

This book assembles in one volume a number of chapters written by actual clinicians working with infants and children and their families. The main focus is on methods and techniques of clinical intervention (e.g., evaluation and treatment strategies) with babies, toddlers, and families facing behavioral and emotional challenges. For this purpose, I have asked the authors to concentrate on what they actually do in their everyday clinical work. How do they understand the difficulties present in the baby or toddler? How do they assess these children? What goes into designing and implementing a program to alleviate their difficulties? These are some of the central questions the contributors address.

Another intention is to present the reader with diverse approaches to clinical work. The contributors practice in different settings with people from various ethnic and cultural backgrounds in several countries, from Japan to Argentina to France. Exchanges with colleagues in the United

States and other countries have made it clear that there are multiple ways to approach problems and that there is much work to do in investigating the best approaches for particular difficulties in a given family. Also, there is a span of models, some applied primarily by home visitors and nurses (although useful for any clinician) and some that require training in psychotherapy and psychodynamic thinking. The case discussions at the end provide a glimpse of further approaches by clinicians and researchers, such as Susan McDonough's interactive guidance technique.

Presenting clinical models of treatment and work with actual babies and families is a difficult endeavor; the idea is not to produce a "cookbook" with prescriptions for what to do in all situations. Rather, the authors have attempted to illustrate their way of thinking, how they understand the problem presented by the child and family, and how they go about trying to help in that situation.

The book is divided into four sections. The first section contains three chapters describing the theoretical background for the real-life disturbances and situations presented later. In the first chapter, J. Miguel Hoffmann, from Buenos Aires, describes "the place for infancy." He points out how difficult it has been for societies to think about the emotional needs of babies, and how tempting it is to think that young children do not feel anything or that early experiences do not matter. He includes his ideas about the development of the self, initiative, and autonomy, and the dangers inherent in that process: submission, compliance, and lack of spontaneity, if not violence. This is a central topic of major concern for all professionals working with the earliest experiences in life.

Efrain Bleiberg, from Topeka, Kansas, then describes the theoretical and clinical implications of trauma during early childhood and its effects on emotional regulation, cognition, and attachment, including potential disruptions of attachment. Trauma leads to distortions in internal working models of relationships, in emotional regulation, and in the experience of oneself and others. Trauma is widely overlooked in the life of young children, perhaps because of the distress it produces in adults to think that infants can be subject to violence, witness major traumatic events, and experience consequences from such events. Bleiberg expands on how early experiences mold the development of the personality and contribute to certain forms of psychopathology later in life.

Peter Fonagy, from London, describes the central notions of reflective self-function and "mind reading" and their correlation with attachment relationships between caregiver and child from infancy. These concepts have profound implications for caregiving practices and their impact on child development. His perspective, from attachment theory, psychoanalysis, and developmental psychology, provides a map that can guide clinicians in observing parent-infant relationships and in assessing the development of the child and of the parent as a caregiver.

The second section presents various schools of parent-infant or infant-parent psychotherapy in a broad sense. In their chapter on maternal role attainment and attachment during pregnancy, JoAnne Solchany, Kristen Sligar, and Kathryn Barnard, from Washington State, illustrate their innovative technique of very early intervention before the child is born. In a moving way, they describe the challenges of working with a population of women who concurrently face multiple stressors while going through pregnancy. Solchany and her colleagues establish a connection with the pregnant woman and her family and attempt to help them connect with the unborn baby by facilitating the psychological work of becoming a parent and of being sensitive to the baby's needs. There is an enormous need for programs that can help prepare parents during pregnancy for the arrival of the baby and the related challenges ahead of them.

Alicia Lieberman, from San Francisco, shares her experiences with attachment disturbances. She describes her understanding of attachment and disruptions of attachment. Using clinical vignettes, she poignantly describes her work with families who have suffered multiple disruptions, disappointments, and marginalization. Many clinicians might find such families "unreachable" and would not think they could be helped. Lieberman describes her techniques for communicating and intervening with families through the baby. She illustrates her concept of "corrective attachment experience" in her work with a family.

The chapter on multimodal parent-infant psychotherapy that I wrote in collaboration with Teresa Lartigue, from Mexico City, describes a method of intervention that can be used with families under severe stress, sometimes called "multiproblem families." These families typically seek mental health consultation for symptoms of distress in the baby, but clinicians soon find that other factors (e.g., parents' individual difficulties, extended family issues, the relationship between partners) have created a complex situation in which the parents no longer feel able to cope. We describe our approach to selecting areas of intervention and techniques, including cognitive and behavioral approaches, with the infant. We also suggest how to teach parents techniques for helping their babies.

A unique perspective on clinical work with infants is offered by Serge Lebovici, from Paris, and J. Armando Barriguete and J. Luis Salinas, from Mexico City, in their description of the therapeutic consultation. The Bobigny School that they represent has been extremely influential in Europe and Latin America. Their work, expanding on the ideas of Winnicott, offers a refreshing perspective on psychodynamics within families and across generations. They also present some novel technical tools.

Their use of the "sacred moment" during sessions and of the body of the therapist as a communication device, as well as the expansion of the concept of empathy, is extremely pertinent to work with infants and parents because much intrafamilial communication takes place through the body, emotions, and nonverbal, nonnarrative means.

Hisako Watanabe, from Japan, describes her approach to the transgenerational transmission of abandonment. Her means of dealing with losses and disruptions in relationships is enriched by certain cultural themes unique to Japan (e.g., the experience of dealing with the aftermath of the atomic bombs). Her work has universal applicability and value. She recognizes the present as related to the past, particularly to past experiences of dealing with relationships, emotional support, and deprivation or frank abandonment. Her description of how she connects with the family, an unassuming and humble approach to understanding the baby and the parents, is impressive and moving.

Alice Eberhart-Wright, a consultant with the Early Head Start program in midwestern United States, also writes on the importance of early intervention. In the United States and other countries, day care for infants is a hotly debated topic, particularly its effect on cognitive, emotional, and social development. Eberhart-Wright focuses on the experiences of day care from the point of view of the infant exposed to multiple caregivers. She addresses the very difficult questions of the effects on infants of changes in caregivers. Many adults, particularly parents, are worried about the consequences of these early disruptions in the child's emotional life. The problem of multiple caregivers affects millions of children but has received little attention in the literature.

The third section of the book is devoted to psychophysiological disturbances in infants. Young children use their body and its functioning to manifest their difficulties. Three areas of particular concern are crying, sleeping, and eating.

Excessive crying is a common problem that worries parents enormously. J. Manuel Sauceda-Garcia, from Mexico City, and I describe some of the most common causes of excessive crying in both very young and older infants. Then we pay particular attention to difficulties in self-regulation. In the second part of the chapter, we describe strategies and techniques for preventing the onset of episodes of crying and sensory overload in the baby, as well as methods for soothing and helping the child with the task of regulating functions and level of excitation. We offer practical suggestions that can be widely applied by health care professionals.

Klaus Minde, from Montreal, eruditely presents the physiology and maturation of sleeping in infancy. After briefly describing the disorders predominantly seen in the clinical setting, he presents intervention strategies to use in dealing with the various difficulties, particularly sleep on-set and sleep maintenance. His chapter is extremely valuable for both its comprehensiveness and its clarity. His approach to dealing with sleep difficulties is humane and sensitive, taking into account the emotions of the child and the parents rather than focusing only on behaviors and on elimination of undesirable ones.

Eating difficulties and failure to thrive are also important concerns of parents that often go unrecognized or untreated until they become severe problems. J. Armando Barriguete and I propose a way of understanding the various phenomena of eating problems and the feeding relationship. We offer various strategies for evaluating the situation and, like Minde, sug-gest the importance of seeing the "total child" and the context in which the child is manifesting the problem. This chapter describes a number of treat-ment strategies that can be used, depending on the diagnostic findings.

The final section of the book features two chapters that describe actual cases of young children in great distress whose families are challenged with multiple difficulties. The first case, presented by Richard Pines, from the midwestern United States, is fairly typical: a young child whose dif-ficult behaviors make him seem a "monster" to his parents. The second case, presented by Charles Millhuff, from Topeka, Kansas, illustrates the sad reality of infant maltreatment, in this instance, a very young infant with a fractured femur.

We were fortunate to have these cases presented to a panel of clini-cians and researchers who gave their opinions about what they thought was happening and what they would suggest as the next steps in assess-ment and treatment. We encouraged panel members to explore their dif-ferences of opinion in hopes of enriching the discussion with multiple and divergent perspectives. The two chapters contain the essence of their points of view and recommendations. This method of presenting clinical material and consulting with experienced clinicians from diverse back-grounds provides an additional, and in some ways unique, opportunity to flesh out more effective assessment and treatment approaches with in-fants and young children and their families.

REFERENCES

Lieberman AF, Wieder S, Fenichel E (eds): The DC:0–3 Casebook: A Guide to the Use of Zero to Three's "Diagnostic Classification of Mental Health and De-velopmental Disorders of Infancy and Early Childhood" in Assessment and Treatment Planning. Washington, DC, Zero to Three, 1997

Zeanah CH Jr. (ed): Handbook of Infant Mental Health, 2nd Edition. New York, Guilford, 2000

Acknowledgments

I want to express my gratitude to the many people who have helped make this work possible. First, I want to recognize the young children and families who place their trust in us and allow us to become a part of their lives. Second, my thanks go to the contributors to the chapters and the case discussions in this book for their generosity and willingness to share their actual theoretical views and clinical approaches. Third, I am thankful to Mary Ann Clifft and Philip R. Beard of the Division of Scientific Publications at the Menninger Clinic for their enormous help with and advice on editorial revisions as well as the formatting and organizing of chapters.

During the past 5 years, I have been very fortunate to have enjoyed the financial support of the Jessie Ball Dupont Foundation, and in particular its representative Ms. Sally Douglass, for helping to fund my clinical and research work. Financial support remains crucial to the research and treatment of infants and toddlers.

I also express my appreciation to Dr. Peter Fonagy, Dr. Efrain Bleiberg, Dr. John Sargent, and Dr. Jon Allen from the Menninger Child and Family Center for making space for infants at the center. Of note, too, is the center's support of this book from the day of its inception. Thanks also go to Dr. Eric Atwood from the Family Service and Guidance Center for his encouragement.

Dr. Marc DesLauriers and Ms. Jayne Roberts of the Menninger Continuing Education Department were also extremely helpful in organizing the conferences where most of the contributors to this volume first gathered to share their wisdom and expertise with participating clinicians. That intellectual venue proved to be part of the impetus for this book.

My appreciation goes as well to Menninger librarians Lois Bogia and Andrea Burgett, and to the rest of the Menninger Professional Library staff, for their help in obtaining resource material and in verifying and reverifying references. The Menninger library and its staff are an oasis in the area of mental health resources.

I am most thankful to my many colleagues and teachers—Dr. William Nathan, Dr. Lucile Ware, and Ms. Marianne Ault-Riché—for their interest in the young child and in families. In addition, Dr. Klaus Minde helped me get started in this field with his advice, generosity, and encouragement. The mentorship and example of such as these have proved to be not only intellectually stimulating but also motivational in my own clinical and research work, as well as in my own professional speaking and writing activities. During the preparation of this book, Dr. Serge Lebovici died. He was a brilliant and kind teacher for generations of mental health professionals in many parts of the world. We will all miss him very much. I also thank Chris Moody, M.S.W., and Linda Helmig, Ph.D., for their help and collaboration in working with babies.

Of special note, too, is the editorial staff of American Psychiatric Publishing, Inc., most especially Ms. Claire Reinburg, former editorial director, whose ongoing encouragement and interest helped keep the project moving along. I also thank Emily Fenichel from Zero to Three for her support through several years.

Throughout the challenging process of compiling this book, I have enjoyed the benefits of the ongoing support and encouragement of Maria-Raquel Morales, my wife and life partner, and our two daughters, Maria-Ximena and Ana-Marcela, to whom this book is dedicated. Without their understanding and patience, this work would not have come to fruition.

Introduction

Peter Fonagy, Ph.D., F.B.A.

In 1999, the Surgeon General of the United States issued a report on mental health and mental illness in which he fully endorsed the significance of psychosocial influences on mental health, notwithstanding the predominantly biological orientation to modern mental health care. His report affirms that "children must be seen in the context of their social environments—family and peer group, as well as that of their larger physical and cultural surroundings" (DHHS 1999, p. 16). It embraces the concept of developmental risk and, in a critical passage, asserts that "childhood is an important time to prevent mental disorder and to promote healthy development. . . . [I]t is logical to try to intervene early in children's lives before problems are established and become refractory" (p. 132). Preventive interventions, it is further asserted, "have been shown to be effective in reducing the impact of risk factors for mental disorders and improving social and emotional development" (p. 18).

Of course, we all know that infancy is a critical developmental stage. Surely, if "the child is father of the man," as the poet William Wordsworth noted in 1807, the infant must be the grandfather. Recent studies of brain development mostly confirm the importance of the first years for neural development (Thompson et al. 2000). Sixty to seventy years ago, Skeels demonstrated that placing infants from orphanages on the wards of mentally retarded adolescents and adults who showed the infants love and attention enhanced the social competence of these infants (Skeels 1966). In addition, they were far more likely to be adopted and go on to live useful lives than those who remained in the orphanages. Countless studies (cross-sectional, longitudinal, and experimental) have since demonstrated the power of early intervention to alter the course of a child's life permanently (Guralnick 1997; Mrazek 1998).

Yet, there is something within the academic community that rebels against this truth, and not long ago, a book could be published with the title *The Myth of the First Three Years* (Bruer 1999). Of course, this controversy is by no means new (e.g., Clarke and Clarke 1976): as recently as 1998, a book that questioned the importance of parents for child development (Harris 1998) received considerable public and scientific acclaim. The influence of those scientists who wish to play down the role of the family environment in favor of genetic factors is increasing at a rate that appears to correspond to the mapping of the human genome. Over the past decade, research in genetics appeared to have all but eliminated the place for a psychosocial account and refuted all theories that advocated the key role of early family experience (see Scarr 1992). There has been a claim that environmentally mediated family influences were inherited and therefore unimportant in themselves (Rowe 1994); if family environment mattered, it was specific to each child, even within the same family (Plomin and Daniels 1987). It has also been suggested that influences, previously considered environmental, were actually genetically mediated (Kendler et al. 1996) and, furthermore, that some genetically influenced aspects of children's behavior may have been responsible for provoking observed negative responses in parents and other people (O'Connor et al. 1998).

How can we square this circle? Do the environmental determinants of early development matter? Or is human infancy a fiction that we have invented to account for previously inexplicable genetic determinants of adult behavior? It is easy to ascribe mental states to the human infant because he or she does not have the verbal capacity to deny our assertions. Have generations of psychosocial theoreticians labored under a profound misapprehension, an attributional bias predisposing us to find cause within our history? The geneticists might reply in the affirmative. But then what do we make of the studies of Romanian orphans (Fisher et al. 1997; O'Connor et al. 2000), in which those who were rescued after the first half-dozen or so months of their lives are still consistently being shown to manifest interpersonal and emotional problems notwithstanding years of secure environmental support? Developmental science has undoubtedly gotten itself into a tangle about the status of early development. Why?

I believe that at the root of the controversy concerning early development is an ignorance about what does or does not take place in the interactions between the infant and the social world. Psychoanalytic theoreticians might have oversold the notion of infancy, attempting to place inexplicable aspects of their adult patients' behavior into what Green (Green 2000) has proudly called "the psychoanalytic infant" (e.g., Bion 1962; Fairbairn 1952/1954; Klein 1933/1948). The infant reconstructed from adulthood, of course, bears few similarities to the infant of observation. Much like Serge Lebovici's concept of the adult's "fantasmatic" baby (Lebovici and Weil-Halpern 1989), in which parents place their fantasies and then determine their transactions with the young child, psychoanalysts have created an infancy unlike the infancy we can observe in behavioral studies (e.g., Stern 1985). Green rejects these studies and claims that they have the potential to destroy the entire psychoanalytic enterprise. He wishes to continue to hide behind the silence of infancy and to entertain claims about early development based on the psychotherapeutic treatment of adult patients. In my view, such an approach risks setting psychoanalysis into disrepute. Fantasy is for the couch, not for science. If we are to advance in our understanding of developmental progression, our understanding must be based on the reality of infancy. We must make infants speak.

This reality-based approach to development is the subject of this book, which brings together theoretical, experimental, and clinical data related to early childhood to help us better understand what actually happens. Setting aside theoretical expectations, what, to paraphrase J. Miguel Hoffmann, is the place of infancy? This book was written by clinicians who have learned—and want to continue learning—about infancy and development from clinical encounters with troubled infants and their families. Their focus is consistent with Freud's epistemology and heritage, but it also points the way to a new and fresh approach to the young child that breaks down many of the barriers of classical psychoanalysis. Working clinically with infants and their families is a rare and precious art. However, its products—solid clinical observations—are the raw material of the science of developmental psychopathology. If the infant is indeed grandfather of the adult, learning about psychosocial influences in adult psychopathology will have to start from ages 0 to 3. The clinicians represented here have both individually and as a group made major contributions to our understanding of not only later mental disturbance but also the developmental processes that lead the child down this path. If we want to understand the moderators of genetic influences, we shall have to understand what takes place in infancy. To help our adult patients, we would do well to observe how the clinician works with the immature mind. There may be skepticism about the significance of early development because of the relative sparsity of normative longitudinal data. The data have not been collected because the process of infancy has, in many ways, not yet been fully understood. This book represents a further step along this road of understanding. At the same time, it is a tribute to the therapeutic creativity and talents of those rare individuals who can offer effective preventive help to the youngest members of our community through theoretical understanding and practical intervention.

REFERENCES

Bion WR: Learning From Experience. New York, Basic Books, 1962

Bruer JT: The Myth of the First Three Years: A New Understanding of Early Development and Lifelong Learning. New York, Free Press, 1999

Clarke AM, Clarke ADB: Early Experience: Myth and Evidence. London, Open Books, 1976

Fairbairn WRD: An Object-Relations Theory of the Personality (1952). New York, Basic Books, 1954

Fisher L, Ames EW, Chisholm K, et al: Problems reported by parents of Romanian orphans adopted to British Columbia. International Journal of Behavioral Development 20:67–82, 1997

Green A: Science and science fiction in infant research, in Clinical and Observational Psychoanalytic Research: Roots of a Controversy. Edited by Sandler J, Sandler A-M, Davies R. London, Karnac Books, 2000, pp 41–72

Guralnick MJ: The Effectiveness of Early Intervention. Baltimore, MD, Paul H Brookes, 1997

Harris JR: The Nurture Assumption: Why Children Turn Out the Way They Do: Parents Matter Less Than You Think and Peers Matter More. New York, Free Press, 1998

Kendler KS, Neale MC, Prescott CA, et al: Childhood parental loss and alcoholism in women: a causal analysis using a twin-family design. Psychol Med 26: 79–95, 1996

Klein M: The early development of conscience in the child (1933), in Contributions to Psycho-Analysis, 1921–1945. Edited by Klein M. London, Hogarth Press, 1948

Lebovici S, Weil-Halpern F: Psychopathologie du Bébé [Infant Psychopathology]. Paris, Presses Universitaires de France, 1989

Mrazek P: Preventing Mental Health and Substance Abuse Problems in Managed Health Care Settings. Alexandria, VA, National Mental Health Association, 1998

O'Connor TG, Deater-Deckard K, Fulker D, et al: Genotype-environment correlations in late childhood and early adolescence: antisocial behavioral problems and coercive parenting. Dev Psychol 34:970–981, 1998

O'Connor TG, Rutter M, Kreppner J: The effects of global severe privation on cognitive competence: extension and longitudinal follow-up. English and Romanian Adoptees Study Team. Child Dev 71(2):376–390, 2000

Plomin R, Daniels D: Why are children in the same family so different from one another? Behav Brain Sci 10:1–16, 1987

Rowe DC: The Limits of Family Influence: Genes, Experience, and Behavior. New York, Guilford, 1994

Scarr S: Developmental theories for the 1990s: development and individual differences. Child Dev 63:1–19, 1992

Skeels HM: Adult Status of Children With Contrasting Early Life Experiences: A Follow-up Study (Monographs of the Society for Research in Child Development, Vol 31, No 3). Chicago, IL, University of Chicago Press, 1966

Stern DN: The Interpersonal World of the Infant: A View From Psychoanalysis and Developmental Psychology. New York, Basic Books, 1985

Thompson PM, Giedd JN, Woods RP, et al: Growth patterns in the developing brain detected by using continuum mechanical tensor maps. Nature 404: 190–193, 2000

U.S. Department of Health and Human Services: Mental Health: A Report of the Surgeon General: Executive Summary. Rockville, MD, National Institute of Mental Health, 1999

I

Theoretical Framework

1

The Place for Infancy

J. Miguel Hoffmann, M.D.

The term *infancy*[1] denotes not only a stage in human development but also a segment of society. In this chapter, I specify, whenever necessary, whether I am referring to the developmental stage or to the group of human beings. Infancy, however, has not yet achieved a place of its own in society, where it could unfold according to its own design, aims, and purposes. The space that should be allotted to infancy has been occupied—and often intruded upon—by adults, who tend to use infants and children as private property, as extensions of themselves, or as instruments of their own expectations, dreams, and desires. These adults include not only the parents but also society as a whole, including its religions and cults, the culture itself, and, certainly, programmed education.

In addition, the nature-versus-nurture controversy has polarized our explanations so much for so long that we have been unable to examine the subject's own contribution. Either we assume determinism from within or we see it coming from outside. Furthermore, we have no theoretical or practical room for random behavior or for purposive, self-designing behavior. Here, I focus on the importance of spontaneity and creative behavior of the infant as it is met by the caregivers.

---

[1] *Infancy* refers to the age group of human beings that differs from other age groups. According to the definition of the World Association for Infant Mental Health (WAIMH), infancy begins at conception and extends to age 3. *Infant* refers to the human being between conception and 3 years of age.

In this chapter, I discuss three main ideas that stem from the work of my colleagues and myself with infants in research and in social programs over the past 14 years:

1. An understanding of human development based on the individual's participation in the process
2. A reformulation of the relationship between individuals and their immediate environment, using the basic philosophy of "to be and let be" as opposed to relationships of submissive compliance
3. The implication of the two previous points for the relationship between individuals and their environment within the cultural context

These three interconnected ideas have clinical relevance as well. Clinicians who deal with infants every day are in a position to recognize the issue of the individuality of the infant as he or she interacts with caregivers and to observe whether such interactions permit the child and caregiver to develop a mutually satisfying partnership. The clinician also has an influence on child-rearing and child-care practices and whether the emotional and developmental needs of the infant and caregiver are taken into account by societies. Some of these fundamental needs and tendencies as they pertain to the individual, the family, and society and culture are examined in the section "Place of Infancy."

A place for infancy develops under normal conditions, first in the mind of the infant's caregivers, then in the psychosocial space of interaction, and finally in the broader social and cultural contexts as these newcomers begin to participate in ways that reach beyond family boundaries. This viewpoint stems from a psychological and psychoanalytic understanding.

PLACE OF INFANCY

What is the space that society makes for infants? By exploring both the microscopic and the macroscopic contexts of the infant as an individual and as part of a group of people, I will present some evidence regarding the claim of misuse or absence of a space for the infant. This examination is necessary to alert those involved with these young children about some ideas and practices we take as commonplace but that may impinge on young children's emotional development and unfolding as human beings.

Impact of Violence on Infants:
Historical and Current Perspectives

Before discussing the impact of violence on children, I will give a brief account of the larger social context sanctioning violence against young children. While entrusted with an assignment to present a report on "The Impact of Violence Upon Infants" to the International Meeting of the International Association of Child and Adolescent Psychiatry and Allied Professions (IACAPAP) (Hoffmann 1994a), I was presented with a whole new reality. Struggling with incredulity, I sought to assemble the pieces of the puzzle of abusive adult behavior toward infants and small children. If reviewing the scientific literature was a traumatic experience for me, reading newspaper accounts was altogether worse. Both sources conveyed the impact of stark images and cruelly crude testimonies. Shocked by contemporary facts, I turned to history, hoping for a better picture from the "good old days." But I found little consolation from the accounts of leading historians of childhood (Aries 1988; Badinter 1980; deMause 1988; Minde and Minde 1986). Killing infants was not even against the law until the fourth century. The enforcement of any infancy protection law took almost another 14 centuries, when the Prussian and Austrian kingdoms issued specific prohibitions against sleeping with infants under the ages of 3 and 5, respectively. These regulations of the late eighteenth century were aimed at the frequent excuse that infants had died from involuntary suffocation when adults shared a bed with them.

In the eighteenth century, inhabitants of Paris would play games by throwing swaddled infants like balls through the air, causing the doctors of Paris hospitals to issue a recommendation to change this practice. Drugging infants into sleep by administering opium was a common practice in Liverpool, with 12,000 doses a week sold for this purpose, just a century and a half ago (Minde and Minde 1986). Sending children ages 8 or 9 to work in another household for 12 or more hours a day was a common practice by upper-middle-class Europeans, not for economic but for "educational" reasons (deMause 1988).

Severe child beating was considered a rare occurrence in the twentieth century, until some Australian doctors in the early 1960s reported on the frequency of repeated bone fractures in hospital admissions for supposedly accidental traumas. The hospital X-ray examinations showed many cases of previous bone fractures of unidentified origin. This report led to the uncovering of a huge and unexpectedly grave scene of home violence, with the main victims being women and infants. Disentangling both forms of domestic violence—against women and against infants—has required a concerted effort, and in most countries this serious problem has not yet been resolved.

In addition to being victims of physical violence, children are often treated as property. For example, they can be rented (e.g., for child prostitution, child work, or child pornography) or sold (e.g., for adoption or as industrial, domestic, or sexual slaves). Children can even be sold for use as "spare parts" in illegal organ transplants. Children are also trained to perform criminal activities, such as transporting drugs or entering private property through small openings for the purpose of stealing.

This list of abuses directed against children could be extended for pages and pages. After reading the UN "Declaration of the Rights of Children," one has to ask: What experiences could have been in the minds of the authors wanting to protect children from so many unbelievable injustices? A child's right and ability to just stay alive physically predominate in the declaration. On the other hand, reading the declaration from a mental health perspective, we see that the dozens of rights that children should have in a modern, sensitive, and caring society are not even insinuated. Just staying alive physically takes center stage in the declaration. Such "pretentious" goals as happiness, the right to creative choices in life, fulfillment in a self-chosen activity, and freedom to form a life project that allows for the proper development of one's own talents and gifts are nowhere mentioned.

How little the infant and the small child count becomes dramatically evident when analyzing the horror stories of great violence in their everyday lives. Atrocities from "simple" neglect continue to receive more attention by the community. The "smaller" violence of the psychological annihilation of infants and young children does not reach the newspapers; it gains attention solely from poets, mental health specialists, and others who dare to take up symbolic violence or the violence of symbolic destructiveness, such as subtle attacks on meaning, personal identity, or the sheer fact of personal existence.[2]

Something similar might be said about the lifelong effects on mental and psychological development of "minor" forms of sexual abuse of children. The excellent account by Lenore Terr (1990) regarding Virginia Woolf as a child abused by her older half-brothers illustrates this point, even more so if we include the interpretation that the famous novelist's death may be at least partly attributed to the unresolved impact of those early experiences.

---

[2]For example, director Ettore Scola's film *The Family* (Italy/France 1987) portrays a grandfather who teases his grandson by asking, "Where is little so-and-so?" while intentionally ignoring the desperate efforts of the child to gain his grandfather's attention. In despair, the child eventually breaks down sobbing.

Infant as Agent

In contrast to the above forms of treatment toward infants and children in general, I present here the view of my colleagues and myself about the infant as an individual. It will help to set in perspective these practices against the developmental needs of the very young child. Although these needs are paramount, they can be easily set aside. Yet, clinicians should take into account developmental needs when assessing a given infant, his or her problems, and the immediate relational context. Also, careful consideration of a young child's needs will help those involved in clinical work to think about how our societies may not take these issues into account. Our research has enabled us to see firsthand an infant's developmental need to be an individual and to examine the different manifestations of the need to express oneself as an individual.

Does the baby have personal initiative? Or is the infant dominated by reflex and reactive activity? Infants have the capacity to determine some of their own behavior. We see the child as an independent agent, endowed with a primitive form of self-determination. Little has been said to date on the origin of this self-determination and about its developmental line.

For the past 14 years, we have collected data on 350 feeding situations of infants ages 4–12 months with their caregivers. The study design (see Hoffmann et al. 1992 for details) allowed us to pinpoint four basic forms of infant initiative; two categories of caregiver response, favorable or restrictive, toward the infant's initiative; and a measure of aversive responses and conflict arising from faulty caregiver-infant interactions.

The pilot study (Hoffmann et al. 1992) of 106 feeding situations produced the following conclusions:

- Infant initiatives evolve over the first year of life both in quantity and in complexity.
- This growth is associated with favorable caregiving responses to the infant's initiatives.
- In the case of a restrictive caregiving response, the quantity and quality of the infant's initiatives diminish.
- In the case of a restrictive response, there is a significant simultaneous increase in aversive responses by the infant, as well as conflict in the caregiver-infant interaction.

These results were validated in a sample of 239 feeding situations (Hoffmann et al. 1998). In a longitudinal follow-up of the same sample of mother-infant pairs, we have been exploring the development of creativity in the child as associated with the quality and quantity of initiatives at 1 year of age. Creativity is determined in a play situation at 24 and 36 months of age.

Initiatives have been defined as the expression of an agency function of the unfolding individual. They are the organization of spontaneous activity emerging from the core self and leading to purposeful action that, in turn, provides experiences that will lead to new initiatives (Hoffmann 1994a, 1994b, 2000). The theoretical value of this model is related to the different types of mental growth attained in experiences developed out of active, participative actions as opposed to passive, compliant experiences. The kind of experiences obtained while relating to the external world and the experiences regarding oneself as the initiator and conductor of the act of experiencing will be very much influenced by the active or passive nature of these experiences.

Clear indicators of an early form of self-will at ages 4–12 months contribute to this picture of a self-initiating, active, participative early human subject. This idea is clearly supported by the signs of distress and struggle in cases where the environmental response is adverse[3] to the infant's initiatives. The baby's aversive reactions seem to be on the level of individual behavior; the infant produces signals of distress, and the caregiver seems not to respond. In the event that the caregiver starts "hitting back" by raising his or her voice, scolding, verbally abusing the child, or even taking clear, more-or-less coercive actions to make the infant comply, we have then an interpersonal conflict in which two individuals are fighting and struggling for control. In our research, both aversive responses and conflict are positively associated with unfavorable caregiver responses and are negatively associated with the qualitative and quantitative development of infant initiatives. This means that the greater the caregiver's opposition to the unfolding of the infant's initiatives, the greater the aversive response by the baby and the greater the conflict between child and caregiver (Hoffmann et al. 1998).

Simultaneously, the greater the opposition to the infant's initiative, the lesser the development of initiatives. On the other hand, the better the caregiver's acceptance of the baby's initiatives, the greater the infant's development and the lower the aversive responses and conflict (Hoffmann 1995b). As Zeldin (1994) stated: "When the children were small, they did what they were told; now as they approach independence, they fill their parents with anxiety" (p. 376). Although this comment could be interpreted in different ways, what Zeldin means is that there is a feeling of potential revenge on the part of formerly

---

[3]Aversive reactions, such as spitting out food, closing the mouth, hitting at the incoming spoon, and jerking and jumping in the chair, increase significantly in cases of adverse environmental responses to the infant's initiatives.

compliant children and grown-up adolescents who have the ability to retaliate.

The value of initiative for the development of human beings is stressed in remarks by Karl Popper (Popper and Lorenz 1985) regarding the interplay between environment and individual contribution: "In a word, it is totally false that we have been *molded* by our environment. It is we who actively *search* for our environment, it is we that *actively mold* our environment" (p. 22; emphasis added). Popper went on to say: "Those beings without initiative, with no curiosity, with no fantasy, are forced to struggle for an ecological niche already taken by someone else; on the contrary, those endowed with initiative can count on ecological niches freshly invented" (p. 27).[4]

To date, we in the developmental field have had a strong tendency toward a deterministic view of human action based on the ideas of instincts and drives as the motorizing forces. The theory of initiative is based on the idea of a thrusting search for experiences emerging from the nuclear self of every newborn—in Popper's words, *inborn activity*. In due time, experiences turn into forces backing new initiatives (Hoffmann 1996a, 1996b).

When one observes[5] an infant struggling with the mother to be able to perform different types of initiatives, one has visual evidence of the importance of these self-initiated behaviors. Three consequences derive from these observations: a) a strong personal adherence to the fate of the initiative, shown in persistence, repetition, and reinitiation; b) a determination to hold one's initiative up against adversity (self-will); and c) the possible choice by the infant of a negative form of initiative—that is, an aversive response (e.g., spitting out food, closing the mouth, turning the head) and a power struggle with the caregiver—if simple persistence is unable to preserve initiative.

I consider the following elements to constitute the closest psychological description of an independent human being:

- Self-initiated behavior (agency function)
- The decision to sustain the initiative in the face of adversity, both determination[6] and self-determination

---

[4]Translation from Spanish by the author.

[5]Aversive reactions can be coded from videotaped meals.

[6]Understood as both "[t]he act of coming to a decision or of fixing or settling a purpose" and "[t]he quality of being resolute; firmness of purpose" (Webster's 1979, p. 497).

- Self-will sustained even against the will of a beloved or needed figure—that is, resiliency to conflict and some degree of autonomy[7]
- Negotiation as a particular form of give-and-take that preserves the relationship while somehow limiting each partner in his or her determination

I think we are witnessing the struggle for a psychological life—for the capacity to be, to become oneself—very early in life. Threats to this process are what make the nursery so noisy as early as 4 or 5 months of life—the furthest back in time our observations have been able to look—and perhaps even earlier. In support of this view are the innumerable accounts of mothers who show a remarkable capacity to identify these early infant strivings to become oneself. By helping out in this process, these mothers earn the intense reward of witnessing the unfolding of a human being becoming a genuine individual, developing personal endowments, and sparkling with creative transformations in play and experimentation.

MYTHS ENCOMPASS ATTITUDES

A number of cultural themes can help us understand our conception of infants and human beings. The themes are important determinants of what families do with their young children and the predominant views of how one should raise them and what traits should be promoted or suppressed. These themes have much meaning for societies, families, and individual infants.

What forces, drives, and motivations make a human being either the necessary, protective, generous, empathic, sensitive caregiver or the *homo lupus hominis* (man, wolf to man)? What determinants are present in the kind of adult who inflicts the different forms of violence in the horror stories noted earlier in this chapter? In psychoanalysis, myths are considered basic condensations of human behavior. The same is to be said for anthropology, especially the type developed by Levi-Strauss (1972), who proposed a structural analysis of myths to extract the basic message.

In psychoanalysis, the myth of Oedipus has been the cornerstone of Freudian theory. This myth view was later questioned. According to Kohut's (1981) interpretation, Freud made a double mistake when he chose the Oedipus complex. The first mistake was a scientific one, namely, he be-

---

[7]"Independence or freedom . . . as of the will or one's actions" (Webster's 1979, p. 929).

gan to interpret the myth from the moment at which Oedipus killed his father, Laius. Freud thus ignored a significant point: In fear of the omen pronounced by the Oracle, the father had been ordered to kill Oedipus while the child was still a small infant. Freud's second mistake, according to Kohut, is the choice of this myth itself. If, instead of the Oedipus story, he had selected the story of Odysseus, the consequences would have been quite different. Very briefly: Odysseus is a young, recently married king having a great time with his beautiful wife, Penelope, and their small son, Telemachus, when he is "drafted" for war against Troy. Unhappy with the idea of leaving his family, Odysseus decides to pretend he is mad and has himself tied to an ox and plow. He screams wildly and behaves like a beast in front of the visiting "draft committee" of three kings. When they turn away in deep sorrow for their lost friend, one of the kings suspects mischief and places Telemachus in the way of the plowing madman. Odysseus then plows in a semicircle in order not to kill his beloved son. This act of protection and fatherly behavior prompts the committee to doubt Odysseus's craziness and he is forced to go to war.

The semicircle that Odysseus plows is identified by Kohut as the essence of mental health. A father in possession of his wits is unable to kill his son for his own benefit; instead, he goes to any length to save and protect his infant or child. Basic mental health on the father's part is thus essential for the child's proper development. This intergenerational attitude of cooperation and helpfulness is the basis for humanity's survival. In the Oedipus hypothesis, there is little chance for survival: the basic attitude is to kill (first, the father seeks to kill the son; then the son actually kills the father). If the attitudes of Laius and Oedipus were pervasive, humanity would not have survived.

What are we to make of these contradictory descriptions? We have to remember that although humankind has survived, we also have sufficient evidence in both historical and contemporary accounts to suggest that the annihilating tendency is present in many parents. Therefore, we might conclude that both myths are rooted in the observation of human behavior. Hence, the Oedipus myth is a valid explanation of the many abuses we observe with astonishment, just as the myth of Odysseus helps explain the heroic forms of parental sacrifice made to secure the infant's survival and thriving.

I propose that a variable mixture of both myths representing basic attitudes in parents guides adult and parental behavior from generation to generation. The myths are sustained by the different forms they take in popular stories, songs, and traditions. Examples include Grimm's Hansel and Gretel; the story of Snow White (with its representational power of the wicked stepmother inside any mother); various child-eating monsters; and the lesser-known story of Correa, the Argentine mother who continued to produce milk for her nursing infant after she died in the desert from thirst and hunger.[8]

Another myth that reveals basic attitudes of adults and culture in general toward infants is the story of Pygmalion. (This myth was also presented in the play of the same name by George Bernard Shaw and in the popular musical *My Fair Lady*.) In the story, Pygmalion, a king of Cyprus, had carved out of ivory a maiden of such beauty that he fell in love with his creation. He begged the gods for help in his despair. Moved by his strong desire and feelings, Aphrodite granted life to the ivory figure, who turned into the woman Galatea. The marriage of Pygmalion to Galatea was his final reward. The conclusion we can draw from this story is that human beings are created out of some sort of inert material, carved and constructed by an artist who finally falls in love with the object of these efforts. At the same time, the gods grant the right to possess the created object, transforming it into a human being by a particular combination of human craftsmanship and effort, plus the devotion and supernatural powers of the gods. Of note is the account by Graves (1965), who conjectures that the Pygmalion myth is related to the establishment of the patrilineal descent of power in the Cyprus monarchy.

In summary, historical and cultural evidence and current social events show that, thus far, little place has been made available for infancy in society. Research results also present a picture of the small infant as being capable of proposing personal initiatives as the way to make his or her experience in life more personal, something chosen. If spontaneity is preserved, each person will reach a greater degree of fulfillment of his or her individual destiny, given one's talents (Hoffmann 2000).

THE EMERGING INDIVIDUAL AND THE IMMEDIATE ENVIRONMENT

If we look at the human infant as an initiative-generating agent, his or her environment is the field for making experiences. But the environment is not only to be experienced; it also shapes the nature of experience itself. One way of shaping the infant's experiences is by how the caregiver sys-

---

[8]In Argentina, the followers of the popular cult of the Difunta Correa have erected a shrine to the "goddess" of alcoholics on the supposed site of the mother's death, as well as numerous images along the roadside where drivers often deposit empty bottles.

tem treats the infant's initiatives. The basic mechanism by which the caregiving system partakes in these events is a three-step process:

1. Reception or detection of the baby's project, which is expressed through the infant's action and organized by the infant's initiative
2. Internal processing in the caregiver
3. Reaction or response by the caregiver

Regarding the first step, reception, we may consider all the thoroughly described maternal perception mechanisms in early developmental accounts as forms of this activity. Some examples are empathy (Kohut 1977, 1981, 1984), intersubjectivity (Trevarthen 1979), attunement (Stern 1985), intuitive parenting (Papousek and Papousek 1995), and reverie (Bion 1962).

Building on Lebovici's (1988, 1991) previous work, I proposed a system of three internal infants in the caregiver (Hoffmann 1995a, 1995b):

1. The infant of fantasy
2. The infant of imagination
3. The infant of perception

The *infant of fantasy* is related to the mother's early developmental history, particularly her relationship with her father, mother, and siblings. It is basically unconscious to the mother.

The *infant of imagination* is first developed during the mother's childhood and adolescence and finally in the exchange with the sexual partner who shares conception and perhaps caregiving. The second, internal baby is clearly more conscious than the infant of fantasy, although it first emerges in the transitional space of the mother during her childhood while playing "Mom" (Hoffmann 1984, 1988). As Erikson (1950) pointed out, such play serves as a preparatory role for future functions. The girl with the doll is getting ready for motherhood, not just working out past traumas or unfinished business in her own development as posited in the more traditional interpretation of psychoanalysis. It is also, as play often is, a creative invention of reality that will, in the sense of a transitional phenomenon (Winnicott 1953/1958), be a creation of what will be needed: mothering capacities.

The third infant, the *infant of perception,* is essentially the baby that presents itself to the caregiver's different senses—sight, hearing, smell, and touch—once the newborn is placed atop the maternal womb or in the caregiver's arms. But even before birth, the infant of perception becomes accessible through deeper, more primitive perceptions—for example, those produced by hormonal changes during early pregnancy; the profoundly unconscious activity of the embryo eating its way into the prepared endometrium; and the changes in cardiac, respiratory, and liver functions long before the fetus kicks the mother's womb from within, creating at around the fourth or fifth month of pregnancy the astonishment and surprise that most mothers remember. (This third infant is different from the other two and is essential for understanding the pivotal focus of this chapter.) Only the perceived baby is capable of contributing to the infant's autonomy.

The infants of fantasy and imagination are the blueprints *in the parent's mind* that predetermine the child's future. The two blueprints, unconscious and preconscious, constitute the parental agenda. The baby's initiative unfolds the infant's program for his or her own agenda. The infant of perception allows the caregiving system to discover the child's own agenda as the infant strives for his or her own experiences. Through the infant of perception, both mother and father can enjoy the freshness of the baby's spontaneity, discovering his or her daily progress once he or she is in contact with the world. This reaching out for experiences by the infant shows up in several forms of temperament but, more essentially, through myriad forms of individual relationship with the environment, including, of course, the caregiving system.

Why would the caregiver react negatively to an infant's initiatives? There may be several reasons. For example, an initiative could be

- Unexpected.
- Considered an obstacle to the caregiver's own project regarding the immediate task with the infant (e.g., feeding).
- Judged as "bad" behavior, conduct, or manners (e.g., "Food is not to be played with").
- Contrary to the internal model held by the caregiver for that particular infant (e.g., "If you want to become a neat surgeon like your grandpa, then you should not be so messy" or "Young ladies who are fit to become a professor like your aunt don't fret so much").
- A painful reminder of something that the caregiver has lost, such as spontaneity, playfulness, or the experience of the richness of life.

The caregiver certainly has many projects for the newborn. Some are conscious; others are hidden under layers of oblivion. The caregiver's own history is present in the educational child-rearing project. The caregiver may expect many of his or her own frustrations to be corrected by the newcomer, who will, in turn, go on to complete a yet-unfulfilled life for himself or herself. Mandates from generation to generation are being handed down. Moral values and prejudices are taught as soon as possible," before it is too late"—both in word and action. Entire symposiums are held in the family during which the newborn, especially a firstborn, is given advice, indications, warnings, and my-own-experience recommendations at high speed and with great pressure exerted by the entrusted caregivers.

The caregiver's history (especially the mother's family traditions, mores, history, and particularities), the culture in which the baby is born, and the specific historical moment of the world are all determinants of environmental pressure against the infant's projects and initiatives, at least against his or her own freedom of action. Thus, there is no scenario imaginable in which the infant's initiative unfolds unquestioned, unharmed, or undisputed. The baby is somehow prepared, or at least that is our interpretation after observing the degree of competency exhibited in handling environmental obstructions by the more than 350 infants we have on videotape. The infant's strategies can be summarized in three types of responses to obstruction:

- Wait and try again later.
- Fight for it, with all means, including negotiation.
- Downgrade one's expectations.

These alternatives are aimed at achieving success, more or less. However, if environmental resistance is nonnegotiable—if there is no strategy to succeed even partially—confrontation becomes unavoidable. The alternative of confrontation, discussed in the next section ("Respect as a Psychological Function in Caregiving"), is a serious complication that threatens different aspects of infantile development. The nature and impact of environmental response to the infant's initiative are unavoidable, often intense, mostly nonconscious, and rooted in personal, familial, and cultural grounds. Environmental response exerts a permanent restriction on the unfolding of the infant's initiative. This response is partly negotiable and is, therefore, a transactional training in mastering reality and human relations. It is also a means for culturalization and familiarization, with all the advantages and disadvantages that both processes imply. The molding process is thus accomplished, but not as a unilateral, unavoidable imposition on the infant. Depending on the quality and quantity of both the infant's initiative and the environmental response, the baby will be able to carve out a greater or lesser degree of selfness. This is the creative conquest of the "ecological niche" referred to by Popper (Popper and Lorenz 1985). The place that a social group acquires in the network of human relationships is not passively allocated; rather it is actively carved out.

The extent to which the infant is pressed for compliance is the single most important environmental factor in early development for evaluating the degree of individuality a human being will be able to attain. Despite the concept of resiliency, there are limits to this corrective potential. An extreme case was noted by Charles Dickens, who said several times that we should stand appalled to know that where we generate disease to strike our children down and entail itself on unborn generations, there also we breed by the same certain process infancy "that knows no innocence, youth without modesty or shame, maturity that is mature in nothing but in suffering and guilt, and blasted old age that is a scandal on the form we bear" (Dickens 1859/1991). Resiliency is perhaps one of the most interesting and underemphasized issues in development, and our understanding of it is still incomplete. But we certainly believe that there are limits to possible corrections after severe strain or trauma, especially in the unfolding of spontaneity.

RESPECT AS A PSYCHOLOGICAL FUNCTION IN CAREGIVING

What is the natural safeguard designed to avoid excesses in the realm of caregiving? What comes out, in practical terms, of the roots of the myth of Odysseus and Telemachus? There is clear evidence that caregivers are capable of allowing their children "to be"—that is, allowing their infants to become determined (not stubborn), creative (not fancy), individualized (not eccentric), and active (not manic) human beings. What mechanism is built into the child-rearing process that warrants a development more or less in accordance with both design and self-designing forces?

The simple word *respect* comes easily to mind. The surprising fact is that this word is charged with all sorts of meanings in dictionaries and in common usage that have little to do with what we are thinking about here. I have elaborated on the use of this word in our culture in other publications (e.g., Hoffmann 1994d). In brief, the word is used mainly in the sense of reverence and is thought of as something that one in a "lower" position offers or owes to someone in a higher position. This definition of respect is clearly not what is meant when it comes to dealing with infants. Fortunately, respect during child rearing is, in fact, understood properly; that is, the caregiver, who is in the higher position, shows respect toward the infant, who is in the lower position. In this context, we understand that higher and lower refer to comparative levels of resources, power, dexterity, and sheer physical force. Respect has, therefore, been defined in a psychological sense in clearly asymmetric situations (e.g., regarding resources, power, and dependency) as the particular attitude that implies acceptance of what is different in the expectations of the one in the position of advantage (Hoffmann 1994d). It is related to tolerance and to the recognition of the other as an independent being. It implies (self-) restraint of power resources. For the recipient, it implies the experience of having fewer impingements to overcome. For the other party, it implies the experience of "letting one be." Respect is a decisive influence on both the primary and future relationships; it is, therefore, a central issue in socialization. Having experienced respect in the passive position predisposes one to the active exercise of this function.

Clearly, what favors respect by the caregiver toward the unfolding infant stems from a combination of the following factors:

- Experiencing respect during one's own upbringing, as well as during the educational process and at the point of entering the social organization (maturity)
- Being supported in the process of child rearing by the concentric circles of caregiving (mother, father, parents, extended family, social and community networks, cultural milieu)
- Having the capacity to process the actual infant as the infant of perception while opposing or neutralizing the infant of fantasy and slowly transmuting the infant of imagination, thus reverting to the tripartite internal model described previously in this chapter

This internal working-through process is of great significance because the conflict in childrearing emerges from the incompatibility between the unconscious and the preconscious infant and the actual, perceived infant. A caregiver's hindrances in accepting an infant's spontaneity arise from having a particular blueprint for the infant's life, elaborated far away from perception and long before the actual appearance of the newcomer, who is born for a destiny planned without his or her participation. When this blueprint is not too strong, one can see the enjoyment the caregiver displays during the unfolding of the infant's capacities, interests, creations, efforts, passion, and determination. Much laughter accompanies the little engineer's constructions or the musician's explorations of the sounds of different objects hit by a spoon. The infant's attempts to communicate the excitement of discovery and the proud discovery of one's self are some of the many meta-learning experiences visible to a sensible caregiver or skilled observer. This evidence does not announce itself with a loud, penetrant impact on the senses. Instead, it is the "small print" of the developmental process, which is unknown to casual observers, unsensible caregivers, or passers-by who wonder what there is to wonder at in child rearing—a messy, nerve-racking process.

ALTERNATIVE UNDERSTANDING OF HUMAN DEVELOPMENT

Human development has often been described as a strongly deterministic process involving genetic endowments and "basic tendencies" (a class term for different forces that explain human behavior through drives, instincts, or motivations). On the other hand, maternal and other environmental influences have been viewed as the visible cause for the origin of human behavior, the Pygmalion side of upbringing. These two basic alternatives have also been framed in the bipolar formulation of nature versus nurture. Little room has been left for chance or casualness, and even less room for an issue once dear to philosophy: free will. Here is a thorny issue without doubt. Nonetheless, free will is again becoming a topic in different realms of the study of human behavior, such as existentialism, both as a philosophical school and in the different forms of therapy derived from it. The concept of free will has never stopped being central to political thought; it is understood as self-determination in both collective and individual terms.

To avoid sliding into a philosophical controversy, I will share here observations of infants' initiatives, sustained by clear signs of self-will expressed by resistance to compliance as early as 5 months of age. The fact that an infant is able to risk disapproval and a reduction in the quality of the interaction with the main caregiver for the sake of completing an initiative is compelling evidence for the existence of an internal force driving the infant.

In psychoanalysis, we have been taught that pleasure-seeking is the big force behind actions. Yet everyday observations do not confirm the universality of pleasure-seeking. More often, an activity is performed with great effort; with expressions of displeasure, rage, and disgust; and with a great deal of painstaking repetition or change in strategy. Of course, pleasure comes in one moment or the other, but not necessarily in sensuous experience.[9]

Cognitive "instincts" have been proposed to account for this desire to explore. For example, one would have an epistemophilic drive to regain the interior of mother or to penetrate the mystery of primary scenes.

---

[9]Kohut (1977) differentiated between pleasure and joy, stating that a treatment could be considered successful when the patient "became capable of experiencing the joy of existence more keenly . . . *even in the absence of pleasure*" (p. 285; emphasis added). In many ways, Kohut made a great effort to distinguish pleasure from joy, with each as a different category of satisfaction.

This instinct is an approximate synthesis of Kleinian formulations (Klein 1950). In Piaget's (1953) account, development brings with it an inevitable quest for understanding and knowledge, which develops in a dialectic form, changing the environment through action that, in turn, changes the internal conception of the outer world, and so forth (Escalona 1968).

Escalona (1968) dedicated a whole chapter to the study of the origins of action, activity, and goal-directedness. She wrote: "Infants seek out stimulation . . . they expend effort to perform behaviors that are their own reward, in the sense that these behaviors take place *even in the presence of obstacles or negative consequences imposed by the environment*" (p. 7; emphasis added).

These concepts were originally formulated by White (1959),[10] who actually proposed the concept of *effectance motivation* as the basic form of motorization beyond instincts and drives. This form of motivation is "persistent in the sense that it regularly occupies the spare waking time between episodes of homeostatic crisis" (p. 321). Piaget (1953) observed his own son, Laurent, at age 4 months performing complex combinations and sequences of movement oriented toward producing changes in the environment. The achievements were then celebrated with laughter. I have been able to observe this behavior in infants during feeding: they are engaged in complex studies of the food's viscosity, temperature, consistency, or whatever experience they are after rather than engaged in seeking the intake of nutritional elements or the satisfaction of an oral zone.

Although I don't want to overemphasize this quest for knowledge, it certainly is an important activity. If explorations are important components, there are at least as many efforts to establish contact with the mother: calling for her attention, searching for her response to certain capacities and new achievements in what has become another classic concept, the "search for mirroring." Both in the work of two Anglo-Saxon psychoanalysts, Winnicott and Kohut, and in that of their French colleague, Lacan (1978), the mirror is an important element in the constitution of the human subject. Differences in approach, however, are quite significant.

Lacan takes as a basis for his theoretical development the studies of the child looking into a real (physical) mirror and thus starting to search for sameness and difference. In the Winnicott-Kohut approach, the mir-

---

[10]In 1980, this issue was taken up from a psychoanalytic point of view by Shapiro and Stern (1989), who pointed out that infants are "stimulus seekers rather than warding them off" (p. 284).

roring is more metaphorical; it is the reaction of the mother to the infant or the child—to behavior, a smile, the infant's looks. For a more complete distinction and for understanding the difference between this primary and secondary mirroring, see discussion by Hoffmann (1995b).

At the same time that experimentation is developing in infants, another complex phenomenon—that of play—arises during the second half of the first year. The nature of play also has been a battleground of theoretical interpretations. Although the task of clarifying this issue is beyond the scope of this chapter, Winnicott (1971/1980) provided a good summary of the idea that play is a complex phenomenon: "It may be very well that we missed something by having these two phenomena (playing and masturbatory activity) so closely linked in our minds" (p. 45).

Thus, it seems difficult to limit explanations of play to one theory, such as instinct, or drive, theory or object relations theory. The latter would explain the importance of play in terms of making contact and searching for interaction, as well as in terms of exploring or more complex experimentation. Play in itself is a complex phenomenon that has resisted explanation by a single theory.

The need for a wider concept led me to propose the theory of initiatives as the first organized form of purposeful activity in human infants. The ultimate nature of these initiatives would lead once again to the cul-de-sac of philosophical considerations unless observation and formulation are understood in their simplest forms. I propose a quality of observed initiatives that could stand in lieu of a philosophical explanation. The quality is spontaneity, which is channeled into the world through initiatives, a first form of organization of different levels of neurological and psychological contributions. These initiatives bear the mark of spontaneity, clearly distinct from induced, compliant, imitated, or reflex behavior. They stem from inside the subject, pressing for release into the world.

This rather simple, phenomenological account of events emphasizes the observed fact of an infant's being capable of exerting a capacity as agent very early in life, a capacity that the infant defends with all his or her lean, emerging might. Those actions created by the spontaneity-initiative axis are clearly emblematic and are defended as a symbol of, or as identical to, the self. Threats to self-initiated action are thus threats to the self. The infant's reactivity is, therefore, as strong as one imagines self-defense to be, depending on the degree of complexity the infant has achieved. It is also possible theoretically to refer to these actions and reactions to environmental impingements as narcissism. Nonetheless, by so doing, we will see that the infant loses the novelty of the observational approach, thus falling into blurring reductionism.

Spontaneity, organized in initiatives, knits together a network of surprisingly dissimilar patterns of behavior, with imaginable variety in experiences for each different set. Again, this is a factor to be stressed, namely, the infinite variety of early human experience possible if each individual infant is left—more or less—to design his or her own successive experiences.

For the sake of illuminating in a different light the coming together of the emerging individual and the caregiving environment, and with an eye on the place allocated to the newcomer infant, I first show the constitution of the two agendas, one for the infant and one for the caregiving system. These agendas may clash and result in conflict, go along with each other, or find ways to engage in give-and-take negotiations. The infant's agenda is determined by the organization of spontaneity through initiative, thus providing the infant with the searched-for experience. Spontaneity is basically a search for experiences in the exchange between the internal and external realities. The environmental agenda is described in a three-layer model.

The Infant's Agenda

- The infant of the maternal unconscious state
- The infant of the mother and the couple's preconscious state
- The infant of perception

Only the third layer in development (the infant of perception) ensures the needed freedom for the infant's unfolding spontaneity. The network of experiences of the world and of oneself provided by those initiatives—transformed first into actions and then into experiences—makes up one's individuality. The particular pattern of the interwoven and infinitely variable experiences, to the extent that they can be had in a reasonably free manner, will be the repertoire of the individual.

Whether there will be some margin of freedom for the baby to choose experiences depends mainly on one environmental function: respect. In this context, I use a definition almost opposed to the common usage of the term, namely, the capacity to check the power the caregiver has to suppress those expressions of the infant that do not fit into the caregiver's agenda. In this understanding of respect, it is really the infant who demands respect, not the adult. Respect is not a matter of giving up or being permissive. Although there is no space here to discuss the semiotic difference, I mention a few orienting signals for each of the following agendas:

The Caregiver's Agenda

- The caregiver's enjoyment in discovering the infant's discoveries
- The touch of novelty permeating a situation that is about to result in struggle or experiencing
- The intensity of the infant's pursuit—even if it is somehow limited by the caregiver

So, rather than giving up, the infant is involved in a very intense search for discovery. For this reason, I once proposed the concept of an encounter between two selves at this merging point in a joint creativity: the infant discovering, the adult finding the way for things to become possible (Hoffmann 1988).[11]

This concept led to a new way of understanding human development from the perspective of the unfolding of individuality as the infant subject motorizes it. The new formulation can be condensed into the simple proposal I made in the introduction ("to be and let be") as opposed to relationships of submissive compliance.

INTERRELATIONSHIP OF UNFOLDING INDIVIDUALITY WITHIN SOCIAL AND CULTURAL CONTEXTS

Keeping within the boundaries of observational elements, I now examine the possible implications of the interface between the microsystem of an individual within the caregiving system and the broader, encompassing environment provided by culture and society. Let us keep in mind that we are exploring the place of infancy, both of the infant as an individual and of the infant as a member of a social group, characterized by a particular situation of dependency, tutelage, and inability to express his or her own will on essential issues in the ways other social groups usually do (e.g., protest, legal action, voting, unionizing, uniting). Those of us in the clinical field know that some of the instruments used by the "bigger ones" are also resources for the infant: hunger strike, violence, self-injury (even self-destruction), and, quite often, passive resistance and civil disobedience (the great power play made popular by Gandhi).

---

[11]The late Michael Basch wrote a 10-page comment (Hoffmann 1988) on this paper, leading to interesting points to be worked out in other publications. I again express my gratitude to this generous teacher.

Consequences of Obstructed Initiatives

So far, I have described the infant as having a spontaneous tendency toward action for the sake of experience within the context of a reactive environment that tends to limit the infant's initiative. These limits may be for the sake of the adult's project for that infant or for the adult's different educational aims for the infant. The interplay between these two forces usually stays within limits that will allow the infant to develop normally. If not, trouble will result.

Where does the problem start? In our sample, there are no infants who show an alarming degree of action that would give the impression of an unmanageable force. Certainly, we see babies endowed with buoyant, effervescent spontaneity who are taxing the caregiver's capacities. Other infants are more contemplative, quiet, and less active, without being depressed or retarded. Temperament is an issue related to the differences in the intensity of spontaneous actions through initiatives.

The problem arises from a particular reactivity of the caregiving environment. As explained previously, the caregiver system has three different infants in the internal world, of which only one, the infant of perception, is close to being identical to the external child. The other two internal infant models are unconscious or preconscious, both created before the actual arrival of the baby. Conflict may, therefore, arise from tension between these internal models and the behavior of the external, redundantly real infant. The smaller the infant of perception, and the stronger the infant of fantasy (the unconscious, historical infant), the greater the contrast will be with the actual, reality-operating baby. Conflict thus arises from a strong, predominantly unconscious infant model in the mind of the caregiver that does not fit the unpredictable, spontaneous, initiative-driven actual child. The infant of imagination, being preconscious, is prone to being transformed for the benefit of the infant of perception through a more or less complex working-through process when the mother is finally able to express her surprise or even her disappointment at the actual child's behavior in conversation with someone such as her partner, her mother, her friend, or her therapist. This process allows for a progressive transformation of the imaginary infant of desires and wishes formed at a conscious-preconscious level. Not so for the unconscious infant of fantasy, who is therefore the prime "troublemaker."

With this origin of conflict in mind, some understanding of the consequences of confrontations is possible. How does a confrontation appear to the eyewitness? First, some actions by the infant do not visibly engage the caregiver. In the feeding situation, for example, the baby will spit out food, shut his or her mouth at the sight of the incoming spoon,

turn the head, hit the spoon, jerk backward in the chair, or start screaming while flailing around and throwing things—a major crisis. Before
there is a response by the caregiver, the infant is somehow giving a solo
performance to signal distress and vent discomfort with some aspect of
the interaction or process. The next step begins as soon as there is a clear
reaction to the infant by the caregiver, a response that may include a
certain degree of "violence." The caregiver may raise his or her voice, become upset, scold the child, or even become physically threatening or
abusive. These actions lead to open conflict. Caregiver and infant confront
each other in a power struggle. The extent and intensity are variable, but
the adult is pressing for compliance. The nature and appropriateness of
the caregiver's response (e.g., a reasonable exercise of authority, an educational must, mother's "bad day") are not being questioned here; it is
simply an overview of events of this nature that happen even frequently.

Our studies have established two categories of such events according
to the gravity of the episode: aversive behavior and interactional events.
Aversive behavior is the solo performance by the infant, a signal of distress about an unfortunate development of events that makes the baby
express disgust. Therefore, it might be seen at the communication level
as a message: "This doesn't fit me." The second category, interactional
events, a two-party issue or fight, is an interactional event with an interactional conflict. It indicates a confrontation between two opposite
projects, two subjects, two wills.

This central point raises the main issue: Infants are subjects endowed
with a project or, in fact, with a whole set of projects running in different
channels from very early on. Inclined to make contact, babies have a
strong interest in the surrounding world that leads them to explore it
thoroughly. They also have the will to persist in difficult and sometimes
quite complex tasks, such as trying to overcome frustration, rage, and im-
potence, and still return to and persist with the same endeavor. During
play, they even have a tendency to make creative transformations: a
spoon becomes a car, a tray becomes a drum, a morsel of food becomes
a fish diving into a glass of water.

A sensible mother perceives most of these investments of her child
and makes space for them, more or less to the satisfaction of the active
infant. Mother and child make a deal whereby they negotiate every inch
of space on a day-by-day basis. Conflict is an expression of what is going
on within their interactions; it indicates that there are two individuals
confronting each other. Can an infant be such at 4 months of age? Yes,
or perhaps even younger. There isn't much observational evidence of
this yet except in cases of clinical complications such as with babies who
suffer from early forms of anorexia, infants who retain their feces, and

perhaps children who are ill with acute respiratory disorders of early infancy. Not wanting to eat, not allowing bowel movements, and perhaps not even breathing—these negative infant initiatives have been pointed out as expressions of a silent confrontation (Debray et al. 1992). Because confrontation is impossible with just one individual, there is thus the possibility of one or more early forms of individuality.

What is the importance of pointing out the existence of early forms of individuality? Individuality is the single most denied fact of infant development. Even those who in recent years have conceptualized the agency function of the early self (Meissner 1986; Stern 1985) have not emphasized the implications of faulty development in this area. From the point of view of psychopathology or of grave social circumstances, an individual can now be understood as being forced to become what is expected of him or her rather than what he or she is designed and desiring to become. A member of a royal family (less inclined each day to bow to those expectations, as the yellow press reports); an inheritor of an economic empire, especially if he or she is the sole child (films such as *Arthur* and *Richie Rich,* which, in reality, are very sad stories, illustrate this situation); the only son of a political leader, destined to become his successor— these are but a few impressive examples of something that happens in less glamorous and notorious forms in the intimacy of many a household. So if we understand that this view of the child happens to parents, why does it happen to professionals as well? or to society as a whole? or to an early culture like Sparta, where "unfit" children were forced to jump off a cliff? Where are the rights of infants and children, except on paper or in the exhausting efforts of a few organizations hoarse from shouting in the desert? Where is written the right of infants to "be and become"? The answer is that infants' and children's rights are still in the making.

Witnessing the struggle of so many infants to be and become might be raising some "unscientific" passion. There should perhaps be a sign posted next to infants: "Careful! Person under construction!" Luckily, after 14 years of observing mother-infant dyads, my colleagues and I have evidence that what predominates is an attitude of letting be, which certainly has nothing to do with the permissiveness defined by Winnicott as a form of abandonment of the person of the infant. Permissiveness forces this little individual to assume self-control, which is far more devastating than maternal control, because it becomes nonnegotiable, acting as it does from within rather than from outside the infant.

So we may speak of different forms of conflict between caregiver and unfolding individual. We propose a basic distinction between:

- *Submissive compliance,* that is, the forced abandonment of the baby's own project or, even more precisely, of the project-generating capacity. In such cases, the infant constructs a facade of the self that is a false, compliant self.
- *Nonsubmissive compliance,* whereby the infant's own project may be postponed, watered down, changed, or even enriched, but not abandoned altogether; certainly, the project-generating capacity is not abandoned.

Both categories are divisible in different degrees, and I have elsewhere offered some explanations for the consequences further down the road to development (Hofffmann 1994b).

Interdependency of Individual and Family in Culture

The relationship of the individual and family within the cultural context is a two-way street:

1. On the outgoing lane is the cultural context being modified by two forms of individual attitudes: a) active-negative attitudes lead to such actions as violent behavior, delinquency, and drug abuse; and b) passive-negative attitudes result in a lack of participation, a failure to act responsibly, and noninterest and apathy. Individuals are being accused of individualism, nihilism, and cynicism. This issue is a great worry for many philosophers, sociologists, and cultural analysts in general. So-called postmodernism has been held responsible as a philosophical (non) attitude.
2. On the incoming lane, from culture toward the individual and the immediate environment (which we may call family), are the many influences held responsible for changes in health and pathology: the role of the media, the influence of ideological and religious systems, the impact of globalization and overpopulation, and the effects of modern forms of "democratic" authoritarianism in the bureaucratic handling of public affairs, to mention but a few issues raised in recent years (Taylor 1992).

I will add a single hint to understanding this puzzle through some conclusions derived from our observations: The interplay between the individual and the family may later influence the interface between the individual and society. The individual going through the educational system gets a taste of what life will be like once he or she enters society as an active member. One proposal has been to accord respectful treatment to the infant as a recognized individual from the very beginning. It is almost a commonsense truth that a person who has not been respected will have a hard time being sensitive to other people's rights and psychosocial space. But the standards by which a respectful upbringing is measured will be incomplete if there is no place for infancy within the minds of caregivers, educators, and society.

How can we say that educated adults have no place for infancy in their minds? Although there is no instrument to measure this, we might do so by appraising how much individuality the infant is credited with, both in word and in action. We might also evaluate how much participation is being sought in any specific situation that involves the infant or small child. Or we might consider how much enjoyment the adult shows in caring for the infant, or how much the caregiver enjoys the little stories that account for a surprising, willful, active, creative infant. Symbolic instruments can help us measure how much to expect a certain institution, society, or culture to respect the individual behind the person. The correct instrument measures the degree to which respect flows from the one (person or institution) in the position of advantage toward the other in the disadvantageous position. For example, if a society, cultural group, or institution is disrespectful toward women, it is hard to imagine that the same society, cultural group, or institution will be respectful toward children and infants. We can replace *women* with *ethnic minority, cultural minority*, or another group in a relatively disadvantaged position vis-à-vis the balance of power. To make it clear, we can measure the place for infancy through positive or negative signs in the family, in the society, or in the cultural group—all interrelated. Therefore, it is difficult, although possible, to find a respectful consideration of individuality within the context of gross negation of freedom to choose as in an authoritarian regime or society.

The reverse side of this issue is that societies and institutions are composed of individuals. The sum of individual traits will make up the composite attitude of the institution or society, as Winnicott (1950/1986) pointed out, according to his "formula" $(100 - [x + y + z])$, where $x =$ antisocial persons, $y =$ indeterminate persons, and $z =$ individuals who are pro-society but anti-individual. Therefore Winnicott estimated that to survive democratically, a society needs 30% mature (or non-x, non-y, and non-z) persons and, by adding a proportion of 20% indeterminate persons (y), reaches a balance level of 50% = 50% that could warrant a democratic culture. A democratic society requires a minimum of 30% mature persons and 20% indeterminate persons to neutralize the number of antisocial persons and those who are pro-society but anti-individual.[12]

---

[12]Winnicott's figures are clearly a metaphorical way of speaking in approximate terms.

Therefore, we count on a certain percentage of mature individuals, a group that does not include those who are pro-society but simultaneously anti-individual. Why is it that we so often hear complaints about the negative social value of individualism? This dilemma might be better resolved very simply by recognizing a great mistake, namely, we often confuse individualism with individuality. Individualism is certainly a negative value, or a nonvalue, inasmuch as it entails a self-centered attitude with little concern for serving common social, community, or cultural needs.

Yet individuality, on the other hand, should be understood as the optimal development of individual endowments, gifts, capacities, and designs. Initiatives, which are the expression of a spontaneous thrust toward the world, are rooted in one's deepest individuality. Initiatives are the way we express ourselves through different channels, such as by relating, knowing, making contact, playing, and thus transforming reality, as well as preparing for new forms of reality. Initiatives not only express and partake of the outer world but also take in that outer world by making experience and, thus, by knowing and transforming oneself. Environmental respect for this process of unfolding one's own individuality is a decisive experience in the necessary acquisition of the capacity to respect other people's projects and expressions.

Not being forced into submissive compliance does not mean that everything is possible for the infant, or that everything must be allowed by the caregiving system. What makes the difference between a submissive infant and a submissive environment is *negotiation*, a commonly observed interaction from very early in the infant's life. Becoming aware of the other's wishes, projects, and needs without giving up one's own is goal-learning during the first year of life that requires the concurrent presence of several functions, including intersubjectivity (Trevarthen 1979), early forms of empathy (Emde 1983),[13] and the pre-representational forms of distinction between self and other (Beebe and Lachmann 1988). Verbal communication is the crowning achievement of a long and successful process of learning to understand what goes on both in one's own mind and in the other's mind. In recent research, many of these issues have become more and more significant for understanding the process of becoming oneself while recognizing the existence of the other as

---

[13]In Emde's (1983) work, early forms of empathy are described during the second year of life; perhaps with new approaches it will become possible to register this capacity before the twelfth month, for which we have some indications in our observations.

a parallel process. Integration of different behavioral sciences is yielding good results. Integration of affects, representations, and neuroperceptual capacities (Mayes and Cohen 1994) allows for a better understanding of the coming about of the infant's capacity to attribute meaning to another's actions.

This return to the explanation of the early relationship is needed to emphasize that without the basic preservation of individuality, there is no form to warrant recognition and respect of others. When the early experience of the unfolding individual is that of a submissive compliance to an inflexible, nonnegotiating caregiving system, the result is the interruption of the goal-learning consequence of becoming oneself.

Conclusion

Becoming oneself, unfolding one's own initiatives, and making those necessary experiences that spontaneous actions are searching for requires a respectful, negotiating, nonpermissive caregiving environment. It provides the setting for different learning processes, including the meta-learning of one's own individuality as different from the other's individuality. This opens up the acquisition of understanding of one's own and the other's behavior, reasons, and desires. It provides the capacity for communication and exchange—the key to more complex future negotiations.

Thus, to become oneself, to be individualized, is the best protection against an isolated, rejecting, self-centered search for unknown experiences. Such a search arises out of a basic dissatisfaction that leads to disavowing both one's own and the other's participation in the common cause and completes the picture of individualism—the pathology of not being able to become oneself.

References

Aries P: Geschichte der Kindheit [History of Childhood]. Munich, Carl Hanse Verlag, 1988

Badinter E: L'amour en plus: l'histoire de l'amour maternel [Love and More: The History of Maternal Love]. Paris, Flammarion, 1980

Basch M: Written commentary on the unpublished paper, Encounters, by JM Hoffmann. Chicago, IL, 1988

Beebe B, Lachmann FM: The contribution of mother-infant mutual influence to the origins of self- and object representations. Psychoanal Psychol 5:305–357, 1988

Bion WR: Learning From Experience. New York, Basic Books, 1962

Debray R, Bernardi R, Hoffmann JM: Initiative and action, passive position, and maternal representations. Unpublished manuscript presented at the Fifth World Congress, World Association for Infant Psychiatry and Allied Disciplines (WAIPAD), Chicago, IL, 1992

deMause L (ed): The History of Childhood: The Untold Story of Child Abuse. New York, Peter Bedrick Books, 1988

Dickens C: Dombey and Son (1859). Oxford, UK, Oxford University Press, 1991

Emde RN: The pre-representational self and the affective core. Psychoanal Study Child 38:165–192, 1983

Erikson EH: Infancy and Society. New York, WW Norton, 1950

Escalona S: The Roots of Individuality. Chicago, IL, Aldine, 1968

Graves R: Griechische Mythologie [Greek Mythology]. Munich, Rowohlt, 1965, pp 189–190

Hoffmann JM: El desarrollo temprano del self [Early development of the self]. Psicoanalisis 6(2–3):261–294, 1984

Hoffmann JM: Encounters. Unpublished manuscript, with a discussion by the late Michael Basch, Chicago, IL, 1988

Hoffmann JM: With boredom, disbelief and failure to respond (panel presentation). Presented at the symposium "The Impact of Violence Upon Infants and Children," Thirteenth International Conference of the International Association of Child and Adolescent Psychiatry and Allied Professions, San Francisco, CA, July 1994a

Hoffmann JM: Nuevo campo [A new field]. Psicoanalisis 16(3):514–551, 1994b

Hoffmann JM: Le Role de L'Initiative dans le Development Emotionnel Precoce, organization du deuxieme semestre [The role of initiative in early emotional development, the second semester of life]. Psychiatrie de l'enfant, XXXVII, 179–213, 1994c

Hoffmann JM: Thinking about respect: some theoretical implications of microanalytic studies of early mother/infant interactions, in Developmental Issues in Child Psychiatry and Psychology 1(2):25–35, 1994d

Hoffmann JM: Espejamiento [Mirroring]. Revista de la Asociacion Argentina de Psicología y Psicoterapia de Grupo, Familia y Pareja 18(1):81–115, 1995a

Hoffmann JM: Making space. Infant Mental Health Journal 16(1):78–88, 1995b

Hoffmann JM: Del Hecho al Dicho [From doing to saying]. Presented at the biannual meeting of the Foundation Colonia del Sacramento, Uruguay, October 1996a

Hoffmann JM: Plenary discussion of Daniel Stern's presentation: therapeutic intervention strategies. Paper presented at the Sixth World Congress of the World Association for Infant Mental Health, Tampere, Finland, July 1996b

Hoffmann JM: There is such a thing as an infant. Infant Mental Health Journal 21:1–11, 2000

Hoffmann JM, Bonomini, P, Morini C, et al: Assessment of the development of initiatives in infants. Paper presented at the Fifth World Congress of the World Association for Infant Mental Health, Chicago, IL, 1992

Hoffmann JM, Popbla LA, Duhalde C: Early stages of initiative and environmental response. Infant Mental Health Journal 19:355–377, 1998

Klein M: The Psychoanalysis of Children. London, Hogarth Press, 1950

Kohut H: The Restoration of the Self. New York, International Universities Press, 1977

Kohut H: On empathy. Paper presented at a conference on self psychology, San Francisco, CA, August 1981

Kohut H: How Does Psychoanalysis Cure? Edited by Goldberg A. Chicago, IL, University of Chicago Press, 1984

Lacan J: Le moi dans la theorie de Freud et dans la technique de la psychanalyse [The ego in Freud's theory and in the psychoanalytic technique], in Le Seminaire II [Seminar II]. Edited by Miller JA. Paris, Seuil, 1978

Lebovici S: La Madre, el Bebe y el Psicoanalista [The Mother, the Baby and the Psychoanalyst]. Buenos Aires, Editorial Paidos, 1988

Lebovici S: La psicoterapia de la interacción madre-bebe [Psychotherapy of the mother-child interaction]. Paper presented at the Second Latin American Congress of the World Association for Infant Mental Health, Buenos Aires, 1991

Levi-Strauss C: Antropologia Estructural [Structural Anthropology]. Buenos Aires, Editorial Eudeba, 1972

Mayes LC, Cohen DJ: Experiencing self and others: contributions from studies of autism to the psychoanalytic theory of social development. J Am Psychoanal Assoc 42(1):191–218,1994

Meissner WW: Can psychoanalysis find its self? J Am Psychoanal Assoc 34(2):379–400, 1986

Minde K, Minde R: Infant Psychiatry: An Introductory Textbook. Edited by Kazdin AE. Beverly Hills, CA, Sage, 1986

Papousek H, Papousek M: Intuititive parenting, in Handbook of Parenting: Biology and Ecology of Parenting, Vol 2. Edited by Bornstein MH. Mahwah, NJ, Erlbaum, 1995, pp 117–136

Piaget J: The Origins of Intelligence in Children. London, Routledge & Kegan, 1953

Popper K, Lorenz K: Die Zükunft is Offen [The Future Is Open]. Munich, R. Pieper & Co, 1985

Shapiro T, Stern D: Establishment of the object in an affective field, in The Course of Life, Vol 1: Infancy, Revised. Edited by Greenspan SI, Pollock GH. Madison, CT, International Universities Press, 1989, pp 271–292

Stern D: The Interpersonal World of the Infant: A View From Psychoanalysis and Developmental Psychology. New York, Basic Books, 1985

Taylor C: The Ethics of Authenticity. Cambridge, MA, Harvard University Press, 1992

Terr L: Who's afraid in Virginia Woolf? Clues to early sexual abuse in literature. Psychoanal Study Child 45:533–546, 1990

Trevarthen CB: Communication and cooperation in early infancy, in Before Speech. Edited by Bullows M. Cambridge, UK, Cambridge University Press, 1979

Webster's New Twentieth Century Dictionary Unabridged, 2nd Edition. New York, Simon & Schuster, 1979

White RW: Motivation reconsidered: the concept of competence. Psychol Rev 66(5):297–333, 1959

Winnicott DW: Transitional objects and transitional phenomena (1953), in Collected Papers: Through Pediatrics to Psycho-Analysis. New York, Basic Books, 1958, pp 229–242

Winnicott DW: Playing: a theoretical statement (1971), in Playing and Reality. Middlesex, UK, Penguin, 1980, pp 44–61

Winnicott DW: Some thoughts on the meaning of the word "democracy" (1950), in Home Is Where We Start From. New York, WW Norton, 1986, pp 239–259

Zeldin T: An Intimate History of Humanity. London, Sinclair-Stevenson, 1994

2

Attachment, Trauma, and Self-Reflection

Implications for Later Psychopathology

Efrain Bleiberg, M.D.

In every nursery there are ghosts. They are the visitors from the unremembered past of the parents; the uninvited guests at the christening. . . . The intruders from the parental past may break through the magic circle in an unguarded moment, and a parent and his child may find themselves reenacting a moment or a scene from another time with another set of characters. (Fraiberg et al. 1975, p. 387)

The classic paper "Ghosts in the Nursery" by Selma Fraiberg and colleagues (1975) evocatively describes how some people's lives are haunted by the ghosts of brutality and insensitivity they encountered in their own childhood and how such maltreatment erupts at unguarded moments when these people become parents and reenact abusive interactions with their own children. Perhaps the most important question raised by Fraiberg et al. concerns resilience: How do some people exposed to abuse contain the ghosts, protecting themselves from severe maladjustment while also protecting their children from the transgenerational transmission of the misery that marred their early life?

Understanding these protective mechanisms is crucial. Socioeconomic pressures and scientific and clinical developments are pushing the mental health field to embrace approaches that emphasize prevention. In this case, the prevention of the patterns of behavior and maladjustment is most important because these acts (violence, self-destructiveness, drug abuse, accident proneness, illegitimate births, and child maltreatment) give rise to the greatest societal distress and greatest consumption of clinical and financial resources. In this chapter, I review the normal and distorted development of the key protective mechanism of *mentalization* or *reflective function* as an outgrowth of the attachment system and its effects on adjustment, particularly in a developmental context of trauma and maltreatment.

ATTACHMENT IN HUMAN AND NONHUMAN PRIMATES

Over the past two decades, a growing body of research has begun to systematically examine the interaction of risk factors and protective mechanisms during the process of generating, organizing, maintaining, and reinforcing patterns of adjustment and maladjustment (Beeghly and Cicchetti 1994; Fonagy et al. 1994). It is beyond the scope of this chapter to examine this burgeoning field in depth (Cicchetti and Cohen 1995). For human beings, however, it is increasingly clear that the crucial protection bestowed by evolution against the maladaptive consequences of biological vulnerability or environmental misfortune occurs within the context of the attachment system.

Developmental and neurobiological research has provided overwhelming support for the notion that the human brain is biologically designed to be organized by social experiences. Moreover, it is *prewired* to recognize, seek out, and crave human stimulation. Indeed, the brain's maturation and its capacity to perform modulating and regulatory functions are contingent on the ongoing presence of a human, interactive environment (Kandel 1998).

The observations of Spitz (1946), Bowlby (1969, 1973, 1980), and others about the distress and dysregulation infants experience in response to separation from their caregivers find support in Kandel's (1983) documentation of the human brain's predisposition to respond to the absence of people by activating the fight-or-flight alarm system. Likewise, the presence of human beings appears to elicit a biologically prepared downregulation of the alarm response. The innate link between separation from caregivers and activation of the fight-or-flight alarm system constitutes the prototype of trauma: evolution has shaped the human brain to interpret and respond to the absence of people as a sign of danger. This response fits well with Bowlby's (1969) observation that, given the helplessness of human infants at birth, nothing guarantees survival so well as the capacity to seek proximity and evoke protection from others.

Humans, of course, are not unique in experiencing distress at separation from their caregivers. All primate infants become distressed in similar situations, and they use a specific cry to evoke their caregivers' protective response. This cry of separation powerfully summons parental involvement in all primates, a response that involves autonomic and limbic-hypothalamic activation (Panksepp et al. 1980).

Although the behavioral and physiological dysregulation of human infants following separation from caregivers is well documented (Field and Reite 1984; Hollenbeck et al. 1980), research on nonhuman primates has allowed a more systematic examination of the long-term effects of such deprivation. Indeed, 50 years of research offers abundant and unequivocal evidence that early disruptions in caregiving reduce the long-term capacity to modulate psychophysiological arousal and cope with social disruptions (Kraemer 1985). Such effects can be linked to abnormal neurochemical responses of catecholamines, cortisol, serotonin, and opioids to subsequent stress (van der Kolk and Fisler 1994).

Beginning with the pioneering work of Harlow and Harlow (1971), evidence has accumulated to show that nonhuman primates separated from their caregivers grow to exhibit grossly abnormal social and sexual behavior. These primates do not produce offspring and will mutilate or kill their babies if artificially inseminated. They become socially withdrawn and unpredictably aggressive, and they develop self-destructive and self-stimulating behavior such as self-clasping, self-sucking, and biting. Of particular interest for the subsequent discussion is the finding that these socially deprived monkeys fail to learn to discriminate social cues, such as facial expressions (Mirsky 1968). Remnants of this deficit persist throughout their lives, despite later exposure to social situations.

Although separation evokes a nearly universal pattern of protest followed by despair and numbing, the age at which protracted separation in monkeys occurs is crucial in determining the intensity of short-term response and the severity of long-term consequences. With some variations, deprivation of caregiving at the end of the first year, roughly equivalent to the third year in human infants, tends to have severe and permanent negative consequences (Suomi 1984).

The consequences, however, are not entirely irreversible. Suomi and Harlow (1972) demonstrated that rearing separated monkeys with peers could eliminate most of the grossly maladaptive behavior caused by isolation. After 3 or 4 years of living with peers, the initially separated monkeys were nearly indistinguishable from normally reared monkeys (Suomi et al. 1974). However, their adaptation was vulnerable under social stress. When complex social discriminations were required, the separated monkeys again became socially inappropriate, either withdrawing or becoming aggressive. They also engaged in stereotypical activities. Even under less stressful conditions, isolated monkeys persistently showed deficits in sexual behavior and ongoing inability to read social cues effectively.

ATTACHMENT AND REFLECTIVE FUNCTION

Research on the effects of disruptions in caregiving on nonhuman primates opens a window onto the significance of attachment in human development. When caregiving is interrupted, human infants, like other primates, go through the stage of *protest* and exhibit agitation, increased arousal, and autonomic activation (Bowlby 1969). After several hours or days, human infants go through the stage Bowlby called *despair*. During this stage, motoric and emotional expression is restricted, REM sleep is decreased, overall sleep is disrupted, and autonomic measures are below the normal baseline (Hollenbeck et al. 1980; van der Kolk and Fisler 1994). The presence and appropriate response of the caregiver are needed to restore optimal levels of behavioral and physiological activation and arousal. Without such response, distress progresses to activation of the fight-or-flight system. Yet infants are obviously limited in their capacity to fight or flee and are thus restricted to a relatively small repertoire of actions to modulate agitation and hyperarousal: gaze aversion, self-sucking, and, particularly, dissociation. By dissociating, infants can enter into trance-like states and perhaps ignore dysphoric or overwhelming input, including internal sensations (Gardner and Olness 1981). Perry (1997) suggests the caregiver's repeated failure to respond to the human infant's signals of distress organizes the infant's developing brain in the direction of a proneness to rapidly trigger the fight-or-flight system, particularly the dissociative component more readily available to infants (Figure 2–1).

The caregiver's capacity to modulate psychophysiological arousal raises the question: What elements of the caregiver's presence or response mediate such regulatory capacity? Stern (1985) called attention to the affect attunement between mothers and their infants—that is, the caregiver's capacity to intuitively grasp the infant's internal states (hunger, agitation, contentment, and playfulness) and respond in a way that conveys to the infant, "I got your message, and I can deal with it or help you deal with it." Stern's research showed the behavior of about half the mothers fit this description of attunement. During these interactions, the heart rates and other physiological measures of mothers and infants paralleled each other.

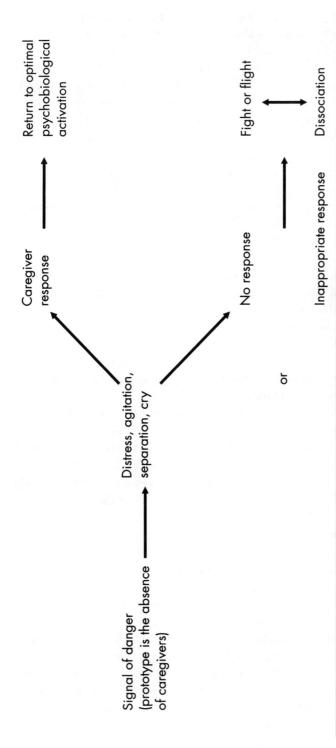

Figure 2–1.   Trauma and caregivers' responses "organize" infant's brain toward organization or toward a proneness to dissociation.

Attuned behavior from caregivers conveys to infants that behind their own behavior are internal mental states (feelings, desires, intentions) making such behavior understandable, meaningful, and predictable. Such a process occurs, for example, when a caregiver makes sense of a baby's crying and fussing and responds with stroking, rocking, feeding, and verbalizations ("Oh, honey, you are so hungry!"). Developmental research is showing such interactions not only change the infant's internal state from agitated and dysphoric to calm and contented but also activate a key inborn capacity: the ability to grasp that mental states underlie human behavior (Fonagy et al. 1991; Gergely and Watson 1996).

When caregivers treat their infants as intentional beings, the infants in turn discover their own behavior, as well as that of others, is intentional. This discovery triggers the unfolding of a biologically prepared ability to interpret the behavior of all agents—themselves and others—in terms of putative internal states. Developmentalists refer to this developmental acquisition as mentalization or reflective function (Fonagy et al. 1991) or as the infant's theory of mind (Baron-Cohen 1994, 1995). This capacity should not be confused with introspection, insight, or the ability to explain our own or other people's motives. It is, instead, the moment-to-moment reading of an interpersonal situation that allows for the mutual adjustments that permit reciprocity in interactions. As Baron-Cohen (1995) and Hobson (1993) demonstrate, the hallmark of autism is precisely the brain-based failure to develop reflective function.

It is beyond the scope of this chapter to examine in detail current ideas about the development of reflective function (see Astington and Jenkins 1995; Baron-Cohen 1994; Fonagy et al. 1993). The biological rootedness of reflective function is apparent in the study of face-to-face exchanges of affective signals during the first 5 months of life (Gergely and Watson 1996; Tronick 1989). Careful analysis of these transactions demonstrates that both caregiver and infant are sensitive to each other's states and both regulate their expression on the basis of the anticipated reaction of the other. This mutual cuing is impossible for autistic infants and for the sense of strangeness and lack of reciprocity reported by their caregivers.

These presymbolic interactions do not involve the infant's grasp of intentionality. Infants process and store their experiences using memories based on unconscious, implicit, procedural memory (Kihlstrom and Hoyt 1990; Schacter 1992; Squire 1987). In contrast to the autobiographical memory system that develops later, procedural memory is nonvoluntary, nondeclarative, and nonreflective, and it is dominated by emotional, impressionistic, motoric, and perceptual information. More importantly, procedural memory, underpinned by its own, relatively homogeneous neurological system, stores the "how to" of the execution of sequences of motor and perceptual strategies in response to specific cues. Thus, the knowledge is context-bound—that is, it is activated by a concrete element such as a physical sensation or visual cue of the context in which the knowledge was acquired, and it is accessible only through performance. It manifests only when the individual performs the skills and operations into which the knowledge is embedded, and it depends on specific sensory and motor systems and on the cerebellum and basal ganglia (Kandel 1998).

The early mental schemas or internal working models of the self in interaction with others are most likely construed as procedural memories that find expression in four patterns of attachment: *secure, anxious/avoidant, anxious/resistant,* and *disorganized/disoriented* (Bowlby 1973). These patterns are classified on the basis of a well-known procedure, the strange situation, in which infants are briefly separated from their caregivers in an unfamiliar environment (Ainsworth et al. 1978). Infants classified as secure readily explore the unfamiliar environment in the caregiver's presence, are distressed during the caregiver's absence, are anxious in the presence of the stranger, but are quickly reassured when the caregiver returns, at which point they promptly resume active exploration. Anxious/avoidant infants show little distress when separated from the caregiver and may avoid the caregiver's efforts to attract their attention or establish contact on reunion. In contrast, anxious/resistant infants appear preoccupied with the caregiver's whereabouts even when the caregiver is present and limit their exploratory activity. These infants are highly distressed by the separation, cannot settle down after the caregiver returns, and continue to cling, cry, and fuss. Finally, disorganized/disoriented infants appear difficult to classify because they are disorganized or disoriented in the caregiver's presence and present a mix of approaching, avoiding, and trance-like behavior (Main and Solomon 1986).

The point here is that an infant's attachment pattern during the first year of life is specifically evoked by a particular caregiver and does not predict the attachment pattern exhibited with other caregivers. Such specificity of context points to the procedural nature of the underlying schemas: Behavioral patterns (crying, exploring, clinging, or avoiding) are triggered by the concrete cue of a particular person but do not generalize to other relationships.

Acquiring the capacity to grasp social cues and "read minds" opens the path for a unique human development: the miracle of symbolic representation (Hobson 1993). There is general agreement that the harmoniousness of the mother-child relationship is a key contributor to the emergence of symbolic thought (Bretherton and Bates 1979). For example, Hobson (1993) draws attention to the phenomenon of social referencing (Campos and Stenberg 1981; Sorce et al. 1985). A 1-year-old confronted with a visual cliff proceeds over the cliff if the caregiver looks relaxed but freezes if the caregiver appears anxious. Hobson points out that the crucial issue in social referencing is the infant's dawning appreciation of the distinction between the concrete world as given and a world in which objects and events can have person-related meanings—the same situation can be either dangerous or inviting. That is, in any situation, the meaning for the infant is not necessarily the meaning for the caregiver.

Because of constitutional abnormalities, autistic children cannot engage in the intersubjective coordination that facilitates understanding people's minds and distinguishing between mental states and things. Thus, they face severe limitations in participating in developmental opportunities that further symbolic development (mainly play, peer interactions, language, and smooth reciprocity with caregivers).

Play and pretend activities foster both understanding of mental states and development of symbolic processing. To play with another person, even in as basic a game as peek-a-boo, requires an exquisite synchronicity of mental states, affect, and tempo lest the play collapse. As play progresses to the realm of pretend, symbolic processing advances. For example, when a 2-year-old chooses a stick as a stand-in for a gun, he or she is conferring a self-selected meaning on the stick (the conception of a gun) alongside the child's recognition of the stick as a thing. When children share their pretend, symbolic meaning with others, they have to simultaneously hold in mind the two realities, pretend and actual, in synchrony with a moment-to-moment reading of the state of mind of the others who share the pretense.

Contacts with peers and siblings also promote mentalization and symbolization (Jenkins and Astington 1996; Perner et al. 1994). In fact, these contacts may be more crucial in building childhood ideals and goals than interactions with parents. Such facilitation is predicated not only on the increased opportunities for pretend play afforded by peers but also on the multiple, pretend and real, roles children must synchronize in more complex social settings. Thus children learn to appreciate the right social cues that signal an opportunity to be a sibling, playmate, rival, child, and so forth.

The central role of language in the acquisition of reflective function and symbolization is well established (Smith 1996). Verbalizations about feelings and the reasons behind people's actions, including early labeling of the infant's actions ("Oh, honey, you are so hungry!"), are linked to the achievement of reflective function (Dunn and Brown 1993; Dunn et al. 1991). But the experience of using language, irrespective of whether it refers to mental states, alerts children to the fact that people are receivers and providers of information conveyed through verbal-symbolic referents.

Perhaps the critical factor in developing children's reflective function is the caregiver's own reflective capacity. The caregiver's ability to read the moment-to-moment changes in the child's mental state appears to be the root of sensitive parenting and the foundation of secure attachment. Securely attached children, in turn, can explore their own and other people's minds and demonstrate their ability through subsequent competence with theory-of-mind tasks (Fonagy et al. 1991).

Through play, pretend, peer interaction, use of language, and intersubjective exchange with sensitive caregivers, the development of the reflective function fuels the growth of symbolic-autobiographical processing and explicit memory. Explicit autobiographical memory is also based on a relatively homogeneous neurological and psychological system. It encodes information accessible to conscious awareness about what things are, compared with the implicit-procedural memory for how to do something. This memory of autobiographical events and factual knowledge requires the input of the hippocampus and the medial temporal lobe. Explicit memories, including autobiographical ones, are amenable to symbolic transformations by separating the symbolic representation or meaning of an object or event from the concrete context in which the knowledge was acquired. This knowledge is not expressed through procedures but through verbal-symbolic referents. Explicit symbolic processing appears designed to create coherent symbolic models—narratives that make sense of the world, other people, and ourselves.

Even at their most rudimentary level during the second and third years of life, symbolic processing and the growing capacity to mentalize allow young children to respond not only to others' behavior but also to their own conception of others' beliefs, feelings, attitudes, desires, hopes, knowledge, imagination, pretense, deceit, plans, intentions, and so on. For example, the child believes the caregiver does not respond because the caregiver is tired. Or the child believes the caregiver is angry and thinks the child is bad because the child wants to hit his or her sibling.

By attributing mental states to themselves and others, children make behavior meaningful and predictable. As they learn to assess the meaning of other people's behavior, they become capable of selecting and activating from the multiple sets of internal working models they have organized on the basis of prior experience the ones best suited to respond adaptively to a particular interpersonal situation. The effect of this capacity to select an internal mediator of behavior—even if this process occurs outside conscious awareness—allows children to transform their whims, urges, and automatic responses to concrete cues into more sustained and active experience of decisions and intentionalities. This development, in turn, enables children to derive a sense of agency about and ownership of their behavior.

As they gain a sense of intentionality and agency, children also begin to integrate wishes, needs, motives, roles, and relationship patterns into a more coherent and continuous sense of self and others. This development, in turn, paves the way for acquisition of the modulating psychological abilities that underlie affect regulation, impulse control, self-monitoring, and the capacity for planning and setting goals, values, and ideals.

TRAUMA, ATTACHMENT, AND REFLECTIVE FUNCTION

Developmental research strongly supports the notion that the human brain has a built-in predisposition toward mastery and the creation of perceptual-experiential coherence and organization. As Emde (1989) remarks, the infant comes into the world "with biologically prepared active propensities and with organized capacities for self-regulation" (p. 38). Stern (1985) also notes the innate tendency of babies to connect in their mind what goes together in reality, that is, to actively create models of reality based on past experience. Bowlby's internal working models are the aggregates of experiences with caregivers that infants organize and use to develop coping strategies (attachment patterns) based on their expectations of caregiver behavior.

It is not surprising that the innate tendency toward mastery and experiential coherence is intimately intertwined with the bias toward attachments. As Greenberg and Mitchell (1983) suggest, human beings have been shaped by evolution to be both self-regulating and field-regulating. We are, as Greenberg and Mitchell assert, fundamentally concerned with both creating and maintaining coherence, mastery, and organization and creating and maintaining sustained connections with others. It appears increasingly clear that the specific way human beings create coherence, mastery, and organization is precisely by grasping social cues and generating meaning out of intersubjective exchanges.

Furthermore, as Stern (1985) points out, infants have a related predisposition to experience a traumatic response and activate the fight-or-flight system when there is a mismatch between the infant's mental model of reality, particularly of himself or herself in relation to others, and the actual interaction or real event (Horowitz 1987). For example, infants respond with obvious distress when shown a videotape of a human face with the sound of the person's voice delayed by even a few hundredths of a millisecond, mismatched with the visual image, and presumably out of sync with their mental model of expected synchronicity between visual and auditory stimuli (Stern 1985).

Freud's early writings described quite well the pathogenic consequences of a disruption in experiential coherence. In "Studies on Hysteria," Breuer and Freud (1893–1895/1955) claimed an event becomes pathogenic when it is incongruous with the "dominant mass of ideas" (p. 116)—the psychic organization that Freud subsequently called the ego—and cannot be integrated and processed through the normal psychological mechanism. Instead, the memory of the event persists unmetabolized, seeking expression through somatic or symptomatic channels.

This early concept set the stage for Freud's later definition of trauma. In *Inhibitions, Symptoms and Anxiety,* Freud (1926/1959) conceptualized trauma as the experience of being overwhelmed by an adaptive demand that renders the ego passive, helpless, and unable to anticipate, cope, and integrate. According to Freud, the essence and meaning of the traumatic situation consists of "the subject's estimation of his own strength compared to the magnitude of the danger and his admission of helplessness" (p. 166). As a corollary, Freud described a self-righting tendency of the ego to turn around such passivity and helplessness to regain activity, control, and integration.

Traumatized individuals, in fact, show impairment in their capacity to integrate traumatic memories and process them through the normal psychological mechanisms of symbolization and encoding of explicit, autobiographical memories. Such memories of terrifying, traumatizing events remain in prolonged, unintegrated storage; are prone to activation by concrete reminders of the trauma (the time of day it occurred, a smell, a physical sensation, a visual cue); and evoke anew the shock, helplessness, hyperarousal, and loneliness of the original trauma (van der Kolk and Fisler 1994). Instead of using affective arousal as a cue to attend to incoming information and select the mental models appropriate to the situation, traumatized individuals respond to arousal evoked by a traumatic reminder as an automatic trigger for fight-or-flight and, as van der Kolk and Fisler (1994) suggest, go immediately "from stimulus to response without being able to make the necessary psychological assessment of the meaning of what is going on" (p. 154).

Because traumatized children and adults suffer from impaired symbolic representation, they lack the capacity to respond flexibly and adaptively to the symbolic, meaningful qualities of their own and other people's behavior. Instead, they find themselves trapped in a fixed pattern of perception and affect-motor responses not amenable to reflection or modulation: the catastrophic response to trauma.

Although all overwhelming life experiences can have pernicious effects, physical and sexual abuse assault children with special destructiveness. These forms of abuse often involve conditions of protracted, if not seemingly inescapable, victimization. This victimization precludes the self-righting tendencies of the normal brain (as described by Freud) from realistically restoring a sense of integration, mastery, and control. That is, the brain is unable to turn around in reality the passivity and helplessness that are the hallmarks of trauma.

Furthermore, the perpetrators of physical and sexual abuse are commonly the same people—the caregivers—on whom children rely to help them develop the symbolic, reflective functions that bring coherence and meaning to experience. Fears of retribution, conflicts of loyalty, and concerns about destroying or bringing shame to the family militate against disclosing and sharing the abuse with others, both within and outside the family, further exacerbating the children's sense of isolation and difficulty in making sense of the abusive events. Feelings of pleasure and specialness mix confusingly with pain, rage, shame, and helplessness, compounding the children's inability to bring coherence to their experience.

An abundance of research demonstrates that children respond more severely to, and are less able to overcome, the effects of trauma perpetrated by parents or other family members (Chu and Dill 1990; Pynoos et al. 1987; Terr 1991). Terr (1991), among others, believes that repeated exposure to physical or sexual abuse, or both, evokes enduring distortions in relationship patterns, subjective experience, sense of self, and coping strategies. For Terr, the defenses and coping mechanisms of children exposed to protracted trauma, which she calls type II trauma, often lead to profound and profoundly maladaptive character changes.

VULNERABILITY AND RESILIENCE: THE PROTECTION OF REFLECTIVE FUNCTION

Yet as Fraiberg et al. (1975) point out, not every abused child grows up to suffer severe maladjustment or becomes an abuser. Although many studies demonstrate that physical and sexual abuse are overrepresented in the background of individuals with severe and persistent psychopathology, particularly those with borderline and antisocial personality disorders (Paris and Zweig-Frank 1997), it is clear that a large percentage—

perhaps even the majority—of survivors of childhood abuse do not grow up to develop persistent patterns of gross maladjustment.

Evidence is accumulating about how reflective function may be the key factor protecting victims of maltreatment from severe maladjustment. The Adult Attachment Interview (AAI; George et al. 1985) has proven to be a remarkably useful instrument for probing the links between attachment experiences in childhood and adult functioning. It is a structured interview that asks the subject to produce and reflect on memories of early attachment experiences and their effects on subsequent functioning. The AAI scoring system classifies individuals as *secure/ autonomous, insecure/dismissing, insecure/preoccupied,* or *unresolved/disorganized* with respect to attachment, loss, or trauma on the basis of the structural qualities (coherence, relevance, completeness, and clarity) of the subject's narrative of early experiences (Main and Goldwyn 1993).

Secure/autonomous individuals value attachment relationships and present them in an internally consistent manner. Their responses are clear, relevant, and succinct. Reflective function—or, as Main calls it, *metacognitive monitoring*—is evident when subjects respond, for example, that their memories might be in error, that the person they are discussing might have a different viewpoint, or that their present beliefs may later change. Such classification is unrelated to whether the childhood experiences are largely positive, difficult, or traumatic.

Insecure/dismissing individuals minimize the importance of attachments, but their narratives are filled with internal contradictions. Insecure/preoccupied subjects, on the other hand, exhibit a confused, angry, or passive preoccupation with attachment figures. Their responses are grammatically entangled, as if they are unable to remain focused on the interviewer's questions once memories are aroused. The unresolved/ disorganized category includes individuals who present cognitive disorganization and disorientation specifically during discussions of potentially traumatic events, such as loss or maltreatment.

A body of research using the AAI is beginning to provide empirical documentation for a notion that clinicians have long understood—namely, that the ability to adaptively overcome adverse, even overwhelming, life events is predicated on the individual's capacity to create a coherent narrative of the experience that gives meaning to the past and allows the person to sustain connections with others. The central mechanism for creating coherent narratives and connecting meaningfully with others is the reflective function: the ability to grasp meaning from interpersonal exchanges, which allows for a flexible reconfiguration of mental representations and limits automatic, unreflective activation of patterns of experience and response.

Rating the reflective capacity indicated in AAI narratives, Fonagy et al. (1991) demonstrated that mothers and fathers with high reflective function were three to four times more likely to have securely attached children. The predictive capacity of reflective function was not affected by the parents' early deprivation. A subsequent study divided mothers according to their degree of childhood deprivation. In this study, all the children of deprived mothers with high reflective function were securely attached to their mothers, while almost none of the children of deprived mothers with low reflective function showed a pattern of secure attachment (Fonagy et al. 1994).

REFLECTIVE FUNCTION, RESPONSE TO TRAUMA, AND PATTERNS OF MALADJUSTMENT

To return to the original question: Why can some individuals develop reflective function despite traumatic events, including maltreatment, while others cannot? It is becoming increasingly compelling to consider that psychobiological alterations prior to a traumatic event, including abuse, shape long-term and acute responses to trauma.

Yehuda (1997) points out that posttraumatic stress disorder (PTSD) occurs only in individuals who present a particular biological response to trauma that is neither typical nor normative. Yehuda's research demonstrates that individuals who develop PTSD show lower-than-normal levels of cortisol, the hormone necessary to terminate the psychobiological response of hyperarousal and autonomic activation following a stressor. It appears that individuals predisposed to PTSD present an enhanced negative feedback inhibition of the hypothalamic-pituitary-adrenal axis. Chronic hyperstimulation of the pituitary leads to pituitary hyporesponsiveness that, in turn, leaves the adrenal receptors (dependent on pituitary input) hypersensitive to stimulation.

Thus, PTSD patients appear biologically predisposed to respond abnormally to stress. They are unable to effectively terminate the brain's response to trauma because of low levels of cortisol and are subsequently hyperresponsive to environmental challenges (traumatic reminders) because of hypersensitive adrenal receptors. Similar abnormalities have been identified in the sympathetic nervous system and in other neuromodulatory systems (McParlane et al. 1993; Murburgh 1994; Shalev et al. 1993) and are consistent with the findings of hypervigilance, increased startle, irritability, and physiological hyperarousal to traumatic reminders characteristic of PTSD patients.

The origins of the biological alteration in the hypothalamic-pituitary-adrenal axis are not clear. But some children may be sensitized to respond catastrophically and with potentially long-term maladaptive consequences to stress and trauma by an unfavorable balance between the constitutional vulnerability of neuromodulatory mechanisms and the protection afforded by reflective function in the context of secure attachments.

As with most aspects of development, the balance between biological vulnerabilities and psychosocial determinants of reflective function development is a bidirectional, transactional process. Certain biological vulnerabilities, such as those in attention-deficit/hyperactivity disorder or learning disorders, may directly limit children's evolving reflective function. For example, these disorders may inherently limit symbolic capacities or disturb the regulation of arousal, as postulated by Yehuda (1997). At the same time, biological factors play an important part in shaping children's experience of themselves and others; their competence and other people's reliability; and the safety or lack thereof in their emotional responses. Such factors also affect their ability to monitor emotional signals from themselves and others, cue others about their internal states, and create reciprocal interactions. Last but not least, biological factors (e.g., irritability, poor adaptability, impulsivity, and overactivity) provoke interpersonal conflicts and caregiver frustration. Thus, biological factors can limit the development of reflective function by generating an environment that fails to promote this function. An inhibiting environment in turn exacerbates the impact of biological vulnerabilities by depriving the individual of social support and the natural protective mechanism of reflective function.

More specifically, the distress of some vulnerable children becomes an overwhelming signal of danger to their caregivers. For caregivers with a history of abuse, this distress acts as a traumatic reminder, evoking in them unmodulated fight-or-flight responses. They feel either compelled to escape their infant's cry or driven to destroy what at that moment appears to be the source of their distress: their own infant. One mother, for example, reported how her baby's cry provoked uncontrollable panic in her, a need to get away, and an overwhelming desire to get the baby to "shut up." She found that she could protect the baby and herself only by locking herself in the bathroom and turning on the shower to muffle the cries of the inconsolable, unattended baby. Weston (1968) confirms this paradigm, noting that 80% of mothers who abused their children gave infants' crying as a reason for the abuse. Typically, however, after the caregiver snaps out of the fight-or-flight mode, he or she replaces the abuse or neglect, or both, with intense, guilt-driven, overstimulating overinvolvement, setting the stage for the disorganized/disoriented pattern of attachment shown by as many as 80% of abused infants and children (Carlsson and Sroufe 1995).

The ghosts from the parental past do intrude at unguarded moments when, under the impact of a reminder of their own childhood trauma, caregivers lose the capacity to process symbolically and maintain reflective function and, instead, find themselves driven to an automatic fight-or-flight response. In effect, the infant's emotional expression triggers in the caregiver a temporary failure to perceive the infant as an intentional, psychological being. Under those circumstances, some children, perhaps those with an unfavorable balance between biological vulnerability and strength of reflective function, cope with the situation by actively retreating from reflective function in response to their own distress. Such a coping strategy evolves out of the children's sense that their distress evokes in the caregiver frightened or frightening behavior or both—that is, behavior that incompletely masks a terrifying internal state: a desire to destroy or escape from the child.

The chaotic and contradictory features of approach and avoidance of the disorganized/disoriented attachment pattern characteristic of abused children may represent not only the children's effort to distance themselves from awareness of their caregiver's terrifying mental states, but also their adaptation to the caregiver's subsequent reengagement. Over time, however, some of these disorganized/disoriented children learn to fraction (Fischer et al. 1990), that is, they split their access to reflective functioning across domains of interpersonal interaction.

Experiencing their own arousal as a danger signal for abandonment, abuse, or the loss of a partner who can experience them as intentional beings, these children become hypervigilant of other people's mental states and overfocus on monitoring their own distress. In emotionally charged interactions or during distress, they withdraw from a mentalizing, reflective stance and instead activate fixed, automatic procedural patterns designed to reestablish a sense of mastery, control, and interpersonal connection.

As a result of the fractionation of their reflective function, they evolve multiple coherent, but unintegrated, subsets of mental representations of themselves in interaction with others. (Some representations are organized by, and encoded in, explicit, autobiographical, reflective means, whereas others are arranged in an implicit, procedural, nonreflective mode.) By retreating from mentalization and instead activating concrete, procedural models, these children restore a sense of activity and control to counter their feelings of helplessness and passivity. They do not wait for trauma to overwhelm their reflective function; rather, they actively retreat from mentalization. In other words, they do not wait for their caregivers to become monsters, that is, people driven by ghosts who can no longer see them as real human beings. Instead, they create concrete, unreflective, rigid mental models of themselves and others through which, in a fixed pattern, they can achieve at least an illusion of coping with overwhelming forces not open to empathy or reflection.

Although these coping strategies afford some semblance of self-righting, the process of activating nonreflective models and withdrawing from a reflective stance leaves children temporarily bereft of the adaptive capacities afforded by reflective function. They struggle to a) maintain a stable and coherent sense of self; b) experience ownership and agency over their behavior; c) self-soothe and otherwise label, contain, and regulate their affective experience; d) create a sense of direction, set self-limits, and tolerate frustration; and e) experience others as intentional, understandable human beings and feel connected to others through the mutual sharing of mental (meaningful) states.

As these children move into school age, particularly adolescence, they face the accompanying demand for more complex social discriminations, an enhanced need to integrate multiple sets of mental representations, and a greater opportunity for emotionally intense interactions and hyperarousal. In this context of increasing psychosocial and psychobiological demands, their proneness to withdraw from reflective function becomes a significant developmental handicap similar to the one experienced by the separated monkeys studied by Suomi et al. (1974).

Adolescence is a time when these youngsters develop coping mechanisms to deal with the experiences of shattered security, subjective dyscontrol, and emotional disconnection linked to the loss of reflective function. These strategies become increasingly rigid and self-perpetuating. The self-righting imperative built into the human brain produces rigid patterns of coping, relating, and organizing subjective experience. These patterns are designed to evoke interpersonal responses that confirm, validate, and reinforce a set of internal convictions and representational models and promote, as much as possible, a sense of control and an ability to still feel connected to others.

Thus, some adolescents transform their sense of periodic subjective dyscontrol (and the associated conviction that misery, passivity, and helplessness will befall them) into the active pursuit of victimization, either self-inflicted or perpetrated by others. Paradoxically, self-victimization induces a secret sense of power and control as these youngsters actively provoke the very trauma they otherwise believe will happen to them.

Some self-victimizing youngsters become particularly adept at creating states of numbness and dissociation whenever they risk becoming overwhelmed or hyperaroused. Terr (1991) describes a boy who coped with his stepfather's brutal beatings by producing a self-hypnotic state in which he visualized himself sitting on his mother's lap while enjoying a picnic at a beautiful park. Although self-hypnosis and other self-induced forms of numbness and dissociation can provide some distance from overwhelmingly painful internal and external stimuli, they can also lead to a terrifying sense of inner deadness. Some youngsters resort to self-mutilation and other forms of parasuicidal behavior to try to restore a sense of being alive, to secure attention and involvement from others, and frequently to express aggression in a concealed way.

Other abused youngsters, particularly boys, express aggression more directly. When faced with experiences of vulnerability, dependency, or helplessness, they desperately attempt to maintain a sense of control by turning others into helpless, intimidated victims (Bleiberg 1988). Perennially haunted by the expectation of being attacked, these youngsters carefully scan the environment for threats. They anticipate that if their shortcomings are revealed and their sense of control is punctured, they will be painfully humiliated and viciously destroyed. They expect the same ruthlessness and lack of compassion from others that they themselves exhibit. For these youngsters, it would appear that dependency on others and efforts to secure protection or comfort from caregivers have led only to greater pain, and physical and psychological survival has seemed predicated on manipulation, toughness, self-reliance, and denial of vulnerability and dependency.

By adolescence and early adulthood, these developmental trends and coping strategies begin to coalesce into persistent patterns of maladjustment. Axis I diagnoses, such as eating disorders and substance abuse disorders, are often incorporated into personality disorders, particularly those in Cluster B or the dramatic personality disorders encompassing the borderline, narcissistic, histrionic, and antisocial personality disorders.

Once they have children of their own, individuals who dealt with abuse by intermittently retreating from reflective function are at enormous risk of becoming abusers themselves, confirming Fraiberg et al.'s (1975) original observation. Children's vulnerability, helplessness, and distress trigger automatic responses of disconnection from the caregiver's own vulnerability, helplessness, and distress. But as Fraiberg et al. point out, those parents who retain an integration of the memories and affects that were part of their own abuse experiences, and retain a reflective function even when presented with traumatic reminders, are far more likely to experience (with conviction and empathy) the pain that parental misattunement can inflict on children.

The factors that permit some people to develop a resilient reflective capacity, even against seemingly large odds, are not entirely clear. A constitutional sturdiness most likely contributes, perhaps in the form of an exceptional innate capacity to develop reflective function (the opposite end of the spectrum from autism) or a greater-than-average capacity to modulate and terminate the alarm response of hyperarousal to stress.

The presence of other people who can respond reflectively to the child also appears to be a critical factor in explaining resilience. In particular, interaction with peers who promote reflective function rather than re-inforce unreflective, impulsive behavior is emerging as a critical factor in explaining differences in outcome. Harris (1998) advances the notion that in both normal and pathological development, peers matter more fundamentally than parents (aside from direct genetic influence) in the shaping of character and personality. Harris cites evidence showing that although African American boys from poor, single-parent, high-risk families commit more delinquent acts than do white boys, when the boys are divided by neighborhood, the effect of coming from a high-risk family largely disappears. African American boys who did not live in the poorest underclass neighborhoods, even if they came from poor single-parent families, were at no greater risk for delinquency than white middle-class boys.

The central point of Harris's observations is that children are not par-ticularly interested in becoming like their parents; they want to be as competent as they can be and accepted as they can be at being children. Given the realities of human development, however, which include rather prolonged maturation and growth contingent on the presence of care-givers, it appears more plausible that parents are essential for activating the crucial capacities on which subsequent development depends, in-cluding the capacity of reflective function.

Reflective function and the associated development of symbolic pro-cess give children, beginning in the second half of the second year and the third year of life, an extraordinary new tool for achieving mastery, integration, and connection with others. Children become increasingly capable of creating a mental representation, which Joffe and Sandler (1967) call the "ideal self." This ideal self is a representation of the self associated with a sense of safety, competence, and satisfaction. The ideal self conjures up the experience of mastery, control, and integration; it involves the ability to meet adaptive demands and maintain attachments with available and responsive others. According to Joffe and Sandler, the ideal self is a composite of a) memories of actual experiences of pleasure, mastery, and attachment; b) fantasies about such experiences (which be-come more elaborated symbolically and more available to serve defensive purposes); and c) the models provided by other people who are loved, feared, or admired.

Children use the representation of the ideal as a blueprint, a road map to reverse states of helplessness and vulnerability and to restore attachments. The ideal self functions as a proximal area of development (Stern 1985)—that is, as a preview of the person the child is about to become. Children are inclined to seek selflike models, particularly peers, to reconfigure their ideal self so that it can continue to function as an effective guide to finding solutions to developmental challenges and life's dilemmas, exploring ways of being in the world and relating to others, and attempting behaviors and attitudes that promise greater mastery, more effective coping, and increased pleasure and adaptation.

Corsaro, as quoted in an article by Gladwell (1998), illustrates how children take their cues from each other and, in the process, make contact with sources that stimulate their reflective function. Corsaro describes watching two 4-year-old girls, Jenny and Betty, playing house in a sandbox, where they are putting sand in pots and teacups. Suddenly a third girl, Debbie, approaches. Corsaro describes how Debbie watches Jenny and Betty for about 5 minutes; then she circles the sandbox and watches again before she moves to the sandbox and reaches for a teacup. Jenny takes the cup away from Debbie and says, "No." Debbie backs away and again watches Jenny and Betty. She then walks over to Betty and says, "We are friends, right, Betty?" Betty, not looking up at Debbie, continues to put sand in the cup and says, "Right." Debbie moves next to Betty, takes a pot and spoon, begins to put sand in the pot, and says, "I am making coffee." "I am making cupcakes," replies Betty. Betty turns to Jenny and says, "We are mothers, right, Jenny?" "Right," says Jenny. Through such interactions, children grasp complex strategies of approach, avoidance, sharing, and competing while picking up cues about the intersubjective meanings being created and exchanged.

Through access to peers who function in such reflective and symbolic fashion, even abused children apparently develop sufficient reflective capacity to overcome the most pernicious long-term consequences of trauma. Even in the face of traumatic reminders, they preserve the ability to create a story about themselves and their past ("Mom was so lonely and scared; she did the best she could") populated by real human beings with meaningful and understandable behavior. Thus, they are in a position to remain attuned and empathic to their own children and to experience them as real, intentional beings rather than as frightening or hated ghosts made of psychological cardboard and evocative only of a compelling need to escape or destroy.

REFERENCES

Ainsworth MDS, Blehar MC, Waters E, et al: Patterns of Attachment: A Psychological Study of the Strange Situation. Hillsdale, NJ, Erlbaum, 1978

Astington J, Jenkins JM: Theory of mind development and social understanding. Cognition and Emotion 9:151–165, 1995

Baron-Cohen S: How to build a baby that can read minds: cognitive mechanisms in mind reading. Current Psychology of Cognition 13:513–552, 1994

Baron-Cohen S: Mindblindness: An Essay on Autism and Theory of Mind. Cambridge, MA, MIT Press, 1995

Beeghly M, Cicchetti D: Child maltreatment, attachment, and the self system: emergence of an internal state lexicon in toddlers at high social risk. Dev Psychopathol 6:5–30, 1994

Bleiberg E: Developmental pathogenesis of narcissistic disorders in children. Bull Menninger Clin 52:3–15, 1988

Bowlby J: Attachment and Loss, Vol 1: Attachment. New York, Basic Books, 1969

Bowlby J: Attachment and Loss, Vol 2: Separation: Anxiety and Anger. New York, Basic Books, 1973

Bowlby J: Attachment and Loss, Vol 3: Loss: Sadness and Depression. New York, Basic Books, 1980

Bretherton I, Bates E: Relationships between cognition, communication, and quality of attachment, in The Emergence of Symbols: Cognition and Communication in Infancy. Edited by Bates E, Benigni L, Bretherton I, et al. New York, Academic Press, 1979, pp 223–270

Breuer J, Freud S: Studies on hysteria (1893–1895), in The Standard Edition of the Complete Psychological Works of Sigmund Freud, Vol 2. Translated and edited by Strachey J. London, Hogarth Press, 1955, pp 1–311

Campos JJ, Stenberg C: Perception, appraisal, and emotion: the onset of social referencing, in Infant Social Cognition: Empirical and Theoretical Considerations. Edited by Lamb ME, Sherrod LR. Hillsdale, NJ, Erlbaum, 1981, pp 273–314

Carlsson E, Sroufe LA: Contribution of attachment theory to developmental psychopathology, in Developmental Psychopathology, Vol 1: Theory and Methods. Edited by Cicchetti D, Cohen DJ. New York, Wiley, 1995, pp 581–617

Chu JA, Dill DL: Dissociative symptoms in relation to childhood physical and sexual abuse. Am J Psychiatry 147:887–892, 1990

Cicchetti D, Cohen D (eds): Developmental Psychopathology. New York, Wiley Interscience, 1995

Dunn J, Brown J: Early conversations about causality: content, pragmatics, and developmental change. British Journal of Developmental Psychology 11:107–123, 1993

Dunn J, Brown J, Beardsall L: Family talk about feeling states and children's later understanding of others' emotions. Dev Psychol 27:448–455, 1991

Emde R: The infant's relationship experience: developmental and affective aspects, in Relationship Disturbances in Early Childhood. Edited by Sameroff A, Emde R. New York, Basic Books, 1989, pp 33–51

Field TM, Reite M: Children's responses to separation from mother during the birth of another child. Child Dev 55:1308–1316, 1984

Fischer KW, Kenny SL, Pipp SL: How cognitive processes and environmental conditions organize discontinuities in the development of abstractions, in Higher Stages of Human Development. Edited by Alexander CN, Langer EJ, et al. New York, Oxford University Press, 1990, pp 162–187

Fonagy P, Steele H, Steele M: Maternal representations of attachment during pregnancy predict the organization of infant-mother attachment at one year of age. Child Dev 62:891–905, 1991

Fonagy P, Steele M, Moran G, et al: Measuring the ghost in the nursery: an empirical study of the relation between parents' mental representations of childhood experiences and their infants' security of attachment. J Am Psychoanal Assoc 41(4):957–989, 1993

Fonagy P, Steele M, Steele H, et al: Theory and practice of resilience. J Child Psychol Psychiatry 35:231–257, 1994

Fraiberg S, Adelson E, Shapiro V: Ghosts in the nursery: a psychoanalytic approach to the problems of impaired infant-mother relationships. Journal of the American Academy of Child Psychiatry 14(3):387–421, 1975

Freud S: Inhibitions, symptoms and anxiety (1926), in The Standard Edition of the Complete Psychological Works of Sigmund Freud, Vol 20. Translated and edited by Strachey J. London, Hogarth Press, 1959, pp 75–175

Gardner GG, Olness K: Hypnosis and Hypnotherapy With Children. New York, Grune & Stratton, 1981

George C, Kaplan N, Main M: The Berkeley Adult Attachment Interview. Unpublished protocol, Department of Psychology, University of California at Berkeley, 1985

Gergely G, Watson JS: The social biofeedback theory of parental affect-mirroring: the development of emotional self-awareness and self-control in infancy. Int J Psychoanal 77:1181–1212, 1996

Gladwell M: Annals of behavior: do parents matter? New Yorker, August 17, 1998, pp 54–65

Greenberg J, Mitchell S: Object Relations in Psychoanalytic Theory. Cambridge, MA, Harvard University Press, 1983

Harlow HF, Harlow MK: Psychopathology in monkeys, in Experimental Psychopathology: Recent Research and Theory. Edited by Kimmel HD. New York, Academic Press, 1971, pp 203–229

Harris J: The Nurture Assumption: Why Children Turn Out the Way They Do. New York, Free Press, 1998

Hobson P: Autism and the Development of Mind. Hillsdale, NJ, Erlbaum, 1993

Hollenbeck AR, Susman FJ, Nannis FD, et al: Children with serious illness: behavioral correlates of separation and isolation. Child Psychiatry Hum Dev 11:3–11, 1980

Horowitz MJ: States of Mind: Configurational Analysis of Individual Personality. New York, Plenum, 1987

Jenkins J, Astington JW: Cognitive factors and family structure associated with theory of mind development in young children. Dev Psychol 32:70–78, 1996

Joffe NG, Sandler J: Some conceptual problems involved in the consideration of disorders of narcissism. Journal of Child Psychotherapy 2(1):56–66, 1967

Kandel ER: From metapsychology to molecular biology: explorations into the nature of anxiety. Am J Psychiatry 140:1277–1293, 1983

Kandel ER: A new intellectual framework for psychiatry. Am J Psychiatry 155:457–469, 1998

Kihlstrom JF, Hoyt IP: Repression, dissociation, and hypnosis, in Repression and Dissociation. Edited by Singer JL. Chicago, IL, University of Chicago Press, 1990, pp 181–208

Kraemer GW: Effects of differences in early social experiences on primate neurobiological-behavioral development, in The Psychobiology of Attachment and Separation. Edited by Reite M, Field T. Orlando, FL, Academic Press, 1985, pp 135–161

Main M, Goldwyn R: Adult Attachment Scoring and Classification System. Unpublished manuscript, Department of Psychology. University of California at Berkeley, 1993

Main M, Solomon J: Discovery of a new, insecure-disorganized/disoriented attachment pattern, in Affective Development in Infancy. Edited by Brazelton TB, Yogman M. Norwood, NJ, Ablex, 1986, pp 95–124

McParlane A, Weber D, Clark R: Abnormal stimulus processing in posttraumatic stress disorder. Biol Psychiatry 34:311–320, 1993

Mirsky IA: Communication of affects in monkeys, in Environmental Influences: Proceedings of a Conference Under the Auspices of the Russell Sage Foundation and Rockefeller University. Edited by Glass DC. New York, Rockefeller University Press, 1968, pp 129–137

Murburgh M (ed): Catecholamine Function in Posttraumatic Stress Disorder: Emerging Concepts. Washington, DC, American Psychiatric Press, 1994

Panksepp J, Meeker R, Bean NJ: The neurochemical control of crying. Pharmacol Biochem Behav 12:437–443, 1980

Paris J, Zweig-Frank H: Parameters of childhood sexual abuse in female patients, in Role of Sexual Abuse in the Etiology of Borderline Personality Disorder. Edited by Zanarini MC. Washington, DC, American Psychiatric Press, 1997, pp 15–28

Perner J, Ruffman T, Leekam SR: Theory of mind is contagious: you catch it from your sibs. Child Dev 65(4):1228–1238, 1994

Perry B: Incubated in terror: neurodevelopmental factors in the "cycle of violence," in Children in a Violent Society. Edited by Osofsky J. New York, Guilford, 1997, pp 124–149

Pynoos R, Frederick C, Nader K, et al: Life threat and posttraumatic states in school-age children. Arch Gen Psychiatry 44:1057–1063, 1987

Schacter DL: Understanding implicit memory: a cognitive neuroscience approach. Am Psychol 47:559–569, 1992

Shalev A, Orr S, Pitman R: Psychophysiologic assessment of traumatic imagery in Israeli civilian patients with posttraumatic stress disorders. Am J Psychiatry 150:620–624, 1993

Smith PK: Language and the evolution of mind-reading, in Theories of Theories of Mind. Edited by Carruthers P, Smith PK. New York, Cambridge University Press, 1996, pp 344–354

Sorce JF, Emde RN, Campos JJ, et al: Maternal emotional signaling: its effect on the visual cliff behavior of 1-year-olds. Dev Psychol 21(1):195–200, 1985

Spitz R: Anaclitic depression: an inquiry into the genesis of psychiatric conditions in early childhood. Psychoanal Study Child 2:313–342, 1946

Squire LR: Memory and Brain. New York, Oxford University Press, 1987

Stern DN: The Interpersonal World of the Infant: A View From Psychoanalysis and Developmental Psychology. New York, Basic Books, 1985

Suomi SJ: The development of affect in rhesus monkeys, in The Psychobiology of Affective Development. Edited by Fox N, Davidson R. Hillsdale, NJ, Erlbaum, 1984, pp 119–159

Suomi SJ, Harlow HF: Social rehabilitation of isolate-reared monkeys. Dev Psychol 6:487–496, 1972

Suomi SJ, Harlow HF, Novak MA: Reversal of social deficits produced by isolation rearing in monkeys. J Hum Evol 3:527–534, 1974

Terr L: Childhood traumas: an outline and overview. Am J Psychiatry 148:10–20, 1991

Tronick E: Emotions and emotional communication in infants. Am Psychol 44:112–119, 1989

van der Kolk B: The body keeps the score: memory and the evolving psychobiology of posttraumatic stress. Harv Rev Psychiatry 1:253–265, 1994

van der Kolk B, Fisler R: Childhood abuse and neglect and loss of self-regulation. Bull Menninger Clin 55(2):145–168, 1994

Weston J: The pathology of child abuse and neglect, in The Battered Child. Edited by Helfer RE, Kempe CH. Chicago, IL, University of Chicago Press, 1968, pp 241–271

Yehuda R: Sensitization of the hypothalamic-pituitary-adrenal axis in posttraumatic stress disorder, in Psychobiology of Posttraumatic Stress Disorder. Edited by Yehuda R, McFarlane A. New York, New York Academy of Sciences, 1997, pp 57–75

3

Understanding of Mental States, Mother-Infant Interaction, and the Development of the Self

Peter Fonagy, Ph.D., F.B.A.

The understanding of mental states and the realities of the interaction between caregivers and infants are important factors in the origin and perpetuation of emotional and behavioral problems in infancy and in disturbances in parent-infant relationships. Here I examine the central role of the concept of reflective function—the predisposition to understand behavior in terms of mental states—in normal development as well as when this development is distorted.

Developmental psychologists have narrowly defined the process of the development of the child's reflective or mentalizing capacity as the child's *theory of mind.* Although at times the theory of mind is described as if it appeared spontaneously—as a normal part of the cognitive progression of the child—the developmental roots of this essential human function lie in the interaction between mother and infant. I shall, therefore, highlight the mechanisms by which this primary relationship leads to the development of a most important human function: the ability to understand others and, consequently, to be able to relate empathically and reciprocally.

Antecedents to the ability to mentalize about other people's states occur before the actual theory of mind is observable or testable (which is not usually possible until the preschool years). The initial intense and constant interaction between baby and mother is the first "template" from which these abilities are exercised and refined.

Mothers who show awareness of the infant's mental states in their day-to-day interactions, event after event, facilitate the acquisition of this capacity in their child by enriching the child's model of the caregiver's actions. In contrast, mothers who act frightened or frightening undermine the development of this capacity. The frightened or frightening mother may compromise the mapping process the infant uses to relate internal experience to observed behavior (manifested by the infant), thus creating a predisposition in the infant to respond with dissociation to later trauma.

A frightening mother is one who at times appears overwhelmed, frustrated, angry, or excessively annoyed by her infant's needs, communications, and dependency. She may inadvertently exhibit behaviors that are scary to her baby, thus leading to a confused perception in the infant. The person who should be secure and soothing to the child can thus be the source of fear and a sense of threat. On the other hand, this same mother may at times appear frightened herself. The infant may trigger memories from her past, even from her childhood, that remind her of someone she fears, or the infant may simply scare her with his or her dependency and neediness or with expressions of anger. These contradictory and alternating interactions are confusing to the baby, whose capacity to process such experiences is limited.

UNDERSTANDING MINDS

The past decade has seen a remarkable growth of interest among developmental psychologists in the child's acquisition of an understanding that human behavior is underpinned by mental states, beliefs, and desires (Morton and Frith 1995). That is, the behavior of a very young child is shaped and informed by the facial expressions, intentions, and beliefs of those around the child. Around age 3, children appear to respond suddenly not only to another person's behavior but also to their conception of that person's beliefs, feelings, attitudes, desires, hopes, knowledge, intentions, and plans (Baron-Cohen 1995). This ability to understand others in a rudimentary way has also been demonstrated to exist in some primates.

Attributing mental states to another person is undoubtedly a useful strategy for the child in that human behavior thus becomes meaningful and predictable. This ability has survival value because in this way the child can learn about the behavior of those surrounding him or her. Also, with repeated experiences, the youngster can develop a "translation" helpful in understanding what other people's behavior indicates and means.

The value of such capacity to understand others is obvious. However, that very capacity is also essential to understanding oneself and to developing an understanding of one's emotions and internal states. This ability also arguably underlies the child's ability to label and find meaning in his or her own psychological experiences.

This internalization of the understanding of minds, emotions, and behaviors is crucial to other developmental abilities. For instance, this capacity may be integral to the child's affect regulation, impulse control, self-monitoring, and self-agency. These are enormous developmental achievements that cannot be taken for granted. As a matter of fact, many children suffer the consequences of being unable to monitor their own behavior and its effect on others. Some do not develop a sense of efficacy and the ability to make a difference or realize their emotions and intentions matter to others or have an effect in their physical and interpersonal world. The regulation of affects has an obvious importance in coping with frustrations and unexpected situations and regulating interpersonal relationships. Understanding one's feelings is a costly developmental gain that unfortunately many children and adults may not quite achieve.

The predisposition to understand behavior—both one's own and that of others—in terms of mental states may be labeled *reflective function* (Fonagy and Target 1997). The notion of reflective function is rooted in the work of Daniel Dennett, who delineated the concept of an intentional stance—that is, the approach to understanding a system not in terms of its physical properties or design but rather in terms of its attribution of beliefs and desires or the assumption that the system is regulated by intentional states (Dennett 1978, 1987). Indeed, there appears to exist, even in the young baby, a tendency to attribute intentions to surrounding phenomena and systems and to expect that systems, even those consisting only of physical objects, will behave rationally.

Although the developmental psychology literature persists in using the rather narrow term *theory of mind* (discussed later in this chapter) to depict the psychological capacity for understanding beliefs and desires, I believe that underlying knowledge of mental states is a much broader capacity that concerns the following developmental achievements:

• Knowledge of the nature of experiences that give rise to particular beliefs and emotions

- The nature of mental experience likely to follow particular experiences
- The expectable transactional relationships between beliefs and emotions in self and other
- The nature of beliefs and feelings characteristic of particular developmental phases and relationships
- Likely constraints on mental experiences imposed by the nature of consciousness
- The interactions between ideas about mental states and the motivational state of the individual

This long list of developmental achievements is related to the reflective functioning of children and, later on, adults. The child comes to understand what kinds of human experiences lead to specific emotions or reactions, first in others, then in himself or herself. This connection, like the connection between beliefs and emotions that occur in the other and in oneself, is an important achievement. What mental contents are associated with which emotions (e.g., a loss of someone loved with sadness, an unexpected occurrence with surprise or fear)?

Thus, reflective function is not the theoretical articulation of behavior in mental state terms nor is it merely introspection. Rather it is an individual's capacity to go beyond immediately known phenomena to respond to behavior in a manner indicating that the individual has "computed," or taken account of, the mental state of the other in organizing his or her actions in relation to that other. It is the view of my colleagues and myself that individuals differ in the extent and the quality of their capacity to reflect on mental states.

It is important to distinguish reflective function from self-reflection, or introspection. Self-reflection defines mental states in terms of consciousness or self-report (Bolton and Hill 1996). Reflective function, on the other hand, refers to the capacity to make sense of behavior and thereby actively regulate it. Reflective function is an *automatic* procedure, unconsciously rather than deliberately invoked, that adds meaning to human action. It is a skill, and an overlearned one at that: the intuitive understanding or realization of what others are going through, of their intentions, and of the meaning of actions is an experiential, not an intellectual, formulation. Reflective functioning is incorporated into representations of relationships, and its pervasive influence lends shape and coherence to self-organization. Knowledge of minds in general is implied in encoded procedures of action, rather than the kind of declarative knowledge implied by introspection.

ACQUISITION OF THEORY OF MIND

Because this chapter is concerned with the acquisition of reflective function and the role of mother-infant interaction in that process, I briefly review below four current theories about the acquisition of theory of mind—a somewhat narrower concept than reflective capacity. The theories considered here emphasize innate learning, past experience, simulation, and social interaction.

- The most prominent approach is that of modularity theorists, who postulate an innate learning mechanism for understanding minds with a specific anatomical location (e.g., Leslie 1994; Segal 1996). This approach postulates that there is a specific "module" within the brain that, on becoming operational, enables the child to understand other minds. It is also speculated that this module is nonfunctioning in autistic children. This model fits within the general model of the mind as composed of multiple modules, each one with a relative specialization, for example, to understand language, express language, and decode symbols in reading.
- Cognitive theorists have suggested that a child evolves a scientific "theory-like" network of independent propositions about the mind on the basis of past experience (e.g., Botterill 1996; Gopnik 1996). This evolution by the child is also called the "theory-theory approach." This approach describes a gradual building of assumptions and understanding about other people based on repeated experiences from which the child learns, one by one, and that eventually become a generalized ability to understand the meanings of the repeated past experiences.
- More socially oriented psychologists have suggested that theory of mind is acquired via a process of simulation of the other's mental state. Some suggest that children learn to make inferences about what they would do in imagined circumstances (e.g., Goldman 1993; Harris 1992). An even more radical version of the simulation idea has been put forward by Gordon (1992), who suggested that the child performs an imagined transformation into the other that does not involve introspection or inference. This approach would simply be an experiential one. Practicing this sort of imitation and being in the shoes of the other allows the child, through his or her own experience, to come to understand the other.
- The last approach is social-interactionist. Some developmentalists argue that the child is socialized into a world of minds because caregivers foster the child's sense of mental self through complex interac-

tional processes. These processes involve behaving toward the infant in a way that eventually leads the child to share the assumption that his or her own behavior and that of others may best be understood in terms of mental states (Astington 1996; Fonagy and Target 1995). In this view, the child's entry into the world of minds is almost a process of apprenticeship whereby caregivers (and senior peers) encourage the child to adopt mentalizing concepts.

What is disappointing about all these theories, except perhaps the last one, is that although they appear to emphasize the social learning aspect of the development of mentalizing, their focus remains at the level of mechanism (the mechanics of how the process of understanding others operates) rather than content (what is being experienced and what it means in what context). Research must go beyond the chronology of acquiring knowledge of minds to consider the child's feelings about the mental states encountered in others. Learning and motivation are closely intertwined. The child may know how the other feels but care little about it. For some youngsters, however, the mental state of the other may be an issue of survival. This issue might be particularly relevant in situations in which the child is likely to be treated with anger or violence. The young child may develop an exquisite perception and understanding of the caregiver's internal states, particularly dangerous ones leading to maltreatment.

The emotional significance of beliefs and desires is likely to determine the development of reflective capacity. In most models, such as the first three described above, the child is considered to be an isolated processor of information, mostly equipped with a biological propensity that subserves biological capacity. Individual differences may exist (e.g., IQ), but they speak to biological differences in brain function rather than to the nature of the child's social environment. In contrast, our approach is that, while those building blocks (anatomical, physiological, neuronal) are necessary, the particulars of the development of reflective functioning are rooted in the actual experiences, interactions, and exchanges between the young child and the caregiver. Therefore, the process is essentially social and transactional.

We know that knowledge of minds is all about content rather than just capacity. The child's emotional relationship with the parent determines which mental states are most important to the child. The acquisition of this capacity is intrinsically intertwined with the family system, uniquely defined by its complex, emotionally and powerfully charged relationships. It is these relationships that necessarily constitute the primary content of early reflective function. Consistent with this perspective, the important pioneering work of Judy Dunn has carefully documented how the quality of parental control, parental talk about emotions, and parental discussions involving affect are closely related to the age at which theory of mind is acquired (Denham et al. 1994; Dunn et al. 1991a, 1991b). Therefore, it makes a difference whether the parents talk about distinct emotions, introduce them in their conversations, and illustrate for the young child the different nuances of emotionality.

To phrase the objections to purely cognitive and imitational theories more formally:

- Biological accounts (i.e., considering emotions as dependent only on the presence of certain circuitry in the brain) cannot explain why social contexts, such as the presence of an older sibling (Jenkins and Astington 1996; Perner et al. 1994), can accelerate the development of reflective function.
- Cognitivist accounts (theories that focus only on when the child can cognitively master the understanding of other minds) cannot incorporate the influence of the nature of the mental state data presented to the child upon which mental state concepts may be built.
- Simulation accounts avoid addressing the question of how children come to think of their own mental states in terms of feelings and desires.
- Even Vygotskian symbolic interactionist accounts ignore the influence of caregiver-child interactions that antedate the development of language. In the Vygotskian view, the social environment is considered an agent to promote development, except that it looks only at the skill acquisition but does not take into account the actual content of the emotional context in which the child develops, particularly in the preverbal stages.

ROOTS OF REFLECTIVE FUNCTION IN MOTHER-INFANT INTERACTION

The mother-infant relationship can be seen as the route for the understanding of mental states, at least within the self, and arguably also within the mother. Between birth and 5 months, the infant engages in face-to-face exchanges of affective signals with caregivers that play a key role in the development of the child's representation of affect (Beebe et al. 1997; Tronick 1989).

There is a rapid, mutually influencing process in which the infant's behavior during time periods of fractions of seconds is predicted by the mother's behavior, and vice versa, on the basis of schemata of the other's anticipated reaction. Interactions at this stage are not mentalistic, or to put it another way, they are not cognitive. Rather, they are emotional and intuitive. The infant is not required to represent the caregiver's thoughts and feelings. However, structures pertinent to the eventual development of the representation of mental states are already present in nascent form.

Two processes are particularly important in mother-infant interactions: representational mapping and the representation of "rational action."

Representational Mapping

Representational mapping evolves between 6 and 18 months of age. During this period, the infant becomes increasingly able to match his or her mental state with that of the caregiver vis-à-vis a third object or person. This mapping is evident, for example, in the child's request for joint attention (Bretherton 1991). Caregiver and child look together at a third object and then may show it to each other or talk about it. The baby looks at the object, then at the caregiver. The baby's realization that they are sharing something is a rudimentary manifestation of the understanding that something is in the mind of the caregiver.

This communication is apparently deliberate, or goal-oriented, because even in the second half of the first year, infants will attempt to repair failed communicative bids (Golinkoff 1986). There is at least rudimentary recognition of awareness and agency in self and the other, which may be underpinned by the intersubjective process of representational mapping (Rogers and Pennington 1991). This process is thought to coordinate representations of self and other and underlies the sharing of affect, attention, and such higher-order aspects of cognition as beliefs. It is difficult to imagine that imitation skills, such as those evidenced in studies of mirroring (Meltzoff and Gopnik 1993), would be possible without a rapidly evolving cognitive structure that maps internal states onto external cues.

Representational mapping may play a critical role in the acquisition of mental state constructs. Elsewhere, we have suggested a model, based on the work of two investigators (Gergely and Watson 1996), that representations of internal states are acquired as part of the mirroring interactions between mother and infant.

The mother, in mirroring the infant's affect, does more than express sympathy—she provides a stimulus that may organize the child's internal experience and provide a label, or symbol, for what he or she is feeling.

The mother's facial representation of the infant's affect is represented by the child and is mapped onto the representation of his or her self-state. This process helps the infant recognize the self as both an agent and an emotional entity.

The mother's response, however empathic and attuned, is never an exact replica of the child's experience, and the caregiver's mirroring can become a higher-order representation of the child's internal experience of affects. In fact, the mirroring might fail if the mother's expression is either too close to or too removed from the infant's experience. Either nonresponsive mothering or overinvolvement, therefore, would yield adverse outcomes. In the first instance, a representation that shares adequate ground with the child's internal experience is simply not available. In the second, the representational potential of the caregiver's reaction is lost because the expression itself becomes a source of emotional arousal rather than a vehicle for containment. The notion of caregiver sensitivity (Ainsworth et al. 1978) boils down to the caregiver's capacity to permit the child's representational mapping of emotion displays and self-experience. We predict that insensitive caregiving retards—and, in the extreme, undermines—the process of organizing self-experience in terms of clusters of responses that will eventually come to be verbally labeled as specific emotions or desires.

Representation of "Rational Action"

The second essential forerunner of mentalizing is the logical structure applied in infancy to the understanding of action. This structure prepares the ground for understanding action in the language of belief and desire. The degree of coordination and anticipatory reaction observed in studies such as those of Beebe and her colleagues requires the infant to have representations of future states (e.g., goals) as explanatory constructs for interpreting the behavior of the other. In other words, it appears that the infant generates some theory of why an object does what it does, what its ultimate goal is, and where it wants to go (a teleological stance).

During the second half of the first year, the infant acquires the capacity to make reference to goals as explanatory entities in the interpretation of behavior based on the principle of rational action (Gergely et al. 1995). The infant appears to adopt a teleological stance in that he or she interprets the behavior of human and nonhuman objects in terms of the observable goals of actions and the reality constraints that pertain at the time. Gergely and Csibra (1997) demonstrated that 9-month-old infants express surprise when nonhuman but moving objects, such as discs in computer-generated displays, appear to act irrationally, not choosing the optimal action, given specific observable goals and reality constraints. These representational structures, although not yet mentalizing, have the potential to become so once representations of future goal states come to be thought of as desires, and when constraints on reality are translated into the belief state of the agent with regard to physical reality rather than to physical reality per se.

The *actual dyadic interactions* between mother and child are a critical factor in the mental model (Johnson-Laird 1983) of action that evolves in the infant. The infant can create a model of rational action only if the caregiver's behavior is predictable and if, by and large, it represents no direct threat to the child's well-being. For example, if the attachment figure's behavior is either frightened or frightening (Main and Hesse 1992), the caregiver's actions will not readily fit the biologically prepared model of rational action into which the infant wishes to assimilate the caregiver's behavior. Frightened responses on the part of the caregiver without readily detectable goal states and reality constraints, such as a frightening object, will puzzle the child. Frightening behavior (e.g., physical threats) will also strain the development of the teleological model. In both reactions (frightened and frightening), the infant may be forced to perceive his or her own actions as the only physical stimulus that might explain the caregiver's unjustified emotional expression.

This model has implications for the clinical phenomena described elsewhere in this book. What the caregiver actually does, the actual exchange of reactions, how emotions are recognized, and the ingredients of maternal sensitivity are factors that powerfully determine the course of the emotional development of the baby. Of course, what the baby actually does is also important. These interactions are not the only factor but are a crucial element in the development of the sense of self, in the child's emotional life, and in the sense of agency and effectiveness.

REFLECTIVE FUNCTION AND CAREGIVER SENSITIVITY

Attachment theorists have recognized for some time that the quality of the mother-infant relationship is an important determinant of the emergence of symbolic thought (e.g., Bretherton et al. 1979). Attachment security is a reasonable marker of the quality of this relationship, particularly of maternal sensitivity (De Wolff and van IJzendoorn 1997). The security in attachment is correlated with how much the mother can perceive, resonate, and respond to the infant's emotional state. A number of studies have demonstrated a relationship between attachment security and the child's capacity to understand mental states (Fonagy and Target

2000; Fonagy et al. 1997a; Meins et al. 1998; Moss et al. 1995). The mother-infant relationship may have a specific role to play in the development of mentalizing capacity.

There are at least two ways of looking at these findings. The first, somewhat less interesting way, might be to suggest that reflective capacity evolves precociously as a consequence of the child's social environment that, in turn, is predicted by secure attachment. Attachment, in turn, is predicted by sensitive maternal caregiving.

How does this evolution happen? There are a number of candidates from the child's social environment. For example, it is possible that joint pretend play or playfulness fosters the understanding of mental states because pretend representations are shared by those engaged in a pretend game (Astington 1996; Leslie 1987). Pretending requires a mental stance involving the symbolic transformation of reality in the presence of, and with a view to, the mind of the other. Independent evidence suggests that securely attached children are more likely to engage in pretend play and, moreover, are more capable of doing so (Main et al. 1985; Slade 1987). This possibility may have implications in terms of psychosocial interventions in infancy. If play is the arena where the emotional life of the child is displayed, and where parents naturally introduce mental states and emotions in people, its therapeutic impact might be used in situations where there is parental insensitivity, disruptions in attachment, trauma, and so forth.

Similarly, another candidate—intense peer group interaction—is likely to provide the child with many opportunities for imagining how play partners are seeing, feeling, and thinking about the world, thereby providing direct exposure to the mentalistic culture of the child's environment (Astington 1996; Lewis et al. 1996). Secure attachment is known to enhance peer competence (Elicker et al. 1992) and social orientation (Park and Waters 1989; Sroufe 1983) and also may have therapeutic implications. In some children with depriving environments, where the parents are unable to provide the experiences of mirroring and affective resonance, a group setting in which there is interaction with other children may supplement this area of development and compensate for the relative deprivation in the home.

Alternatively, talking and language may be the principal conveyors of mental state constructs (Harris 1996; Smith 1996), with secure attachment in children predicting greater fluency in conversations (Bretherton et al. 1990; Cassidy 1988). From this point of view, active exchanges of exposure to language between child and caregiver might promote the development of these mental functions.

An alternative approach, which I favor, might explain the correlation between attachment and the infant's acquisition of mentalizing capacity in terms of the nature of the child's experience with a caregiver during the first year of life. There is evidence that mothers who are more likely to invoke mental states in describing their own childhood attachment relationships rear children who are more likely to be securely attached to them (Fonagy et al. 1991). These children also manifest superior mind-reading ability (after verbal fluency is controlled for) at 5½ years. We found that the mother's mentalizing ability, as measured before the birth of the child, was directly related to the child's reflective capacity, even when we controlled for verbal ability and the child's security of attachment. This finding suggests that the mother's capacity to envision the child as a mental entity during the first year of life may enrich the infant's teleological models and representational mapping.

The acquisition of reflective capacity is thus part of an intersubjective process between the infant and the caregiver. The infant is oriented to creating a model of the caregiver's behavior. The child attempts to map that behavior onto his or her own mental states. The caregiver, whose behavior during these interactions clearly reflects concern for the mental states of the infant, forces the child to create a model of his or her own experience in mental state terms. This mapping process highlights the importance of the first year of life and the realities of interactions between the caregivers and baby. Thus, what happens in that period lays the foundation for the development of sensitivity—that is, the ability to think about one's own internal states in relation to the mental states of other people.

Gradually, by mapping subjective experience to observable behavior, the infant assumes that his or her own behavior may be best understood through the assumption of ideas, beliefs, feelings, and wishes. They determine not only the infant's actions but also the reactions of others. In possession of this awareness, the child may then gradually extend these constructs to models for understanding the reactions of others. The sensitive—or, more precisely, the reflective—caregiver behaves in a way that creates contingencies between the child's internal and external experiences. For the most part, actions by the infant elicit a response contingent on the message conveyed by the infant. In light of interactions with the mother, and given an internal state of belief or desire within the child, the infant concludes that the mother's reactions may be understood as rational.

CONCLUSION

In normal development, the caregiver unconsciously and pervasively ascribes a mental state to the infant, which is reflected in the caregiver's

behavior. She treats the infant as a mental agent, which the infant ultimately perceives. The child's perception is then mapped onto his or her
internal states and is used in the elaboration of the infant's teleological
models. This process is likely to be mundane. Whenever the caregiver
acts in a way that is not predictable on the basis of observable end results
and the constraints of physical reality, the infant's teleological model is
enriched.

To take a single example, an 11-month-old infant sitting in a high
chair may be pointing to a glass of water. The mother reaches down and
hands the infant some silver foil. The observer may be puzzled. Yet the
mother responded accurately to the infant's desire. She had noticed that
the infant had been playing with the silver foil, knocked it off the chair
accidentally, lost sight of it, and was now pointing at something else that
was shiny in order to signal a need. The mother's reaction in this context
may be thought of as strengthening the infant's awareness of internal
states.

Children's development and perception of mental states in themselves, and later in others, depend on their observations of their mother's
representation of them. They are able to conceive of mental states in
themselves to the extent that the caregiver's behavior implies such states.
Thus, mental state concepts are inherently intersubjective. Proximity-
seeking by securely attached children may index their expectation that
the caregiver will recognize their internal states. Avoidant children may
shun the mental states of the other because their attempts at mapping
the caregiver's behavior onto their own internal experience generally
yield a poor match. Resistant children may be focused on their own states
of distress to the exclusion of close intersubjective exchanges. Disorganized attachment may indicate children's hypervigilance to the caregiver's
behavior, but it occurs at the cost of preserving adequate attentional resources for the necessary representational mapping. Thus, representations of internal states never fully develop.

The explanation above illustrates some possibilities in terms of the
style of attachment representations of the baby vis à vis the primary caregiver. What happens in more problematic situations, such as when disruptions in attachment and emotional trauma occur?

Exploration of the mental state of a sensitive caregiver in these interactions enables children to find in the caregiver's mind an image of self
as motivated by beliefs, feelings, and intentions. Disorganized infants,
even those who develop the skill of mind reading, fail to integrate this
ability with self-organization. In addition to committing disproportion-
ate attentional resources to understanding a frightening or frightened
parent, disorganized infants have few reliably contingent experiences to

draw on. Moreover, a disorganized child's exploration of the caregiver's mind is further inhibited by intense anxiety, provoked, at least partially, by the caregiver's malevolent attitude toward the child.

In traumatized children, intense emotion and associated conflict lead to a partial failure of the integration between internal and external reality. These infants lack the physical capacity to resort to a fight-or-flight response in the face of anxiety. Their only available coping strategy is a mental separation from internal experience, an abandonment of representational mapping. Clinicians working with traumatized patients may recognize this response as akin to dissociation. There are undoubtedly similarities between the behaviors manifested by disorganized infants and the dissociative responses of traumatized patients (Fonagy 1998; Liotti 1995; Main and Morgan 1996). Dissociation is the converse of mentalizing. In the disassociation model, my colleagues and I suggest that mother-infant interactions characterized by the mother's persistent nonresponsiveness create a vulnerability in the infant to respond to later trauma by abandoning the capacity or wish to consider mental states in self and other. This vulnerability is evident in traumatized individuals with symptoms of severe personality disorder, particularly borderline psychopathology or violent criminal behavior (Fonagy et al. 1997b; Steele et al. 1996).

One of the implications of this theory would be the early recognition of the processes of dissociation, emotional trauma, and frightening caregiver-infant interactions. Intervening early and alleviating these experiences might have a protective effect for the baby and for the working model of relationships that the infant will develop and use more or less throughout life.

REFERENCES

Ainsworth MDS, Blehar MC, Waters E, et al: Patterns of Attachment: A Psychological Study of the Strange Situation. Hillsdale, NJ, Erlbaum, 1978

Astington J: What is theoretical about the child's theory of mind? A Vygotskian view of its development, in Theories of Theories of Mind. Edited by Carruthers P, Smith PK. Cambridge, UK, Cambridge University Press, 1996, pp 185–199

Baron-Cohen S: Mindblindness: An Essay on Autism and Theory of Mind. Cambridge, MA, Bradford/MIT Press, 1995

Beebe B, Lachmann F, Jaffe J: Mother-infant interaction structures and presymbolic self and object representations. Psychoanalytic Dialogues 7:133–182, 1997

Bolton D, Hill J: Mind, Meaning, and Mental Disorder: The Nature of Causal Explanation in Psychology and Psychiatry. Oxford, UK, Oxford University Press, 1996

Botterill G: Folk psychology and theoretical status, in Theories of Theories of Mind. Edited by Carruthers P, Smith PK. Cambridge, UK, Cambridge University Press, 1996, pp 105–118

Bretherton I: Intentional communication and the development of an understanding of mind, in Children's Theories of Mind: Mental States and Social Understanding. Edited by Frye D, Moore C, et al. Hillsdale, NJ, Erlbaum, 1991, pp 49–75

Bretherton I, Bates E, Benigni L, et al: Relationships between cognition, communication, and quality of attachment, in The Emergence of Symbols: Cognition and Communication in Infancy. Edited by Bates E, Benigni L, Bretherton I, et al. New York, Academic Press, 1979, pp 223–270

Bretherton I, Ridgeway D, Cassidy J: Assessing internal working models of the attachment relationship: an attachment story completion task for 3-year-olds, in Attachment in the Preschool Years: Theory, Research, and Intervention. Edited by Greenberg MT, Cicchetti D, Cummings EM. Chicago, IL, University of Chicago Press, 1990, pp 273–308

Cassidy J: Child-mother attachment and the self in six-year-olds. Child Dev 59: 121–134, 1988

Denham SA, Zoller D, Couchoud EA: Socialization of preschoolers' emotion understanding. Dev Psychol 30:928–936, 1994

Dennett DC: Brainstorms: Philosophical Essays on Mind and Psychology. Montgomery, VT, Bradford, 1978

Dennett DC: The Intentional Stance. Cambridge, MA, MIT Press, 1987

De Wolff MS, van IJzendoorn MH: Sensitivity and attachment: a meta-analysis on parental antecedents of infant attachment. Child Dev 68:571–591, 1997

Dunn J, Brown J, Beardsall L: Family talk about feeling states and children's later understanding of others' emotions. Dev Psychol 27:448–455, 1991a

Dunn J, Brown J, Somkowski C, et al: Young children's understanding of other people's feelings and beliefs: individual differences and their antecedents. Child Dev 62:1352–1366, 1991b

Elicker J, Englund M, Sroufe LA: Predicting peer competence and peer relationships in childhood from early parent-child relationships, in Family Peer Relationships: Modes of Linkage. Edited by Parke RD, Ladd GW. Hillsdale, NJ, Erlbaum, pp 77–106, 1992

Fonagy P: Attachment theory approach to treatment of the difficult patient. Bull Menninger Clin 62:147–169, 1998

Fonagy P, Target M: Towards understanding violence: the use of the body and the role of the father. Int J Psychoanal 76:487–502, 1995

Fonagy P, Target M: Attachment and reflective function: their role in self-organization. Dev Psychopathol 9:679–700, 1997

Fonagy P, Target M: The place of psychodynamic theory in developmental psychopathology. Dev Psychopathol 12:407–425, 2000

Fonagy P, Steele M, Steele H, et al: The capacity for understanding mental states: the reflective self in parent and child and its significance for security of attachment. Infant Mental Health Journal 12:201–218, 1991

Fonagy P, Redfern S, Charman T: The relationship between belief-desire reasoning and a projective measure of attachment security (SAT). British Journal of Developmental Psychology 15:51–61, 1997a

Fonagy P, Target M, Steele M, et al: Morality, disruptive behavior, borderline personality disorder, crime, and their relationships to security of attachment, in Attachment and Psychopathology. Edited by Atkinson L, Zucker KJ. New York, Guilford, 1997b, pp 223–274

Gergely G, Csibra G: Teleological reasoning in infancy: the infant's naive theory of rational action: a reply to Premack and Premack. Cognition 63:227–233, 1997

Gergely G, Watson J: The social biofeedback model of parental affect-mirroring. Int J Psychoanal 77:1181–1212, 1996

Gergely G, Nadasdy Z, Csibra G, et al: Taking the intentional stance at 12 months of age. Cognition 56:165–193, 1995

Goldman AI: Philosophical Applications of Cognitive Science. Boulder, CO, Westview Press, 1993

Golinkoff RM: "I beg your pardon?" The preverbal negotiation of failed messages. Journal of Child Language 13(3):455–476, 1986

Gopnik A: Theories and modules: creation myths, developmental realities, and Neurath's boat, in Theories of Theories of Mind. Edited by Carruthers P, Smith PK. Cambridge, UK, Cambridge University Press, 1996, pp 169–183

Gordon RM: Simulation theory: objections and misconceptions. Mind and Language 7:11–34, 1992

Harris PL: From simulation to folk psychology: the case for development. Mind and Language 7:120–144, 1992

Harris P: Desires, beliefs, and language, in Theories of Theories of Mind. Edited by Carruthers P, Smith PK. Cambridge, UK, Cambridge University Press, 1996, pp 200–211

Jenkins JM, Astington JW: Cognitive factors and family structure associated with theory of mind development in young children. Dev Psychol 32:70–78, 1996

Johnson-Laird PN: Mental Models: Towards a Cognitive Science of Language, Inference and Consciousness. Cambridge, UK, Cambridge University Press, 1983

Leslie AM: Pretense and representation: the origins of 'theory of mind.' Psychol Rev 94:412–426, 1987

Leslie AM: Tomm and Toby: core architecture and domain specificity, in Mapping the Mind: Domain Specificity in Cognition and Culture. Edited by Hirschfeld LA, Gelman SA. New York, Cambridge University Press, 1994, pp 119–148

Lewis C, Freeman NH, Kyriakidou C, et al: Social influences on false belief access: specific sibling influences or general apprenticeship? Child Dev 67:2930–2947, 1996

Liotti G: Disorganized/disoriented attachment in the psychotherapy of the dissociative disorders, in Attachment Theory: Social, Developmental, and Clinical Perspectives. Edited by Goldberg S, Muir R, Kerr J. Hillsdale, NJ, Analytic Press, 1995, pp 343–363

Main M, Hesse E: Disorganized/disoriented infant behavior in the Strange Situation, lapses in the monitoring of reasoning and discourse during the parent's Adult Attachment Interview, and dissociative states, in Attachment and Psychoanalysis. Edited by Ammaniti M, Stern D. Rome, Gius, Latereza & Figli, 1992, pp 86–140

Main M, Morgan H: Disorganization and disorientation in infant Strange Situation behavior: phenotypic resemblance to dissociative states, in Handbook of Dissociation: Theoretical, Empirical, and Clinical Perspectives. Edited by Michelson LK, Ray WJ. New York, Plenum, 1996, pp 107–138

Main M, Kaplan N, Cassidy J: Security in infancy, childhood and adulthood: a move to the level of representation, in Growing Points of Attachment: Theory and Research (Monographs of the Society for Research in Child Development, Vol 50). Edited by Bretherton I, Waters E. Chicago, IL, University of Chicago Press, 1985, pp 66–104

Meins E, Fernyhough C, Russell J, et al: Security of attachment as a predictor of symbolic and mentalising abilities: a longitudinal study. Social Development 7:1–24, 1998

Meltzoff A, Gopnik A: The role of imitation in understanding persons and developing a theory of mind, in Understanding Other Minds: Perspectives From Autism. Edited by Baron-Cohen S, Tager-Flusberg H, Cohen DJ. New York, Oxford University Press, 1993, pp 335–366

Morton J, Frith U: Causal modeling: a structural approach to developmental psychology, in Developmental Psychopathology, Vol 1: Theory and Methods. Edited by Cicchetti D, Cohen DJ. New York, John Wiley, 1995, pp 357–390

Moss E, Parent S, Gosselin C: Attachment and theory of mind: cognitive and metacognitive correlates of attachment during the preschool period. Paper presented at the biennial meeting of the Society for Research in Child Development, Indianapolis, IN, March–April 1995

Park K, Waters E: Security of attachment and preschool friendships. Child Dev 60:1076–1081, 1989

Perner J, Ruffman T, Leekman SR: Theory of mind is contagious: you catch it from your sibs. Child Dev 65:1228–1238, 1994

Rogers S, Pennington B: A theoretical approach to the deficits in infantile autism. Dev Psychopathol 3:137–162, 1991

Segal G: The modularity of theory of mind, in Theories of Theories of Mind. Edited by Carruthers P, Smith PK. Cambridge, UK, Cambridge University Press, 1996, pp 141–157

Slade A: Quality of attachment and early symbolic play. Dev Psychol 23:78–85, 1987

Smith PK: Language and the evolution of mind-reading, in Theories of Theories of Mind. Edited by Carruthers P, Smith PK. Cambridge, UK, Cambridge University Press, 1996, pp 344–354

Sroufe LA: Infant-caregiver attachment and patterns of adaptation in preschool: the roots of maladaptation and competence, in Development and Policy Concerning Children With Special Needs. Edited by Perlmutter M. Hillsdale, NJ, Erlbaum, 1983, pp 41–81

Steele H, Steele M, Fonagy P: Associations among attachment classifications of mothers, fathers, and their infants: evidence for a relationship-specific perspective. Child Dev 67:541–555, 1996

Tronick E: Emotions and emotional communication in infants. Am Psychol 44: 112–119, 1989

II

Therapeutic Approaches to Relationships and Their Disturbances

4

Promoting Maternal Role Attainment and Attachment During Pregnancy

The Parent-Child Communication Coaching Program

JoAnne Solchany, R.N., Ph.D.
Kristen Sligar, R.N., M.S.N.
Kathryn E. Barnard, R.N., Ph.D.

Throughout the past 50 years, we have witnessed advancement after advancement in the fields of reproductive health and childbearing. Reports of frozen embryos, artificial insemination, surrogate mothering, superfertility drugs, and the surge of multiple births, including twins, triplets, and even septuplets, have become commonplace in the media. Research on the best clinical practices to support positive pregnancy outcomes has been intense. What is best for the baby? What is best for the mother? How about the father?

However, one question, in spite of its importance, has rarely been asked from an empirical and research-based point of view: How does what occurs during pregnancy affect later parent-child relationships? With all the attention devoted to improving pregnancy outcomes, it is interesting that we have virtually ignored the emotional and psychological work done during pregnancy. Pregnancy produces intense physical and emotional changes in a woman that have been shown to be related to later medical outcomes. Culpepper and Jack (1993) stated not only that there is evidence that psychological interventions undertaken in pregnancy, or even prior to conception, have a significant influence on pregnancy outcomes, but also that medical and physical interventions may be ineffective for some women unless the psychological issues are also addressed.

The significance of the psychological and emotional journey of the pregnant woman has long been acknowledged. Mercer (1995), building on the theories of Rubin (1984), asserted that women in pregnancy begin cognitive restructuring, which is necessary to take on the maternal role. Bibring et al. (1961) likened the woman's transformations during pregnancy to the changes associated with puberty or menopause. They noted that all three life stages are periods of crisis "involving profound endocrine and general somatic as well as psychological changes" (p. 12). They referred to these crisis periods as turning points in the woman's life, at which she has the opportunity to grow, mature, resolve past issues, and move forward to a new developmental place. Bailey and Hailey (1986) indicated that pregnancy can be characterized most consistently as a period of anxiety. They related this anxiety to the woman's efforts to resolve past conflicts with previous mother figures and to take on her new identity as a mother. Lederman (1996) described the period of pregnancy as facilitating a paradigm shift: a woman with a child is forced to view the world differently than does a woman without a child. Finally, Affonso and Sheptak (1989) applied Taylor's theoretical orientation of cognitive processes that become activated during threatening situations (real or perceived). They described the three components of this model as clearly paralleling the cognitive processes present in pregnancy: searching for meaning, regaining a sense of mastery, and sustaining self-enhancement amid the stressors of pregnancy.

Pregnancy is a developmental transition that provides the woman with a chance for self-realization and an opportunity for new growth (Rosenthal and O'Grady 1985). This opportunity for growth involves dealing with new conflicts that develop and revisiting old issues from the past that seem to reawaken during pregnancy. Existing issues to be dealt with often include relationships with family of origin and past models of mothering, while new issues may include accepting the idea of parenting a child and assuming the mothering role. The degree to which a woman is able to deal with these issues depends to a large extent on her coping mechanisms, her history of loving and warm relationships, her personality and lifestyle, her experience of being nurtured, and the care and support of family, friends, and professionals in her world (Rosenthal and O'Grady 1985).

Once we accept that pregnancy involves a host of emotional and psychological—as well as physical—changes for the woman, we next need to consider how the work of the woman during pregnancy affects her later attitude toward her baby. If a pregnant woman goes through a psychological reorganization and is unsuccessful at navigating this reorganization, how does that contribute to the development of her relationship with her infant? What if the woman's preparation for a baby through her fantasy and practice fails to adequately prepare her for the reality of having a helpless baby dependent on her? Bibring and her colleagues (1961) asserted that the disequilibrium between the emotional and psychological work done in pregnancy and the emotional and psychological impact of transitioning to the role and responsibilities of a mother with a child may be partly responsible for some early mother-infant disturbances. They also suggested that this disequilibrium may lay the groundwork for a cycle of mutually induced frustrations and sensitive reactions, later leading to dysfunctional patterns of mother-child interaction that may span more than the mother and child's lifetimes, for a transgenerational impact as well.

In our Early Head Start (EHS) program for high-risk mothers with the University of Washington, we decided to embrace this period of psychological and emotional reorganization during pregnancy. We developed a series of interventions called the Parent-Child Communication Coaching (PCCC) program, part of which was implemented during pregnancy. This program was designed to promote improved mother-child attachment outcomes. In this chapter, we describe the psychological work of pregnancy, the PCCC program, the difficulties and successes we experienced, and our recommendations for future pregnancy intervention programs.

THE PSYCHOLOGICAL COURSE OF PREGNANCY

Many factors go into the development of the mother-child relationship. It is important to remember that the relationship between mother and child begins long before the birth of the child, probably even before its conception. This relationship originates in the woman's fantasies and in her relationships with other significant figures in her life, beginning with her own mother. Who were the woman's role models? How nurturing and loving were those relationships? What kind of relationships with a life partner existed before this point in time?

The literature on the psychological work of pregnancy and on the impact of this work on the mother-infant relationship spans decades and represents a rich diversity of disciplines and theoretical underpinnings. It has described the psychological and emotional work of pregnancy as occurring in a maze of stages, phases, domains, or dimensions. Although this approach makes for interesting reading, it also makes it difficult to summarize the literature logically and coherently. For purposes of this chapter, and to simplify the literature to be more applicable to practice, the most basic levels of emotional and psychological work during pregnancy are described here. The progression through these levels, however, is not linear. Instead, the levels should be seen as a layering of mastered, semimastered, and unresolved levels. Each level can build on other levels; partially mastered levels can still lay the groundwork for mastery of other levels. These levels include acceptance of the pregnancy, development of a fantasy baby, development of mothering behaviors, redefinition of self, and reworking of relationships.

Acceptance of the Pregnancy

Before any work can be done during a pregnancy, the woman first needs to acknowledge and accept the fact that she is indeed pregnant. Lederman (1996) related acceptance of the pregnancy to the woman's level of adaptation within this period and to her transition to motherhood. Mercer (1995) added fetal attachment to the equation, stating that acceptance, adaptation, and attachment are all strongly interrelated. Ballou (1978) asserted that early acceptance can be a good predictor of the woman's postpartum adjustment to motherhood. Failure to accept the pregnancy can have serious consequences. While a full denial of the pregnancy is rare (Maldonado-Durán et al. 2000), a partial rejection can be fairly common. It may involve ambivalence or conflict about being pregnant, which is frequently expressed in the first trimester (Cohen 1966). This denial most often occurs unconsciously (Rosenthal and O'Grady 1985), and the seriousness of the denial may increase over time. Davidoff and O'Grady (1985) described the denial of pregnancy as one of the key factors in neonaticide.

Acceptance of the pregnancy should become easier as time progresses and the woman undergoes a series of bodily changes to accommodate the growing fetus. Bibring et al. (1961) stated that the occurrence of quickening produces an "undeniable" acknowledgment of the baby growing inside the mother. Kemp and Page (1987) also related prenatal attachment to the advent of quickening. Carter-Jessop (1981) found that pregnant women who were taught to interact with their fetuses through recognizing body parts and stroking the abdomen developed a higher level of maternal-infant attachment before birth. Finally, Ballou (1978) described a relationship of a woman's recognition of her pregnancy and the child within her to the beginnings of a relationship with that child. In other words, the more aware the woman becomes of her child-to-be, the more apt she will be to develop a positive nurturing relationship with the child.

The meaning of the pregnancy for a woman often determines how well she accepts the pregnancy. Pregnancy can mean different things to different women, depending on their stage in life, their desire for a child, the response of significant others, and the cultural meaning of being pregnant. Rosenthal and O'Grady (1985) differentiated between the wish for a baby or child and the wish to be pregnant. A pregnancy can be desired for many reasons: a woman's "biological clock is running out," the woman has been told that having children may be doubtful if not impossible, she wants confirmation that her body can reproduce, or she may even desire to leave a piece of herself in the world. Rosenthal and O'Grady (1985) also discussed issues related to adolescent pregnancy, such as rebellion against parents, peer pressure, desire to be loved, sexual identity issues, or desire to hold on to a specific partner. One study of adolescent mothers found that in the year prior to conception, a significant number had experienced a major loss (Rosenthal 1977). Finally, pregnancy can also be seen as a "public statement of a woman's sexual activity," which can be experienced by the woman as a source of pride or embarrassment (Rosenthal and O'Grady 1985, p. 50).

Acceptance of the pregnancy is important not only for the mother herself but also for her network of friends, family, and significant others (Rubin 1984). If the woman does not have other people in her life who support her pregnancy, it will be more difficult for her to accept it in a positive light. The woman needs to "make a place" in her world for her child-to-be, but she can do so only if the people around her allow and support her endeavors.

Development of a Fantasy Baby

The development of a fantasy baby or an internal working model of the baby-to-be has been shown to be extremely influential in a mother's later relationship with her baby. A fantasy baby is the idea of a baby the mother creates in her mind, through internal imagery and fantasy. A tool developed by Zeanah et al. (1994) called the Working Model of the Child Interview (WMCI) is an interview that elicits, explores, and classifies parents' mental representations of their child. Benoit et al. (1997) found not only that prenatal outcomes on the WMCI predicted Strange Situation attachment outcomes at 12 months' postpartum but also that there was a stability in the prenatal mental representations of the child and the postpartum representations at 12 months. These findings suggest that much of the work that goes into the development of a relationship and attachment occurs before birth. It therefore seems important to help the pregnant mother lay some of the groundwork for her later relationship with her child.

Ballou (1978) stated that women prepare to mother their child through daydreaming and fantasizing about their baby. In fact, she found that failure to conceptualize the baby-to-be in warm and protective ways before birth often contributed negatively to the postpartum relationship. Sherwen (1987) found that mothers who rehearsed mentally around the baby-to-be and mothering adapted better to motherhood. Cohen (1966) also supported the notion that in the psychologically healthy woman, attachment to the baby begins long before the baby is born. Finally, Cranley (1993) found that attributing characteristics and intentions to the fetus played an important role in fetal attachment and maternal bonding.

Development of Mothering Behavior

It is critical for women to practice the role of mother and to begin thinking about it in a multidimensional manner. Women accomplish part of this practice through the use of the same imagery and fantasy that they use for relating to their baby. They imagine themselves as a mother or parent. Just as a mother fantasizes about what her baby will be like, she also fantasizes about what kind of mother she will be and what kind of behaviors she will have to develop (Ballou 1978; Lederman 1996; Rubin 1984; Zeanah et al. 1994). Muller and Ferketich (1992) found that the ability to imagine oneself as a parent was important in fetal attachment. Mercer (1995) pointed out that mothers use night dreaming as a way to resolve concerns over assuming the mothering role.

Rubin (1967, 1984) identified the development of mothering behaviors to involve the cognitive operation she called "replication" (Mercer 1995). Replication is seen as mimicry and role-playing—that is, women look to other experienced mothers and to experts for information on caring for an infant. Pregnant women become interested in young children and may even seek opportunities to practice caring for a baby through babysitting. Rubin described the work in replication as reducing a woman's anxiety, decreasing her uncertainty about her behavior, and validating her ability to be a mother.

Redefinition of Self

A woman without child is not the same as a woman with child. Not only does a woman need to develop a new repertoire of behaviors to be able to care for her baby-to-be, but she must also negotiate an entire shift in how she views herself. This redefinition of self occurs throughout the pregnancy and into the postpartum period. It involves both a taking in of new ideas of who she needs to become and a letting go of old thoughts of who she can no longer be.

Rubin (1970) described pregnant women as experiencing a loosening of their cognitive structures, which allows them to think about who they are and what kind of person they want to be. She identified pregnancy as a period of searching and self-questioning, when some aspects of the self are identified as "a good fit" but others are abandoned. Rubin also identified grief as an important piece of the cognitive work for the pregnant woman (Mercer 1995; Rubin 1984). The woman needs to identify components of herself that are incompatible with her new role as mother-to-be. She needs to let go of these and grieve for the pieces of self that were part of who she was for a long time. This identity reorganization can be a difficult, almost impossible step for many women, especially those at the stage of life when they are just defining who they are (e.g., the adolescent or the woman who has never had a clear definition of self).

This redefinition of self can be conceptualized as the development of a *mother ego,* that is, the transformation of the ego or identity to incorporate the idea of becoming a mother. The idea of the mother ego can be thought of from two perspectives, either as part of a larger whole or as a total transformation of the woman's self-identity. Becoming a mother does not erase who the woman is in her other roles, such as self-as-lover, self-as-friend, and self-as-daughter. The self-as-mother, or the mother ego, develops as a response to becoming a mother and as a way of preparing to mother a child.

The second perspective, the transformed self-identity, requires acknowledgment, and ultimately some grief work, that the woman without child will soon become the woman with child. The woman will never be able to go back to the identity of woman without child regardless of the outcome with this particular child. Once she has created a baby and that child has inhabited a space in her womb, this event can never be erased; it is a permanent transformation of her self or ego. The degree to which this transformation takes place and how much the woman actually incorporates the role of mother into her self-identity depend on multiple factors, such as her emotional and cognitive ability, her support system, and the quality of past relationships.

For some women, the development of a mother ego becomes their entire self; for others, it is part of a larger whole. A good example of this transformation is a woman we were seeing for another study, in which we interviewed women with 6-month-old infants. We asked these women what having a child at this point in their lives meant to them. This particular woman, a professional (nurse) in her mid-30s working in labor and delivery, responded very emotionally, immediately breaking down into tears. She said that although she loved her daughter more than anything, not a day went by that she did not grieve for her "previous life." She was an attentive, engaged, high-quality mother, yet she was able to identify and verbalize the loss of her previous identity as woman-without-child and the incorporation of her new mother ego.

As part of redefining one's self, a woman must also begin to differentiate herself from her own mother or mother figure (Ballou 1978). Ballou (1978) suggested that if a woman is going to accept the dependency of her child-to-be, then she must to some extent accept her own sense of dependency on her mother or mother substitute. Kemp and Page (1987) also spoke to this issue, suggesting that women, during pregnancy, need to constantly readjust to a changing image of themselves. They begin to develop a mental model of themselves as capable of being a mother and of mothering children. During this period, women also begin to incorporate the idea of another person joining the family, making it necessary to begin exploring who they are in relationship with this new person, their soon-to-be-born child.

Reworking of Relationships

As a woman adapts to the idea of becoming a mother, she begins to examine her previous and present relationships. As her pregnancy progresses, all of her important relationships undergo a restructuring (Mercer 1995). One of our EHS program mothers, demonstrating excellent self-awareness, summarized this link to her parents when she said, "You can't really separate yourself from your parents . . . entirely, when you are having and raising your own children." Although all a woman's early attachment relationships are important, the two most significant ones discussed in the literature are her relationships with her own mother or mother substitute and with her spouse or partner.

By developing a deeper understanding of her relationship with her mother, the mother-to-be can begin to construct the relationship she will have with her child (Benedek 1970; Deutsch 1945). In order to relate to her child, the woman must access her early sense of her mother (Benedek 1970). Benedek believes that a woman's relationships with her mother and with her own child are set in a context of dependency. Rosenthal and O'Grady (1985) stated that when a woman's relationship with her mother has been good and adequate, it becomes a helpful connection for the woman; on the other hand, if the woman's relationship with her mother has been disturbed or inadequate, she may not only fear that she too will be an inadequate mother but also face an increased risk for peripartum depression.

Bibring and colleagues (1961) found that women sensed changes in their own reactions to their mothers from the very beginning of pregnancy. Women reported rethinking childhood conflicts and other experiences with their mothers, which led them to abandon their previous judgments and solutions and to replace them with a variety of new ways of identifying with their mothers. Bibring and colleagues (1961) termed this process maturational resolution. Women look at their own life experiences with their mothers (Lederman 1996). They begin to ask themselves questions about their mother-daughter relationship and its quality, and about how much of that relationship they want to either discard or carry over into their relationship with their child-to-be. This transgenerational transmission from mother to daughter and then to baby was also noted by Ballou (1978). In fact, she found that positive identification from mother to daughter was passed on just as often as was poor identification. She also noted that the "occurrence of a matriarchal line of controlling, rejecting mothers was not uncommon" (p. 4).

The degree to which the woman is able to satisfactorily rework her relationship with her mother depends on many factors. Lederman (1996) found four components to be the most important:

1. The availability of the woman's mother
2. The mother's reaction to the pregnancy, especially her acceptance of her grandchild-to-be
3. The mother's respect for her daughter's autonomy, as demonstrated by the transition from parent-child to adult-adult
4. The mother's willingness to reminisce with her daughter and share with her examples of her own childbearing and parenting experiences

If a woman's relationship with her mother is so dysfunctional or unsalvageable that she is unable to do this psychological and emotional work, that failure may contribute to a decrease in maternal competency (Ballou 1978). Women who reported not feeling adequately mothered themselves demonstrated difficulty empathizing with and meeting their child's dependency needs (Ballou 1978).

If a woman's mother is unwilling or unable to be available for reworking the mother-daughter relationship, the husband or partner must become a stand-in for that psychological function (Ballou 1978). This situation can be very confusing because the woman also undergoes a reworking of her relationship with her partner during pregnancy. The relaxed defenses during pregnancy stir up both old and present psychological conflicts for the woman, which then require her to reevaluate her marital relationship. The woman faces the task of replacing her mother's role in her life with that of her husband or partner. Although some of this work has most likely been done prior to pregnancy, the intensity of the work progresses throughout the pregnancy (Bibring 1959).

Bibring and colleagues (1961) captured some of the psychological work the woman does and how it is woven into the progressive development of the woman's relationship with her child. They described a woman as initially bonding with the man she loves, then out of that love wishing for a child. In this early stage, she begins the developmental shift from a woman without child to a mother. "She shifts from being a single, circumscribed self-contained organism to reproducing herself and her love object (her husband) in a child who will from then on remain an object outside herself" (p. 17). The relationship she develops with her child will not only be different and separate from any of her earlier relationships but also remain unique from any of her future relationships. This mother-child relationship will emerge from a synthesis of the woman's relationship with her actual child as a separate and distinct person, her relationship with the child as the love object representing her husband, and her relationship with the child representing the mother herself.

The husband or partner also needs to be available to fulfill some basic needs of the woman during pregnancy. He needs to be emotionally available and be able to demonstrate empathy for the progressive pregnancy (Lederman 1996). The woman also needs to see her husband as flexible, cooperative, trustworthy, and reliable (Lederman 1996). Furthermore, he needs to be able to be in touch with the feminine aspects of his personality (Bibring 1959). The husband's ability to meet these needs for his wife in turn allows her to be empathetic and thoughtful of his developing needs as a father (Lederman 1996).

THE PSYCHOLOGICAL WORK OF PREGNANCY AND HIGH-RISK POPULATIONS

The psychological work of pregnancy clearly goes beyond everyday consciousness into the deeper levels of the unconscious, specifically into the areas of early attachments and the internal working models developed throughout childhood. It is the nature of these earliest of relationships that forges our egos (Wilkinson 1996). The strength and stability of the ego then provide the support that women need to do the emotional work demanded of them in pregnancy. What if the woman's early relationships were inconsistent, toxic, or empty? What happens when a woman's attachments were unreliable, dangerous, or even nonexistent? When this has been the woman's experience, it is believed that the woman will have developed a weak or fractured ego. In the case of a young adolescent mother, her ego may also be immature and developmentally compensatory—trying to fill the void left incomplete because of a neglectful or troublesome childhood.

When a woman with a weakened or fragile ego has to navigate the psychological work of pregnancy, several events may transpire. First, the ego may not be strong enough to sustain the idea of a pregnancy, to develop a vision of incorporating a child into one's life, or to rework the relationship with self, mother, or others. Second, the woman may not have adequate early memories or experiences to capitalize on so that she can do the work required of pregnancy. In fact, she may have emotionally survived her childhood by holding on to fragments of relationships, constructing idealized fantasies of nurturing figures, and pushing the pieces of relationships and attachments that cannot be tolerated or understood into deep areas of the unconscious. Third, when certain memories become reactivated, especially those around maternal relationships, the emotional content rising into consciousness may be painful and overwhelming, leading to an emotional crisis in the mother-to-be. Finally, all these issues become complications and deterrents to the woman's early attempts to recognize her baby-to-be, to make a place for the child in her world, and to see herself as a mother with the ability to care for and nurture a child—in other words, the development of her mother ego. The woman's ego must go through a transformation that incorporates her past significant caregiver relationships, whether or not they were nurturing.

The population of pregnant women we intervened with included women of poverty. Through Adult Attachment Interviews, we learned that while some women had exceptional families of origin who lovingly cared for and protected them, many had a history of abuse, neglect, deprivation of early mother or other attachment figures, and early relationships riddled with inconsistency, unpredictability, trauma, and chaos. Many demonstrated moderate to severe difficulty in developing and maintaining any type of positive relationship. Some also had birthed children prior to this pregnancy from whom they were now separated because of death, failure to protect from abuse, intervention from Child Protective Services, or their own personal decision that they were not ready or able to function as a mother at that particular time in life. Some women had custody of their previous children; however, their relationships with these children were often problematic in that nurturing was limited or absent and the relationship was permeated with inconsistency and anger. Furthermore, many of the women we worked with did not have their own mothers or mother substitutes readily available to provide them with the means to adequately rework their mother-daughter relationships. In addition, many were also without a husband or partner who might act as a mediator for the relationship work. Our goal was to develop a set of interventions designed to facilitate, encourage, and support the development of an identity of self as mother and the development of a healthy, positive, nurturing relationship between mother and baby-to-be. It is this program we describe here.

THE PARENT-CHILD COMMUNICATION COACHING PROGRAM

The PCCC pregnancy intervention was one part of a set of age-specific interventions that began during pregnancy and continued through the second year of the child's life. The intent of the PCCC program was to improve parent-child relationships, which were measured in the outcomes of parent-child interaction and child attachment. The primary themes of the pregnancy intervention were maternal tasks of recognizing the fetus, gaining acceptance for the infant within the family, and trying on the maternal role. Three sections of the intervention were designed to be introduced during pregnancy: Baby Kicks and Wiggles (KW), Support Network (SN), and Attachment and Motherhood (AM). A fourth section, involving the cloth baby carrier, was to be introduced prenatally or early postpartum. The intervention we report here was evaluated through a joint effort by the Kent Children's Home Society and the South King County Families First EHS program and researchers at the University of Washington.

The intervention was designed to be carried out by home visitors who saw mothers on a weekly basis if the mother was not working and on a monthly basis if she was working. The PCCC pregnancy intervention was implemented by home visitors of the Kent Children's Home Society and the South King County EHS program. The typical home visitor held a bachelor's degree in early childhood education, child development, or a related field and had a minimum of five years' experience in early childhood education settings or in child and family development programs. The activity sheets outlining the intervention for all phases of the PCCC program were developed through the collaborative effort of the university research team (JoAnne Solchany, Kathryn Barnard, and Susan Spieker), the home visitors, and the Seattle-King County Public Health Nurses. Selected examples from the protocol are presented in this chapter. (The entire pregnancy program is being revised for later publication.)

Sample: Early Head Start Mothers

The women and children of South King County who were eligible for the EHS intervention met the poverty income level necessary for enrollment and lived in a rural-suburban area south of Seattle. This geographical area has the lowest per capita income in the county, as well as the highest incidence of child abuse and neglect. Compared with the rest of the county, South King County has more low-birth-weight infants, more hospitalizations for children ages 1 to 4, more Medicaid childbirth hospitalizations, more single heads of households living in poverty, more inadequately immunized children, and more families experiencing alcohol and substance abuse problems.

The mothers enrolled in the program were more likely than the general population to have a history of insecure attachment relationships, which may complicate the development of secure maternal-infant attachment (Main et al. 1985). In addition, 60% of the women enrolled in Kent EHS met criteria of the Center for Epidemiologic Studies Depression Scale (Eaton and Kessler 1981) during their pregnancy.

Pregnancy Intervention and Its Implementation

Unlike any prenatal program documented in the literature, the PCCC intervention (Barnard et al. 1996) aimed to address the maternal-infant attachment process, as well as to facilitate accomplishment of the tasks of pregnancy as previously described. The three objectives of the intervention were based on Rubin's (1984) theoretical framework of the developmental tasks of pregnancy: to help the pregnant woman a) recognize her fetus, b) gain support for her infant within the family, and c) explore the maternal role. Accomplishing these tasks may facilitate incorporation of the maternal role, enhance maternal-infant attachment, and encourage use of a support system (Koniak-Griffin 1993; Mercer 1985; Rubin 1984). We will now discuss how the PCCC program facilitated achievement of the three objectives, as reported by home visitors in this EHS program. One of the authors (KS) obtained this information by interviewing the home visitors after the pregnancy period was over for all subjects.

Recognizing the Fetus

The design of the KW protocol focused on recognition of the fetus through three interventions: 1) the Fetal Movement Count, 2) the Movement Interpretations Questionnaire (MIQ) (Figure 4–1), and 3) My Baby Predictions (Figure 4–2). In the Fetal Movement Count, mothers are asked to count the number of movements they perceive during a specified short period of time. The MIQ is intended to elucidate the perceptions and attributions of the future mother regarding the baby's movements. My Baby Predictions attempts to help the woman visualize and name her fantasies, wishes, and perhaps fears regarding her future baby.

---

1. How would you describe your baby's kicks today? (vigorous, slow-moving, sharp, rhythmical, hard, etc.)
2. What do you think your baby's body position and location were today?
3. What do you think your baby was feeling today when you felt him/her move? Explain.
4. Have you had a day during this past week when you felt your baby's movements showed that he/she was excited or upset? How could you tell?
5. Have you noticed any specific activity that brings on an increase in kicking or movement? Explain.
6. Do you notice your baby's movement increasing or decreasing at certain times of the day?
7. Do you think your baby responds to voices, sounds, or music? Explain.
8. Have family members or friends been able to feel the baby move? What was their reaction?

Figure 4–1.   Movement Interpretation Questionnaire.

Home visitors indicated that the Fetal Movement Counts themselves did not significantly influence the mothers' perceptions of the fetus as an individual. However, the counts did serve as a foundation for the next step of the KW intervention, the MIQ. The MIQ helped some mothers draw a connection between the movements and the reality of the fetus as an individual. For both adolescent and adult mothers, the MIQ worked as a catalyst. "The light bulb went on," one home visitor said. As Rubin (1984) and Stainton (1990) wrote, interaction with the fetus solidifies the reality of the fetus for the mother. Encouraging mothers to play interactive games with the fetus, such as pushing back when the fetus kicks or shining a flashlight at the mother's abdomen to elicit a response, may further this function. The counts and the MIQ were rarely completed by mothers as homework; however, completing the activities during the visit allowed the home visitor to act as a witness and to celebrate the event.

Boy or girl _____

Hair color _____

Long hair, short hair, or bald _____

Weight _____

Length _____

Eye color _____

Date of birth _____

Time of birth _____

Unusual traits or characteristics _____

My baby will look a little like _____

What other predictions can you make about your baby?_____

Figure 4–2.   My Baby Predictions.

This support was beneficial for women without partners or supportive peers. Despite positive results with some mothers, the MIQ was difficult to implement, which may reflect clients' difficulty describing emotions or drawing attention to their own body. This resistance may be the result of a variety of contributing factors, such as clients' cognitive development, attachment history, or history of abuse (Bohn and Holz 1996).

Implementation of My Baby Predictions also encouraged recognition of the fetus and promoted fantasy about the anticipated child by mothers as well as fathers. By sealing the completed My Baby Predictions in an envelope to be revealed postpartum, home visitors created a game out of the activity and added a celebratory aspect to recognition of the anticipated child.

Gaining Support for the Infant Within the Family

In Rubin's (1984) theoretical framework, the father of the baby and the family of the mother are the sources of motivation, supportive strength, confidence, resourcefulness, and creativity for the childbearing woman. Many of the EHS mothers did not have partners or family and were in need not only of emotional resources but also of more concrete resources. Although the SN activity was sometimes used as a means of discussing ways to inform family members about the pregnancy, the activity was more often used as a tool to elucidate multifaceted sources of support, including instrumental, informational, and emotional. The home visitor essentially used a graphic style (circles, squares, branching system) to have the mother record those she considered part of her support system.

Implementation of the SN protocol also helped expand mothers' perceptions of available resources. This written activity provided a visual map of the mother's resources, and a form with telephone numbers created a means through which to access that support. Many mothers in the program posted the completed form next to their telephones. When there were gaps in clients' resource network, home visitors informed mothers about available community resources. Thus, the resulting discussion served as a means of widening perceptions of the support available for the mother and infant within both the family and the community.

Reaching out for help and accepting assistance was difficult for a number of mothers. With the SN protocol, home visitors attempted to impress on mothers that requesting and accepting help is expected and necessary. Completing the Birth Plan also helped mothers identify their support people, specifically for labor and delivery. The activity served as a rehearsal for decision making and accessing support for the anticipated child. Because many of the EHS mothers had a primarily reactive mode of decision making, the Birth Plan provided a new and rare opportunity for deliberate decision making and planning. The Birth Plan is part of the later section of the program (attachment), but it involves eliciting assistance from support persons.

Exploring the Maternal Role

According to Rubin (1984), exploring potential role models is the primary and predominant mode of incorporating the separate valued and esteemed elements that the pregnant woman has observed in other women who are mothers. Discussion of relationship qualities, which the mother chooses to emulate or avoid, was introduced by the SN activity. The AM protocol involved four parts: 1) Attachment Moments, 2) Roles of Motherhood, 3) Birth Plan, and 4) Family Traditions and From Me to You. These activities further promoted exploration of the maternal role.

The Roles of Motherhood activity (Figure 4–3) was used as a tool to discuss the maternal characteristics to which the client would like her child or children to be exposed. Home visitors said that the discussion of roles was fairly easy to move through. Many clients agreed with the categories of maternal roles, although they did not always experience their own mothers in those roles. One home visitor said, "They would look at it and say, 'Oh, my mom didn't snuggle and cuddle me,'" which led to discussion about what kind of environment the client wanted to create for her baby. The protocol also prompted one mother who had a limited support network to explore print and video resources on motherhood at the library. The Roles of Motherhood activity was also useful for adult

Mother as protector
- Saves from people who might hurt them
- Saves from household dangers
- Saves from health risks
- Saves during travel

Mothers are responsible for keeping their children safe from dangers of any kind.

Mother as nurturer
- Snuggles and cuddles
- Hugs and kisses
- Kisses "booboos"
- Nurtures baby and self

Nurturing is a way of sharing love, care, and warmth from one person to another.

Mother as provider
- Gives nourishment
- Provides warm and safe place to sleep
- Makes home feel positive
- Provides medical care
- Provides fresh air

Mothers have the greatest responsibility for making sure their infant is provided for.

Mother as educator
- Makes safety rules
- Teaches the qualities of a good person
- Interacts to teach communication
- Models patience and understanding

Mothers teach children through example, actions, words, and direct coaching. This process is ongoing throughout the parent-child relationship.

Mother as pillar of strength
- Buffers intense emotions
- Soothes tears
- Provides security
- Provides stability for out-of-control feelings

Babies are not born with the ability to deal with intense emotions—positive or negative. They learn this skill through observation, practice, and maturity. Until this ability matures, mothers become the buffers or holders for intense feelings.

Mother as woman
- Takes care of herself
- Balances self needs with baby needs
- Nurtures self
- Doesn't judge self harshly
- Maintains a sense of humor
- Conserves and prioritizes time & energy

Motherhood can be a wonderful part of being a woman. It should be celebrated. Mothers should never forget, however, the woman inside.

Figure 4–3.   Roles of Motherhood teaching handout.

mothers, postpartum. For example, one home visitor used this activity to highlight how the client was already fulfilling the maternal role.

Several mothers found the concepts of the Roles of Motherhood too difficult or abstract to discuss. When asked to identify the roles of mother, they had a hard time articulating them. Home visitors used a variety of approaches to communicate these ideas and concepts. They found that one way to facilitate dialogue was using examples of people the mother had known during her childhood. Discussions were more successful when the home visitors related the concepts to mothers' own experience. This seemed to make the concepts more concrete and understandable for some mothers. The mother's firsthand experiences were found to be much more meaningful than discussing observed role models, such as friends or media persona. For clients who had difficulty describing the roles they hoped to fill in their child's life, collage and painting served as a supplemental and alternative means of communication.

The Roles of Motherhood discussion was particularly valuable with adolescent mothers who had not accepted the maternal role by the postpartum period. For example, when asked to sign the home visit form under "parent's signature," one 16-year-old client routinely handed the form to her own mother. This client admitted to the home visitor that she did not feel ready to accept her new role. After her baby was born, the young mother said that it felt like she was babysitting and that the actual parents would arrive soon to take the newborn home with them. The Roles activity helped open up discussion about this new mother's roles and responsibilities.

The cloth baby carrier provided early success in the new maternal role. For many mothers, the use of the cloth baby carrier consistently helped to calm and quiet the newborn, providing the new mothers with an opportunity to enjoy a feeling of competency. Cloth baby carriers also helped fathers feel both more comfortable when holding the small newborn and successful in quieting the child. The cloth baby carrier was a helpful solution for one adolescent mother who lived with her boyfriend's family. The grandmother discouraged the adolescent parents from holding the baby as frequently as they wanted when the baby cried. By carrying the baby in the cloth baby carrier, they were able to hold and calm the infant without being criticized by the grandmother.

The Attachment, Attachment Moments, and Family Traditions activities, which explored concepts such as the nature of attachment, were a valuable contribution to the clients' newly forming maternal role. The initial question "Why should I think about motherhood?" established the groundwork for discussion about attachment. These activities served as opportunities to discuss the environment that clients hoped to create for their children. The discussion also helped to persuade some mothers that nurturing and loving their infants cannot lead to a spoiled child.

The Attachment protocol aimed to divide the concept of attachment into a number of small, easy-to-understand, usable, concrete, interactive behaviors, such as caressing the pregnant belly, cuddling, soothing, singing, and gazing. Attachment was defined as a process of developing affectionate ties between mother and child on the basis of the increasing accumulation of smaller Attachment Moments or behaviors. Sensitivity and responsiveness by the mother were also stressed. The concept of each Attachment Moment adding to the relationship was discussed metaphorically to suggest a more solid base, giving rise to a stronger and more stable relationship.

Two additional activities, From Me to You and Family Traditions, encouraged the mother to think of ways to welcome her child into her world and to help her transition into motherhood. From Me to You gave the mother several options of creating a gift for her baby-to-be. One idea was to create a cassette tape of favorite lullabies or of the mother singing or telling a story. The mother was encouraged to begin playing this tape while the baby was still in utero and to continue playing it for the baby after birth.

Family Traditions encouraged mothers to consciously design and facilitate traditions and customs unique to them and their babies. These celebrations could be built around welcoming the baby or, for the mother, around making the transition into the role of mother. An example of an activity to welcome the baby is beginning a collection box, with treasures such as a special rock for stability or a button from the shirt that the mother wore to the hospital to symbolize her love for her baby. One adolescent mother decided to create a cookbook of her mother's best recipes. This idea emerged from a discussion about this client's mother and her positive attributes, which included cooking. Having a tea party with valued friends who can share stories of the mother's life might also help the mother make the transition into the maternal role.

These activities also allowed mothers and fathers to describe their wishes for the child by writing letters to the anticipated newborn. Discussing family traditions also led to planning for the child's future and for the client's future desired roles. Mothers whose own childhood had been too chaotic for holiday traditions had an opportunity to describe their hopes of being able to celebrate special occasions with their child. The home visits seemed to create a rare opportunity for the mother to consider issues that she might not otherwise have thought of or that she may have given a low priority.

Intervention as Structure for Discussion

Implementation of a consistent, non-crisis-driven pregnancy intervention emerged as something of value in itself. Home visitors said that mothers became more receptive to visits and protocols over time. Also, the discussion became more relaxed and activities became easier to introduce. Concrete and hands-on activities worked best initially, followed by gradual introduction of more abstract ideas. One home visitor explained that mothers were simply unaccustomed to discussing ideas such as those included in the PCCC program, and that over time mothers developed skills and comfort for such discussions. An additional benefit also emerged: mothers told home visitors that they felt more comfortable talking to their prenatal care providers as a direct result of the home visits and conversation.

Other Issues

Special Needs of Adolescent Mothers

The home visitors' comments correlated with the professional literature, which suggests that adolescents face heightened barriers to maternal role attainment as a function of their developmental stage (Julian 1983; Mercer 1985, 1990; Williams-Burgess et al. 1995). All home visitors described working with adolescent clients as challenging. Discussing abstract ideas, such as the concept of attachment, was particularly difficult. Activities that referred to the mother's body, and, by extension, to the fetus within her body, were also challenging. "The younger they were, the harder it was for them to talk about what was happening in their bodies," one home visitor said. Another home visitor worked with two clients who had difficulty with the MIQ questions. For instance, "What do you think your baby was feeling today?" was difficult to answer because neither adolescent was able to describe her feelings about the pregnancy itself. Home visitors used the strategies of illustrating abstract ideas with concrete examples, such as making collages or painting, and of introducing protocols gradually. The comments of home visitors also reflected their different expectations of the maternal relationship with an adolescent; for instance, the home visitors believed that trust between them and the adolescent mothers would build slowly.

Mercer (1990) found that pregnant adolescents require more time to achieve the maternal role than do mature women. Adolescents are also particularly dependent on role models to accomplish developmental tasks. A good self-image and a sense of competence in the new situation are important variables for the adolescent client (Diehl 1997; Mercer 1990). In orienting new home visitors to this intervention, combining the home visitors' suggestions with Mercer's findings could facilitate a more effective intervention with adolescent clients.

Father Involvement

Although only a fraction of fathers were accessible during home visits, the home visitors described an openness on the part of the pregnant women to attempt encouraging involvement of the fathers who demonstrated even low levels of interest in the PCCC intervention. Fathers participated in the Fetal Movement Counts and My Baby Predictions, and they helped to complete the SN forms. "Roles of Fatherhood" were improvised, and some fathers helped create projects for the child, such as letters or videos. Fathers also helped with the Birth Plan and, in some cases, used the cloth baby carrier.

Home visitors suggested enhancing father participation by being open, flexible, and creative. They also suggested adjusting the written language of the protocol and possibly adding optional forms to be included when fathers were accessible. The support systems literature suggests that maternal role attainment is strengthened by the father's support of the mother during pregnancy (Burke and Liston 1994; Crnic et al. 1983;

Zachariah 1994). Also, children benefit when fathers are consistently involved (O'Hara 1998; Parke 1995; Pleck 1997). The growing body of literature on fatherhood is beginning to identify needs of fathers as they assume paternal identity (Malnory 1996; Parke 1995; Pleck 1997). The literature also suggests that fathers who are interested in participating have typically felt excluded in maternal-and-infant–focused intervention programs (Jordan 1990; O'Hara 1998).

In the context of the PCCC pregnancy intervention, home visitors expressed an interest in encouraging the connectedness of fathers with their families. The fathers' efforts may be enhanced through the home visitors' increased awareness of their own biases, assumptions, and use of language (O'Hara 1998). Such efforts have the potential benefit of enriching the experience of the child and the mother, as well as the father.

Need for Mental Health Referral

Approximately 60% of the clients involved in the Kent EHS pilot program met depression criteria at intake, according to the Center for Epidemiologic Studies Depression Scale (Eaton and Kessler 1981). Also, as previously mentioned, many clients had a difficult childhood history. Some clients stated simply that they felt they did not have a mother as a child themselves. It is not surprising, then, that the protocols exploring each client's support network and encouraging reflection on her relationship history and wishes for change might aggravate the pain of past losses, abuse, or neglect. AM discussion stirred memories of difficult issues during childhood and previous pregnancies. Also, one client's labor and delivery experience brought molestation issues to the surface. Other women requested mental health referrals independently as they entered the program. These findings support the view of pregnancy as not only a period of openness and reflection but also a time that can reactivate losses for each woman (Rubin 1984; St.-Andre 1993). Considering the complex challenges faced by families of EHS, mental health treatment may be warranted for each receptive client during this unique but finite window of opportunity.

Resistance

Pregnancy has been identified as a time of philosophizing and a time of openness to new ideas (Rubin 1984). Although home visitors' reports reflect a degree of openness among some clients, for many clients such openness was not present. It is unclear whether this reticence to communicate was the result of mental health issues, chaos, a cultural barrier, or limited verbal skills. Home visitors commonly described some resistance that was evident on a number of levels.

Client resistance to completing projects independently was common. Some mothers just seemed to need more one-on-one support and often would be willing to complete activities with the home visitor during home visits, such as counting fetal movements in the KW protocol. A more challenging scenario was client reluctance to map out the SN; this response was interpreted by home visitors as an unwillingness to acknowledge the limited nature of their support systems. A third form of client resistance—inability to describe abstract ideas or emotions—may have reflected a lack of comfort, skill, or experience in doing so.

Finally, individual home visitors expressed some resistance to particular protocols. This resistance was perhaps a function of discomfort with the particular activity or the expectation of a client's resistance. Home visitor skepticism about the goal of the activities was not evident. Home visitors who expressed doubts about the effectiveness of their interventions were often less experienced. In contrast, those who used a more persistent, assertive technique seemed less doubtful about their own efficacy and often possessed greater experience.

EFFECTIVENESS OF PREGNANCY INTERVENTIONS

Despite challenges in implementing activities with many mothers, all home visitors recommended continued use of the PCCC pregnancy intervention. Their criticism of the protocols and their recommendations for improvements were fairly specific, which suggests that amendments are feasible. Although no quantitative data on the impact of the PCCC pregnancy intervention are currently available, the home visitors' comments indicate that implementation of the intervention increased mothers' recognition of the fetus, facilitated identification of mothers' support systems, supported exploration of the maternal role, and, in addition, encouraged fathers' involvement, promoted relationship building with home visitors, and increased mothers' comfort in communicating with health care professionals.

There is evidence from past empirical work and theory that pregnancy is an important time for developing the capacity for mothering. Rubin's (1967) original observations of pregnant women lead us to assert that this is the natural work of the woman herself and it does not require direction from health care providers. However, it remains an open question as to whether women who have not had adequate mothering themselves, or who are in conflict about their pregnancy, need guidance in recognizing the fetus, gaining support within the family, and exploring the maternal role and attachment.

We have found that an attempt to focus the "at-risk" mother on preparing for the maternal role is generally well received by mothers. We have also found that home visitors without specific training in the psychological state of women during pregnancy can implement the planned activities with the mothers in EHS. The specific issues around attachment and the mothering role were the ones most likely to elicit the women's past negative experiences with their own childhood history. The home visitors reported that having more skills in dealing with their distressed feelings would have allowed the women themselves to gain more understanding of their past. Ideally, providers of maternity services should be more aware of the psychological work of women during pregnancy. As a result, true primary prevention of mental health problems in parenting and early parent-child relationships would be more easily accomplished.

Primary obstetrical providers should focus on identifying women with a poor relationship history, particularly those who have early experiences of unresolved loss or trauma. Measures such as the Impact of Events Scale (Horowitz 1986) can be quite helpful in discovering such experiences. These women need to have the normal process of preparing for mothering facilitated for them so that they do prepare for taking on the maternal role. We know that a high number of current pregnancies are not planned (40%–60%) and that a significant number are not even wanted by the last trimester (10%–15%) (Lederman and Miller 1998). It seems only logical to incorporate primary maternity services into preventive mental health efforts such as the ones described in this chapter.

CONCLUSION

The actual birth of a baby takes only about one day. No other day in a woman's life comes loaded with as much vulnerability, pain, emotional stress, exhaustion, possible physical injury or death, and permanent role change—from woman without child to mother of a new human being (Simkin 1996). The maternal tasks that the woman progresses through are thought to be universal, but how she approaches these tasks and how she demonstrates them behaviorally reflect her cultural and specific life situation (Mercer 1995). Her journey through pregnancy and the psychological work she accomplishes will be guided by many factors, including her own personality structure, her ability to adjust to and resolve emotional conflict, her particular life setting, and the quality of her family constellation (Bibring et al. 1961), as well as the support she receives from care providers.

What kind of impact can the quality of the mother's navigation through her psychological work of pregnancy have on the parent-child relationship and the lifetime trajectory of a child? The answer to this question is not clear. First, a child's life is filled with opportunities and obstacles, and we know that no singular event is directly responsible for later lifetime outcomes. Second, we are really just beginning to address the importance of this period for the developing parent-child relationship, as well as for lifetime trajectories. Pregnancy, infancy, and early childhood have been explored only minimally; more quality research needs to take place. What we do know about these periods, however, is intriguing. In an elaboration of Fraiberg's (1975) concept of "ghosts in the nursery," which referred to parental projections of past experiences, Karr-Morse and Wiley (1997) wrote about the phenomenon of "ghosts from the nursery," which links certain distressing womb experiences and poorly established relationships in infancy and early childhood to the development of a trajectory toward violent behavior. Other researchers have supported the close relationship between womb and early infant experience and later behavioral and relationship outcomes (Piontelli 1987, 1992; Zeanah et al. 1994). Although the direct pathways establishing this relationship are still being debated, the significance of the link is widely accepted.

It is clear from the evidence that the period of pregnancy is a rich time for psychological change. Primary health care providers attending to the woman's pregnancy should keep in mind such possibilities. Psychological care providers should also be aware of the psychological vulnerability that surfaces in pregnancy. Although it can be a time of psychological growth and opportunity, pregnancy can just as easily awaken demons long laid to rest by the mother-to-be as she moves into a fragile, overwhelming, frightening, and even dangerous psychological space. Caring for the mother psychologically during and after pregnancy can lay one more brick in the foundation of the mother-child relationship that can provide solid support for the child throughout life.

REFERENCES

Affonso DD, Sheptak S: Maternal cognitive themes during pregnancy. Matern Child Nurs J 18(2):147–166, 1989

Bailey LA, Hailey BJ: The psychological experience of pregnancy. Int J Psychiatry Med 16(3):263–274, 1986

Ballou JW: The Psychology of Pregnancy. Lexington, MA, Lexington Books, 1978

Barnard K, Spieker J, Morisset C: Grant proposal submitted to Administration on Child, Youth and Families, Early Head Start Research Partnerships, 1996

Benedek T: The psychobiology of pregnancy, in Parenthood: Its Psychology and Psychopathology. Edited by Anthony EJ, Benedek T. Boston, MA, Little, Brown, 1970, pp 137–152

Benoit D, Parker KCH, Zeanah CH: Mothers' internal representations of their infants during pregnancy: stability over time and association with infants' attachment classifications at 12 months. J Child Psychol Psychiatry 38(3):307–313, 1997

Bibring GL: Some considerations of the psychological processes in pregnancy. Psychoanal Study Child 14:113–121, 1959

Bibring GL, Dwyer TF, Huntington DS, et al: A study of psychological processes in pregnancy and of the earliest mother-child relationship. Psychoanal Study Child 16:9–72, 1961

Bohn D, Holz K: Sequelae of abuse: health effects of childhood sexual abuse, domestic battering, and rape. Journal of Nurse-Midwifery 41(6):442–456, 1996

Burke P, Liston W: Adolescent mothers' perceptions of social support and the impact of parenting on their lives. Pediatr Nurs 20(6):593–599, 1994

Carter-Jessop L: Promoting maternal attachment through prenatal intervention. Maternal and Child Nursing 6:107–112, 1981

Cohen MB: Personal identity and sexual identity. Psychiatry 29:1–12, 1966

Cranley MS: The origins of the mother-child relationship: a review. Physical and Occupational Therapy in Pediatrics 12(2–3):39–51, 1993

Crnic K, Greenberg M, Ragozin N, et al: Effects of social support on mothers of premature and full-term infants. Child Dev 54:209–217, 1983

Culpepper L, Jack B: Psychosocial issues in pregnancy. Prim Care 20(3):599–619, 1993

Davidoff R, O'Grady JP: Disorders of mother-infant attachment, in Obstetrics: Psychological and Psychiatric Syndromes. Edited by O'Grady JP, Rosenthal M. New York, Elsevier, 1985, pp 181–195

Deutsch H: Psychology of Women. New York, Grune & Stratton, 1945

Diehl K: Adolescent mothers: what produces positive mother-infant interaction? Maternal and Child Nursing 22:89–95, 1997

Eaton WW, Kessler LG: Rates of symptoms of depression in a national sample. Am J Epidemiol 114(4):528–538, 1981

Fraiberg S, Adelson E, Shapiro V: Ghosts in the nursery: a psychoanalytic approach to the problems of impaired infant-mother relationships. J Am Acad Child Psychiatry 14(3):387–421, 1975

Horowitz MJ: Stress Response Syndromes. Northvale, NJ, Jason Aronson, 1986

Jordan P: Laboring for relevance: expectant and new fatherhood. Nurs Res 39:11–36, 1990

Julian C: A comparison of perceived and demonstrated maternal role competence of adolescent mothers. Issues Health Care Women 4:223–236, 1983

Karr-Morse R, Wiley MS: Ghosts From the Nursery: Tracing the Roots of Violence. New York, Atlantic Monthly Press, 1997

Kemp VH, Page C: Maternal self-esteem and prenatal attachment in high-risk pregnancy. Maternal-Child Nursing Journal 16(3):195–206, 1987

Koniak-Griffin D: Maternal role attainment image. J Nurs Scholarsh 25:257–262, 1993

Lederman RP: Psychosocial Adaptation in Pregnancy: Assessment of Seven Dimensions of Maternal Development. New York, Springer, 1996

Lederman R, Miller DS: Adaptation to pregnancy in three different ethnic groups: Latin-American, African-American, and Anglo-American. Canadian Journal of Nursing Research 30(3):37–51, 1998

Main M, Kaplan N, Cassidy J: Security in infancy, childhood, and adulthood: a move to the level of representation. Monogr Soc Res Child Dev 50:66–104, 1985

Maldonado-Durán JM, Lartigue T, Feintuch M: Perinatal psychiatry: infant mental health interventions during pregnancy. Bull Menninger Clin 64:317–343, 2000

Malnory M: Developmental care of the pregnant couple. J Obstet Gynecol Neonatal Nurs 25:525–532, 1996

Mercer R: The process of maternal role attainment over the first year. Nurs Res 34:198–204, 1985

Mercer R: Parents at Risk. New York, Springer, 1990

Mercer R: Becoming a Mother: Research on Maternal Identity From Rubin to the Present (Focus on Women Series, Vol 18). New York, Springer, 1995

Muller ME, Ferketich S: Assessing the validity of the dimensions of prenatal attachment. Matern Child Nurs J 20(1):1–10, 1992

O'Hara N: Working with fathers in home visitation, in Within Our Reach: Effective Home-Based Strategies for Family Support. Symposium conducted at the meeting of the Department of Social Services Western Region Annual Conference, San Francisco, CA, April 1998

Parke R: Fathers and families, in Handbook of Parenting, Vol 3: Status and Social Conditions of Parenting. Edited by Bornstein M. Mahwah, NJ, Erlbaum, 1995, pp 27–61

Piontelli A: Infant observation before birth. Int J Psychoanal 68(4):453–463, 1987

Piontelli A: From Fetus to Child. London, Tavistock/Routledge, 1992

Pleck J: Paternal involvement: levels, sources, and consequences, in The Role of the Father in Child Development. Edited by Bornstein M. New York, Wiley, 1997, pp 66–103

Rosenthal M: Sexual counseling and interviewing. Prim Care 4:291–299, 1977

Rosenthal M, O'Grady JP: Psychological adjustments to pregnancy, in Obstetrics: Psychological and Psychiatric Syndromes. Edited by O'Grady JP, Rosenthal M. New York, Elsevier, 1985, pp 47–63

Rubin R: Attainment of the maternal role, Part II: models and referents. Nurs Res 16:324–346, 1967

Rubin R: Cognitive style in pregnancy. Am J Nurs 70:502–508, 1970

Rubin R: Maternal Identity and the Maternal Experience. New York, Springer, 1984

Sherwen LN: Psychosocial Dimensions of the Pregnant Family. New York, Springer, 1987

Simkin P: The experience of maternity in a woman's life. J Obstet Gynecol Neonatal Nurs 25(3):247–252, 1996

Stainton M: Parents' awareness of their unborn infant in the third trimester. Birth 17(2):92–96, 1990

St.-Andre M: Psychotherapy during pregnancy: opportunities and challenges. Am J Psychother 47(4):572–590, 1993

Wilkinson T: Persephone Returns. Berkeley, CA, Pagemill Press, 1996

Williams-Burgess C, Vines S, Ditulio M: The parent-baby venture program: prevention of child abuse. J Child Adolesc Psychiatr Nurs 8(3):15–23, 1995

Zachariah R: Mother-daughter and husband-wife well-being during pregnancy. Clinical Nursing Research 3(4):371–392, 1994

Zeanah CH, Benoit D, Hirshberg L, et al: Mothers' representations of their infants are concordant with infant attachment classifications. Developmental Issues in Psychiatry and Psychology 1:1–14, 1994

5

Treatment of Attachment Disorders in Infant-Parent Psychotherapy

Alicia F. Lieberman, Ph.D.

The importance of relationships and attachment in the emotional life of children and adults is being increasingly recognized today. Unfortunately, many children experience disruptions in their relationships with caregivers, for example, by losing contact with their parents, by being taken out of the home, or by enduring a lack of involvement on the part of a parent who is present. These disruptions and losses exact a major toll on the emotional life of youngsters. In this chapter, I focus on disorders of attachment in infancy, how they develop, and what can be done to treat them.

I have come to appreciate the importance of these disorders through clinical work with marginalized families who often have little access to health care, including mental health services. Given the multiple stressors that these impoverished families experience (e.g., financial problems, housing difficulties, mental health disorders, and high neighborhood crime), their young children are at great risk for suffering the effects of these conditions and for having childhood experiences with a very negative impact.

One feature of our clinical work in infant-parent psychotherapy at San Francisco General Hospital is that we often conduct treatment through home visits. Many families with whom we work have few resources; they not only lack emotional resources but also often have no way to come in for an office visit. Sometimes families do not see why they should come to an office, or once there, they may not feel welcome or comfortable. So we reach out to them and try to enter their lives through the experience of their motherhood or fatherhood. We also try to gain an understanding of the experience of the child living within such a family.

About 70% of the families we treat are headed by a single mother. Unfortunately, that does not necessarily mean that in the remaining 30% a father is present, in the usual sense of the word. The father may be part of the family only periodically or erratically.

The figure of the father is extraordinarily important in the life of a child, whether he is physically present or not. In fact, on many occasions, his absence can be as powerful as his presence. Or, he is present in the life of the child by the fact of his absence. Despite the importance of this relationship, it is the mother-infant relationship that has been the focus of attachment theory and attachment problems. This same tendency is encountered in our own work and our thinking about families, even when we try to correct the imbalance by focusing also on the importance of the father, whether present or absent physically in the life of the child.

In any case, it is remarkable that the mother-infant relationship has long been recognized as pivotal in shaping personality development. Many statements could be offered in support of this view, such as the one by Donald Winnicott, who said that "there is no such thing as a baby" (Winnicott 1958, p. 99). Winnicott meant that babies do not exist outside the mothering they receive—that a baby can really be understood only within the context of the mother-child relationship. Sigmund Freud also captured this insight in his impassioned statement that the mother-child relationship is "unique, without parallel, laid down unalterably for a whole lifetime and the first and . . . the strongest love object . . . the prototype of all later love relations—for both sexes" (Freud 1940/1964, p. 188).

It is, therefore, not surprising that the mother-infant relationship has long been considered the primary influence in the promotion of mental health or, alternatively, in the genesis of psychopathology in the young child (Boris and Zeanah 1999). The role of the father as an equal contributor, as a mediator, or as a corrective presence in the attachment relationship and in working models of relationships for the child is just now being acknowledged. This awareness is long overdue.

The quality of the earliest relationships can be said to lay down a model or template for future relationships in the emotional life of first the child and later the adult. The Adult Attachment Interview (Main et al. 1985), for instance, attempts to investigate the vestiges of the earliest relationships and trace their outcome in the present life of the adult: What are the working models of adult relationships? How sensitive can a person— mother or father—be, particularly regarding children's emotions and behaviors? Does the adult have an internal *secure base* that allows for exploration of the world and integration of memories from childhood, as well as integration of early feelings and experiences?

Indeed, early life occurrences, whether involving continuity of contact with caregivers or disruptions and losses, have a powerful impact on the internal world of the child (who eventually may also become a parent). Early attachment experiences influence the child's capacity to establish a secure, dependent relationship with the parent.

ATTACHMENT DISTURBANCES

In the context of these powerful and primary relationships, disorders of attachment can be defined as deviations from the optimal pattern of relationships between a child under 3 years of age and his or her mother or caregiving figure (Lieberman and Zeanah 1995). Negative experiences during this period of life may lead to a distortion of the emotional components of the mother-infant relationship, which may contribute to the infant's feelings of insecurity, dissatisfaction, avoidance of intimacy, dependency, and emotional closeness not only toward the parent but also in future relationships with other people, particularly intimate relationships.

Attachment disruptions may lead the child to disavow feelings and their importance as though the child has "closed the door" to the perception of feelings, emotional states, and feared emotional intimacy and dependency on others. Disturbances in the attachment relationship may lead, for instance, to a premature sense of pseudo-independence, pseudo-autonomy, and the feeling of being completely alone in the world. It is as though the child does not feel the need for anyone in the sense of depending emotionally on others.

The definition of disorders of attachment discussed in the previous paragraph seems straightforward enough, but it conceals several sources of possible controversy. For example: How does one define a mother figure? How are different attachments organized in the child's mind, and is there a hierarchy of attachment figures with one figure clearly preferred? Can fathers or surrogate caregivers qualify as attachment figures on a par with mothers? Our position is that they certainly can.

Attachment patterns are influenced by individual differences and by cultural patterns and mores. The unique characteristics of each child and each parent or caregiver may color the quality of the relationship and the enduring attachment. A child with a difficult temperament may affect the parent's perceptions and emotional reactions, whereas a very rhythmic and easy baby may be able to give more emotional rewards to the parent, perhaps in turn facilitating sensitivity to the child's needs.

Social mores and customs, which exert a powerful influence on child rearing and caregiving values, have an impact on our understanding of normality. Culture helps determine the ideal features of the child, how much dependency to tolerate (or encourage) in the infant, and how to respond to the baby's signals of distress. Culture also helps determine matters such as whether the mother and child will have experiences of separation, whether someone else will take care of the baby in addition to the parents,[1] and whether the child should soothe himself or herself or expect the parent to provide continuous soothing.

In a multicultural society such as the United States, these questions are critical. For instance, we are constantly grappling with the question of when a particular child-rearing pattern we see in family after family is adaptive within the cultural mores and social values of a minority culture. Another central—but not easily answered—question is what to do when the parenting style is a maladaptive but understandable response to family circumstances that should not be there in the first place (e.g., poverty, community violence, neighborhood dangerousness, overcrowding). One might ask whether a child-rearing style that prepares children to deal with the possibility or even likelihood of community violence or economic deprivation should aim to toughen them up or make them more insensitive so that they can better cope with the realities of that world.

In addition to cultural and subcultural factors determining variations in the patterns of child rearing and relating, physical or organic factors may also affect the infant. These factors may have an impact on the quality of the child's relationships and, therefore, on his or her mental health, for example, when a child has a life-threatening disease or a physical malformation. In the former situation, the parents' fear of losing their baby could make them constantly fearful, causing them to try to protect their child from experiencing frustration. They may even overprotect the infant from experiencing any anxiety at all.

Another question is whether any disorder in infancy might have an impact on the quality of the child's attachment to primary caregivers and,

---

[1]See Chapter 9, this volume, by Alice Eberhart-Wright, for discussion of the effects of multiple caregivers.

therefore, be considered a disruption in attachment in one way or another. For example, is an infant who is anxious or depressed also suffering at the same time from an attachment disruption or even a disorder? How can one disentangle the problems of anxiety or depression in the infant from the quality and nature of the relationship between the child and parents? Conversely, could a problem in the relationship with the primary caregiver play a causal role in determining depression and anxiety? Or, to put it differently, can we diagnose pathology in an infant without assessing the quality of the child's primary relationship?

I do not attempt to answer all these questions in this chapter. They can be thought of as a framework for further examining and discussing the nature of attachments and their relationship to emotional and behavioral disturbances in the infant. Instead, I focus on situations in which the primary difficulty is precisely one with attachments and relationships between parents and infants.

CLASSIFICATION

The appearance of the *Diagnostic Classification of Mental Health and Developmental Disorders of Infancy and Early Childhood* (Zero to Three 1994) was a great step forward in thinking about different mental health disturbances, disorders, and diagnoses in infancy. Chaired by Stanley Greenspan and including clinicians from several disciplines with different areas of expertise, the task force had to devise the classification. The classification, therefore, is the result of expert consensus and not primarily the result of empirical studies. The task force worked for about 5 years to produce the first version, and revisions are envisioned as new knowledge accumulates. Although the classification is a very bold step forward, we still have a lot to learn.

This classification system attempts to describe and order a number of emotional and behavioral difficulties exhibited by infants. One chapter is devoted to attachment disorders. The construct of attachment disorder is useful in identifying the emotional disorder that results when a child is not given the opportunity to attach because of the lack of a potential attachment figure. Essentially, in this framework, an attachment disorder is conceptualized as a constellation or pattern that the child develops in order to cope with the absence of a stable, persistent, and sensitive mother or father figure.

The most widely used current diagnostic categories of attachment disorder are those described in DSM-IV-TR (American Psychiatric Association 2000) and ICD-10 (World Health Organization 1992), which refer to these problems as reactive attachment disorders. This is also the term used in the Zero to Three diagnostic manual: The main criterion for the diagnosis is a severe and pervasive disturbance of social relatedness in the child vis-à-vis the primary caregivers. According to these three manuals, attachment disorders are manifested in two main patterns, each having a different causal mechanism: withdrawal and indiscriminate sociability.

In the first pattern, the baby withdraws from social interaction. The disturbance is thought to stem from neglect of the child's need for human contact, failure to attend to his or her other emotional needs, and gross general deprivation. The child, without contingent responses from another person, gives up and withdraws. This withdrawal is accompanied by hypervigilance, including a suspicious attitude toward people in general, and it may lead to delays in those functions that require significant social input in order to develop (e.g., language, emotional control, reciprocity).

The second pattern, indiscriminate sociability, looks quite different. In this subtype, the child does not seem to differentiate between adults and seeks proximity and physical contact with anyone who is momentarily available. It is chilling to see children who show this pattern. For example, they may approach a strange adult who comes into the room as if that person were a cherished love object, but when the person leaves, these children show no reaction. They are ready to go on to the next stranger who comes in, and they show no noticeable change in affect from person to person (Albus and Dozier 1999). Such infants often do not show any difference in affective reactions toward people they know or do not know. This pattern is thought to result from exposure to multiple caregivers and losses of caregivers. One person is lost and another is substituted, and this pattern repeats itself. Eventually, children in this situation develop psychological defenses to cope with such disruptions; the defenses involve suppressing anxiety and fear and acting as if people were interchangeable.

Despite the reality of the existence of these two very severe patterns in infants and young children who have endured a major interruption of contact with attachment figures, the descriptions of these patterns do not encompass other situations. For example, they do not address the problem of an existing and ongoing relationship (e.g., a current attachment) that is strongly pathological in nature. We should try to understand further the effects of this kind of attachment on the evolving structure of the child's personality.

In connection with attachment issues, it is necessary to mention that the Zero to Three diagnostic classification manual has one unique feature. It not only incorporates the traditional definition of a disorder in the child in Axis I, which denotes the precise disorder in the child as an individual (e.g., depression, traumatic stress syndrome, anxiety), but it also goes further. It has a second axis that addresses the quality of the relationship between the infant and the primary caregivers. Thus, one can look simultaneously at the disorder and at any relationships in which the infant is embedded. The clinician then assesses the degree of harmony or, alternatively, pathology in each relationship. This diagnostic process is a step forward, compared with other classification systems. Nevertheless, following Winnicott's thinking, one could go as far as saying that there is no such thing as a mental health disorder of infancy without a subsequent attachment disruption, disturbance, or disorder. This interrelatedness occurs because the infant's problems always emerge within, depend on, and have an impact on a social context.

From this perspective, our team, together with Charles Zeanah Jr., is attempting to develop and test the validity of the construction of additional specific disorders of attachment (Lieberman and Zeanah 1995; Zeanah et al. 1993). We have proposed three major categories or groups of attachment disturbance: 1) lack of attachment, 2) disordered attachment, and 3) disrupted attachment.

In the first category, lack of attachment, the infant does not demonstrate normal attachment, that is, a reliable preference for an adult caregiver. The child does not even have an attachment figure. In this sense, this category is the same as a reactive attachment disorder described in DSM-IV-R and the Zero to Three classification.

We have, however, added two other categories. The second one, disordered attachment, indicates that attachments exist but have a pathological nature. They lack the predominant feelings of closeness, intimacy, pleasure, and synchronicity between parent and child that characterize healthy attachments. Disordered attachments are characterized by pervasive conflicts resulting from feelings of anger, fear, and anxiety in the relationship with the parent or primary caregiver. These emotions are not necessarily expressed directly; they may be masked by defenses such as avoidance, transformation of affect, fighting, inhibitions, and the development of a precocious sense of competence or reliance on oneself.

It is necessary to remember the work of Selma Fraiberg, who in 1981 described the early psychological defenses of infancy (Fraiberg 1987). Before her work, traditional psychoanalytic wisdom held that psychological defenses could not develop before the development of the ego and that the ego did not develop until the third or fourth year of life. Before then, everything in the psychic apparatus was pre-ego. Fraiberg had the audacity to cut through that stodgy theoretical structure. She had the courage to write about her observations in the clinical situation: namely, there are defenses even in the first year of life.[2]

In the third category, disrupted attachment disorder, the child experiences grief, bereavement, and mourning in relation to the loss of the attachment figure. We find that the loss of a primary attachment figure is inherently pathogenic because very young children do not yet have either the personality structure or the cognitive and emotional resources to cope adaptively with such loss. Even when the child is eventually able to transfer the attachment bond to a new caregiver, fear of abandonment, anxiety reactions, depression, and other forms of vulnerability to loss are likely to persist and to color the child's new attachment relationships.

To elaborate, I draw on our experience in infant-parent psychotherapy in San Francisco General Hospital. Part of this work involves consulting with child protective services on very difficult and dramatic situations. We have often encountered staff of child protective agencies, and even mental health clinicians, who believe that a given child will quickly and easily reattach to another, formerly unknown person after the loss of an attachment figure. This presumption suggests a certain interchangeability between people.

In contrast, our impression is that the new attachment is influenced by a fear that another loss will occur. Children learn from experience: if they go through one loss, they will anticipate another. Our working model of attachments does not embrace the theory that such children will be able to turn off their feelings as they would a water faucet or piece of machinery, and then when they are placed elsewhere turn the system back on again without any consequences or sequelae. Indeed, it is extraordinary to observe situations in which children are placed with little forethought in foster care with different families, one after the other, with the personnel making these decisions totally confident that the children already are or will become resilient enough to reattach again and again.

We often encounter situations in which an infant is referred for an evaluation after experiencing the threat of violence or actual aggression from an attachment figure against the child or against another attachment figure (Lieberman and Van Horn 1998). As a consequence, and in addition to these painful experiences, the child may have undergone several placements. Our view is that there is little empirical validity for the theory of easy reattachment after object loss. Although this perspective does not imply

---

[2]From a theoretical point of view, it would be interesting to speculate on what would happen to the theory of ego formation if one had to take into account the existence of defensive operations this early in life, but such is not the main focus here.

that the child can never reestablish a trusting relationship, it emphasizes the importance of realizing the seriousness and devastating effects of disruptions in attachment relationships. These experiences should be viewed as traumatic and taken very seriously. The baby and the toddler are both particularly vulnerable to such losses and their effects. When children cannot explain their experiences or feelings verbally, it is often assumed that such reactions and feelings do not exist. However, it is precisely the inability to communicate and symbolize unmanageable emotions that contributes to their long-term destructive effects on development.

Disorders of attachment in infancy have three main sources: 1) constitutional vulnerabilities in the infant, 2) emotional liabilities in the parents, and 3) "poorness of fit" (Thomas and Chess 1977) between infant and parent. Constitutional vulnerabilities may be inherent in given infants, either because they have a diagnosable disorder, such as those that Greenspan and Wieder (1993) called regulatory disorders, or because, although without a diagnosable disorder, they are temperamentally difficult. Vulnerabilities may include irregular patterns of eating and sleeping, resistance to being cuddled, and a low threshold of reactivity that prompts the baby to overreact to even moderate stimulation and then to become fussy and difficult to console. Such vulnerabilities may overwhelm the parents' caregiving resources and may contribute to failure in the infant's relationship with the primary caregiver.

It is important to realize that constitutional vulnerabilities do not necessarily evolve into attachment disorders. They need a contribution from the caregiving environment. However, these vulnerabilities make infants very challenging to care for, so parents may misunderstand the meaning of a child's responses (e.g., crying, arching back, resisting being cuddled or touched, waking up multiple times during the night) and then respond in a way that the infant perceives as overwhelming or even painful. In turn, the child's response is further compromised and becomes maladaptive, reinforcing a cycle of mutual alienation and anger that can eventually become a disorder of attachment.

The second source of attachment disorders is parental emotional liabilities that interfere with caregiving. These challenges may have their origin in emotional disturbances such as depression. Several mental disorders, including severe depression, bipolar disorder, severe personality disorders, and posttraumatic stress disorder, may correlate with additional psychosocial stressors. These liabilities are frequently associated with problems such as family disruption, socioeconomic problems, difficulties in adult relationships, or a combination of all these elements.

Such risk factors predispose parents to misperceive or misreact to a child's behavior: The adult may attribute to the infant certain capacities, abilities, intentions, and motivations that are inaccurate or developmentally inappropriate. In clinical work, we often hear mothers describe their 1-year-olds as deliberately pursuing a course of action to antagonize them: "He knows precisely what he's doing and he won't stop himself. . . . He just wants to do it to get my goat." This misperception is clearly a worrisome attribution of defiance or "badness" to the baby, which may become part of the core of how the baby starts thinking about himself or herself.

The third source of disorders of attachment is the extremely useful term "poorness of fit," coined by Alexander Thomas and Stella Chess (1977). It refers, among other things, to a poor synchrony between the parents' style and who the baby is constitutionally. For example, a baby may be slow to respond, muted in his or her signals, and passive, whereas the mother moves fast, wants life to be exciting, and is always in a hurry. As a result of this poorness of fit, the mother feels totally bored by her baby.

Despite this mismatch or dysynchrony, parents who are flexible and adaptable can compensate for the poorness of fit by, for instance, modifying their expectations or caregiving practices to "fit" the situation better. The parent may also enlist the help of other caregivers to alleviate the situation. For example, a mother with whom we recently worked could not stand how slowly her baby took the bottle. Fortunately, the baby's father was like the child. The father loved to hold the baby and just gaze into space or gaze into the baby's face. He enjoyed feeding the baby, and the two of them would spend hours together. The father feeding the baby was a very nice way for the father to cope with something that the mother could not do well, and it conserved her patience for times when the child needed her in other ways and in activities that could not be delegated to the father because he was not there.

In situations with less adaptability or when the baby's constitutional vulnerabilities are more severe, the situation may become extremely difficult for both the caregiver and baby to tolerate. When there are additional difficulties such as the emotional problems and socioeconomic stressors mentioned previously, modifications and adjustments become even less likely. In the most problematic situations, even the therapist may struggle. If it seems that every intervention the therapist attempts to improve the parent-child relationship works against that goal, the therapist will need to muster as much patience as possible to stay with the program without acting out and giving up.

TREATMENT STRATEGIES

I will now review the question of treatment, in particular the method of infant-parent psychotherapy that I have found to be most useful and effective. This method is an intervention developed by Selma Fraiberg before she moved it to the infant-parent program at the University of California, San Francisco.

There is a strong and understandable tendency to associate infant-parent psychotherapy with Selma Fraiberg's work described in the article "Ghosts in the Nursery" (Fraiberg et al. 1975). Fraiberg coined this phrase more than two decades ago to refer to the child's engulfment by the unconscious expectations and attributions of the parents or caregivers. The phrase refers to being caught in the parents' unresolved psychological conflicts. Fraiberg also used this term as shorthand for the transgenerational transmission of attachment patterns or disorders, as well as mental health problems.

The powerful image of ghosts in the nursery captured the imagination of many clinicians, almost to the point of the concrete. Some time ago, I was approached by an experienced and wonderful neonatologist, who asked me, "These ghosts in the nursery, do they really exist?" The question illustrates how tangible those ghosts have become in the minds of many people. In trying to describe how to treat disorders of attachment, it is paramount to address the issue of whether the ghosts really exist.

The ghosts are a way of referring to the baby's role in the family that, among many other things, is the unconscious representative of attachment figures from the parents' own past. When the baby acquires this meaning for a parent, the infant stands not only for who he or she is, but also for somebody else who is often unnamed. The baby may thus become the target of a negative transference through which the parent repeats unacknowledged and unexorcised pain, anger, and disappointment experienced in earlier relationships.

In other words, the parents' internal representation of the infant and their experience of the baby's behavior become distorted by their own past experience—by what they bring to the parenting situation. For example, a baby's cry is not perceived as a call for help but rather as an angry accusation that the parent is doing nothing right and deserves strong criticism for ineptness. In this way, a baby is not just a baby. Instead, the baby is also perceived as a tyrant who probably existed somewhere in the parents' past and is being revisited through the baby.

When parents actually feel this way, they are unlikely to attend wholeheartedly to a distressed baby no matter how much others (e.g., therapists) try to persuade them to do so. The parents are likely to either ignore the baby or respond out of guilt feelings, a sense of duty, or a desire to please the people who are urging the parents to take this course of action. But none of these alternatives is likely to work in the long run, or even in the short run, because the unconscious parental conflicts about the baby will always find another avenue of expression when the first way of expressing those negative feelings is blocked.

Infant-parent psychotherapy was developed as an attempt to correct, soften, or modify parental misperceptions and to increase empathy and continuous pleasure in the relationship between baby and one or more caregivers. The most readily recognized aspect of infant-parent psychotherapy is the process of helping parents understand their own overly intense and pervasive ambivalence toward, or actual rejection of, the child that may lead to abuse or neglect of the baby in light of the parents' own negative experience. It should be stressed (see Chapter 3, this volume) that these painful childhood experiences are often repressed and not readily accessible to the conscious mind of the parent. Alternatively, they may be denied or not remembered at all because nothing of childhood is remembered. Another possibility is that the adult may remember the actual experiences and can recall them intellectually or cognitively but may be unable to process them affectively; in other words, there is dissociation from the corresponding feelings. As Bleiberg notes in Chapter 2 of this book, parents may remember, but they do not feel what they remember.

This particular component of infant-parent psychotherapy, the effort to connect the present with the past and to search for the linkages between how early experiences affect current experiences, has led to the perception of therapists as "ghostbusters." In trying to free the baby from the haunting parental past, infant-parent psychotherapy ultimately seeks to help parents come to terms with their own childhood rather than acting it out through the child.

In classical infant-parent psychotherapy and in our work today, the baby is usually present during the sessions. In other words, we do not ask the parents to talk about their past in the absence of the baby. The baby's presence is very powerful in helping to understand and capture the parental conflicts in all their emotional intensity and immediacy. This immediacy is often more vivid when the therapy is conducted in the family home. The therapeutic process unfolds in the natural environment of the baby's own space. The therapist attempts to create a favorable environment for evoking those images, memories, and feelings. At the same time, current interactions between parent and infant continue to unfold. We are really seeing what takes place in those relationships and how they usually tend to happen even when we are not there.

It must be said that this kind of work can also be done successfully in the office, but the home adds a level of immediacy that is quite valuable in itself. In essence, the therapeutic work encourages the parents to speak about themselves and their baby in their own way—that is, in their own free associative way—except that in this circumstance, free associa-tion consists not only of words but also of actions. This is because while the parents are talking to us, they are also relating to the baby.

As the parents speak, we look at their behavior and what they are do-ing with the baby. At the same time, the baby's response to their actions constitutes itself into a parallel form of communication. Indeed, there are really two levels of interaction occurring: the level of behavior and the level of verbalization. The therapist tries to understand the extent to which whatever the parents say about themselves, the baby, and the baby's earlier life is echoed by their behavior toward the child. Some-times there is quite a contrast between what a parent is saying and what a parent is doing. Clinicians who observe this contrast will try to under-stand it, perhaps as a conflict within the parent between different percep-tions, wishes, and emotions.

For example, young parents may talk about how incredibly rejecting they feel toward their baby, how fed up they are with being parents, or even how they sometimes would like to kill their baby. Nevertheless, their behavior toward their child seems to be unfailingly empathic. One is left with the puzzle of what all this means. Are the parents unaware of how good their parenting really is on an overt, behavioral level? Are they let-ting us know that this empathy is only part of the picture and that they are unconsciously asking the therapist to not be deceived by it? Perhaps the parents are asking the therapist to pay attention to what they are say-ing and hoping it is taken seriously.

At times, what a parent is saying may be so unsettling that the therapist takes refuge in what the parent is doing. A therapy supervisee recently said, "Oh, that's not really true, she [the baby's mother] really is wonder-ful toward the baby." The therapist feels pulled to try to reassure the par-ents. However, if the reassurance is given prematurely, the parent may feel unheard or misunderstood.

The therapist has a responsibility to be there—with the parents and the infant—in both forms of communication (with words and with ac-tion). In this sense, the infant-parent psychotherapist definitely needs Theodore Reik's (1948) proverbial third ear, a hovering attention by the therapist used to capture and sense unspoken themes in the patient's narrative. Moreover, one could say that the therapist also needs a "fourth ear" to capture the baby's experience and ascertain how it may or may not fit with the parent's ongoing narrative and behavior.

In other words, the baby gives us the whole picture—either consistent with or totally different from that offered by the parent—of how things are at home. Thus, the therapist should pay as much attention to the baby as to the parent's words and actions. At times, the enormous difficulty posed by the task of having to divide attention between a very needy parent and a very needy baby is in itself an important clue to existing problems. The therapist, as an emotionally involved participant, is able to feel this tension or conflict between the needs of each member of the dyad or triad.

To illustrate the technique and themes used in the therapeutic process, I refer to an example and quote from a session. To highlight the points I have mentioned, the quotations are taken from a session in which the baby has not yet been born, thus allowing full concentration on the internal world of the parents. Even so, the baby is present in a certain way, not yet there to make peremptory demands, but there in the fantasy and reverie of the parents-to-be.

Case Study

Shawn and Eva were a couple recovering from a criminal lifestyle and chronic drug addiction. They were also struggling with anger toward their unborn baby because she was in a breech position and might require a cesarean section instead of a normal delivery. At the time of the consultation, the due date was about 3 weeks away. So there was a certain urgency to the situation.

Shawn, the father-to-be, was seen in the following terms (to make the description more vivid, I quote verbatim from therapy notes):

> Shawn continued to talk with great gusto about his life—mixing bravado with anguish—as he gave me one chilling example after another of the violence and the constant fear of being killed. These young people had been gang members earlier in their lives. Upon hearing this narration for a while and given that the baby's delivery was almost imminent, I felt it was time to make a link to the baby. I commented that the past seemed to be coming back with great force. I said that having a baby often did that: "It forces people to remember their past because they need to prepare for the future." Shawn replied that he had been thinking a great deal about becoming a father, and he added that there was some news that made him think even harder. When I asked what the news was, he said that the future baby had had her "medical checkup."
>
> Eva, who was also present, had been told that the baby was in a breech position and that a C-section might be needed unless the baby turned around. Shawn said, "I keep telling that little asshole to get his ass in gear or I'll kick the shit out of him." I said, "Likely, with that kind of warning, the kid would be too scared to move, I would imagine." They laughed and then Eva said, rather too sweetly perhaps (I emphasize here because Eva harbors a lot of anger that she is not letting herself show me): "I tell the baby it's either this C-section or his bicycle, that we don't have the money for both."

In spite of the laughter and Eva's attempt at minimization, it was clear that this was a serious topic, i.e., their frustration and anger toward the current situation. One could easily speculate that these parents might become violent toward their child. There was plenty in their history that they had already told me to indicate they were capable of a great deal of cruelty. Although it was not yet an immediate reality, it was an important topic to pursue, partly because it reflected the parents' distorted perception of the unborn baby as willfully inflicting pain on them.

The parents' intense attributions and comments about their life history led me to seek a door (opened by the couple) for preventive intervention before violence actually occurred. A central goal of our program is to practice prevention, which often works much better than treatment. I, therefore, asked them what they thought about physical punishment. Both of them said something like: "Of course, it is the natural way of teaching a child how to behave. How else are you going to teach them?" I said, "I don't see it that way," and asked them whether they themselves had been physically punished when they were growing up. As I expected, they both said, "Yeah, of course, we've been." I asked them how they felt at the time. Giving me a triumphant grin, Eva said, "I don't remember. See, I forget, I don't even remember. It's not any big deal; don't make such a big deal out of it." Shawn said more or less the same thing. This parental response was the equivalent of my being told, "You are just hopelessly naïve."

This conversation was unsettling, but I managed to say, "You know, I'm not surprised that you don't remember. I kind of thought that you wouldn't remember. I think that the reason children don't remember what they felt when they were hit is because they feel so much anger and fear that they try to forget those feelings as soon as they can." There was a long silence, then Shawn turned to Eva and said, "Maybe that's why I feel the way I feel toward my parents, hon." I asked, "What is that, Shawn? I don't know how you feel about your parents." He then told me that both of his parents were alcoholics and had treated him brutally. He remembered, in particular, an episode when he was 5 or 6 years old when he had broken a window while throwing dirt clods with a friend. Shawn's father had hit him with a tree branch until Shawn's legs were bloody. Describing this scene, Shawn said, "At first I cried, but then the pain turned into hatred and I stopped crying. I did not want to show any feelings. My father kept hitting me harder and harder and screaming at me, 'Cry, for God's sake! Cry!' But I refused to cry. That is the last time I remember crying in front of anybody. I stopped and I never did it again. From then on, I only felt rage. He didn't even let me explain . . . that bastard!"

Shawn remained silent for a while, his eyes reddened. Trying to compose himself, he then said, "I don't understand why I was so scared at first and then I could only feel anger." I said, "Maybe it was easier to be angry than scared. . . . You were so frightened and there was nobody there to help you feel less scared. You had to help yourself and maybe you used your rage to protect yourself from your fear." Shawn's eyes filled with tears and then this huge, heavily bearded, and profusely tattooed man sobbed like a child for a few minutes. He said in a chilled voice, "And I've been carrying that rage inside me ever since. I never could do anything else with it." After he regained some composure, Shawn looked at Eva and shyly asked her how he had started talking about his childhood.

To her credit, Eva remembered and said that they had been talking about spanking the baby so that it would get in the right position and Eva would not then need a C-section. Again, there was a silence and I said to Shawn, "Now I can understand better how you feel about Eva having a C-section. You have been hurt so much, and now it's hard to think that the woman you love can be hurt like that and there is no way you can protect her. Thinking of Eva's pain made you so scared that, once again, it's easier to feel the rage." Shawn's eyes again filled with tears, and he sobbed for a few minutes. He then put his foot on Eva's chair and Eva rubbed his foot gently. Eva then said, "We will not let it happen, honey. This baby is still going to turn around." They talked quietly to each other for a few minutes lightly, trying to reassure each other.

I suggested, "I think you are trying very hard to find new ways of raising your child to get over your own childhood and the way you were raised, to raise a child that will not have the same memories that you have and that are so hard on you." Shawn sighed and said, "Yeah, that's exactly true. And, boy, is it hard."

In the next sessions, we continued talking about how hard the situation was. The subsequent progress was interesting because a session like the one I just described gives the therapist a feeling of "Ah! We're on safe ground now." There has been an insight and a linking of the past and the present, so there is an anticipation that the parents will do better from now on. But it's not that simple. The parents' defenses keep coming back. The defenses have been there all their lives, and they do not disappear magically following one successful interpretation. In the next sessions, the anger that was directed at the baby was now turned on the doctors.

Shawn began talking about how he was going to beat up the doctors if they started doing things he disapproved of. He said he was going to be in the delivery room, and if they gave him any grief or if they did not stand to attention when he told them what he wanted, he was just going to "grab their heads." He said that he had spent his life "grabbing people's heads," and it wasn't going to be hard to do it again if he needed to protect his wife. I suggested, "Would you let me be an intermediary between you and the doctors?" They said, "Sure." After the session was over, I went over (across the hall) to the obstetrics and gynecological clinic and, without betraying confidentiality, talked to the doctors about the family. I talked about the concerns that the couple had and also about their impulse control. Doctors in a hospital like ours are very used to understanding such hints. They see the results of violence every day, so one doesn't need to go into great detail to convey a message. There is a saying in Spanish: *Al buen entendedor pocas palabras le bastan.* It means: "To the one who understands well, a few words are enough. You don't need to elaborate and elaborate."

The doctors and I designed a plan to prevent the delivery situation from getting to the point where they and the father would get into a power struggle. Fortunately, after we made the plan, the baby turned around and the delivery went well. The therapeutic work continued, and the child is now in primary school and her mother is doing well. The daughter has never been hit or abused. The work really did what it was supposed to do.

Discussion

This therapy case has three main components of infant-parent psychotherapy:

1. Linking the past with the present to increase the parents' awareness of their own conflicts.
2. Applying didactic developmental guidance to talk about the needs of babies in a way that respects the individuality and uniqueness of each child. Conversely, it means not talking according to a preestablished schedule about what the baby "should" be doing week by week but, instead, talking about what is happening in the relationship between parent and baby in the presence of the therapist.
3. Not hesitating to take action in the real world to change potentially destructive situations; in this case, it was the work with the doctors in the sessions that followed the initial consultation.

One of the most interesting or exciting aspects of infant-parent psychotherapy is that insight can be used effectively with parents who are not the typical candidates for psychoanalytically oriented psychotherapy. Both Shawn and Eva suffered from pervasive and serious characterological disorders, yet they were able, again and again, to use insight to learn more about themselves and to become good-enough parents of their child.

As this case illustrates, the effort to banish psychic ghosts is clinically and intellectually compelling, but often it is not enough to just offer interpretations of the ghosts from the past. It is particularly true in the context of poor or deprived social and economic conditions such as those that affect large segments of the population today, and likely to increase in the current political climate.

To put it another way, today's ghosts often have no nursery to haunt. They are reduced to invading the grand corridors of residential hotels or overcrowded apartments. They are lucky if they have a nursery. Large numbers of parents increasingly carry not only the burden of their past but also the day-to-day humiliations of powerlessness and loss of dignity in the face of deteriorating socioeconomic conditions and vanishing supports. Racial and cultural minorities are particularly affected, and babies raised in these circumstances become ready scapegoats for their parents because their developmentally appropriate needs and demands compound the already unbearable internal and external stresses experienced by the parents.

This is the point where the other therapeutic modalities used in infant-parent psychotherapy become relevant. We can no longer afford to conceptualize treatment or parenting independently of the sociocultural and economic context in which it takes place. As the Spanish sociologist José Ortega y Gasset (1957/1994) wrote memorably, "*Yo soy yo y mi circunstancia*" ("I am myself and my circumstances"). In Ortega y Gasset's thinking, an individual's quality of functioning, sense of self, and possibilities for achievement and fulfillment—indeed, the person's very morality—are intricately shaped and inseparably linked, moment by moment and day by day, to the political, socioeconomic, cultural, and family conditions in which he or she lives. Ortega y Gasset not only anticipated Winnicott's (1958) famous statement that "there is no such thing as a baby" (p. 99), but he also applied this principle more broadly and, I believe, more accurately. He was, in essence, saying, "There is no such thing as an individual." Some may consider this viewpoint too radical, but the notion of the person in the context of his or her circumstances remains a powerful reminder of social belongingness and its influence on personality development and daily functioning.

In infant-parent psychotherapy, these considerations influence how we think of a family's predicament as we assess what is clinically needed. Even the process of arriving at an accurate diagnosis of the parent's psychopathology is strongly influenced by the socioeconomic context. For example, when parents have a steady income, live in a safe neighborhood, and have ready access to appropriate medical care and adequate schooling—and are not culturally marginalized—then we feel that the diagnosis is probably accurate and even useful. But what about a young mother who lives in very traumatic conditions? How do we know whether she's suffering from posttraumatic stress syndrome as a result of repeated experiences of violence, or whether she has a borderline personality disorder, perhaps with early trauma as a significant etiological factor? Does the father suffer from organic brain syndrome, or is he exhibiting transitory symptoms of drug abuse or withdrawal? In another case, does the parent have a schizoid personality organization, or are we simply seeing a complex transference reaction of avoidance and withdrawal from us, his mental health workers, based on the parent's previous negative experiences with the helping professions or the child protective system?

These are extremely important but difficult questions. How we answer them will affect our assessment and the prognosis for infant-parent psychotherapy. Despite these problems, a diagnosis that is as accurate as possible is essential to making informed clinical decisions, particularly in relation to issues of focus and timing.

For example, mothers with serious narcissistic disorders are often unable to tolerate the therapist's attention to their baby. If one arrives at the conclusion that a mother suffers from this condition, then it would be necessary to be very tactful and incredibly benign. Any attention paid to the baby could be experienced as abandonment, rejection, or criticism of the mother's parenting.

In this context, the appropriate therapeutic response might be to focus on the mother, even though we might feel we are abandoning the baby, and provide her with all the attention, support, and unconditional acceptance she needs. This therapeutic stance might well continue for many months and make us feel very anxious or even feel that we are not doing anything for the baby. The important thing to remember is that we cannot forget the infant; we need to keep looking at the baby and keep trying to understand the relationship between the mother and her child. When we really forget the baby, he or she is abandoned. But if we keep the baby in mind and listen to the mother with the baby in mind, we are not colluding with the mother. For these mothers, improvement in their psychological functioning and in their relationship with their baby may come not from an exploration of conflict, not from the elegant psychological linking of past and present, but, instead, primarily from changes in their sense of self as a result of the therapist's initial and continuing empathic availability.

Parents who are depressed, who have concrete thinking styles and impoverished egos, or who are not particularly intelligent may need expressions of sympathy and support conveyed through actions rather than words. I want to emphasize that this need pertains not only to parents who are not particularly intelligent, although they are the easiest ones to identify, but also to parents who are totally bombarded by sociocultural misery and who do not, with good reason, trust words. They may really need concrete assistance—for example, driving them to an appointment, helping them fill out forms, accompanying them to grocery shopping, helping them handle laundry, or interceding on their behalf during bureaucratic tangles with "the system." For them, such practical interventions make the therapist's abstract offer of help more real.

Parents with severely impoverished egos, or who are very needy and in poor circumstances, often do not perceive themselves as people who could be likable or deserving of care and attention. Discovering that the therapist thinks highly enough of them to make an effort on their behalf can become the first step in making them realize that relationships can be helpful and rewarding rather than abusive, disappointing, or burdensome. This realization, in turn, is an important condition in enabling parents to become more positively invested in their own babies.

As therapists, we may find ourselves unwilling or unable to provide such concrete assistance. We may not have the time, the energy, or the possibility of spending 2 hours with this patient because we need to see another patient. All kinds of circumstances intervene and therapists cannot be everything to everyone. It seems that our first duty as good-enough therapists is to become increasingly aware of what we can and cannot offer so that we do not feel guilty, overwhelmed, or stretched too thin. Nevertheless, it is still useful to know that concrete assistance is a worthy therapeutic modality that, when used well, can open the door to the possibility of substantial and lasting psychological change. I mention this possibility so that we do not disparage concrete assistance just because we don't feel up to giving it. It really is worth doing, and it can lead to many important consequences.

Each modality of treatment described by Selma Fraiberg as a component of infant-parent psychotherapy applies to treatment: insight-oriented interpretations, didactic developmental guidance, crisis intervention, emotional support, and concrete assistance with problems of living. One common ingredient of all these essential interventions is the relationship with the therapist.

To paraphrase Franz Alexander, who talked about the corrective emotional experience, there is such a thing as a corrective attachment experience. This concept conveys the irreplaceable emotional power of the therapist's supportive, accepting, and empathic attitude. The corrective attachment experience enables parents to experience the therapy from someone who will join with them to find solutions to internal and external issues and conflicts. The therapist's attitude and behavior contrast with the parents' conscious or unconscious expectations of abandonment, punishment, criticism, or ridicule, which is what they are used to and what they expect. But if the therapist consistently tries to contradict these expectations through an accepting response, a new beginning may be possible.

In the course of the therapeutic process, the parent's internal representations of self change and become more benign, allowing for a new and fresh relationship vis-à-vis the baby. In one study, we provided infant-parent psychotherapy to a group of Latino immigrant mothers and their infants from Mexico and Central America (Lieberman et al. 1991). These new immigrants, in the United States for less than 5 years, were extremely deprived in terms of their current circumstances. Many had tremendous experiences of abuse, neglect, and deprivation in childhood and throughout life. When we assessed this group of mothers and their babies, we identified the attachment pattern of the infant using the Strange Situation (Ainsworth et al. 1978) and classified the children according to these four commonly identified patterns: 1) secure attachment, 2) anxious attachment, 3) avoidant or resistant, or 4) disorganized.

Parents who were assigned at random to an intervention group received 1 year of infant-parent psychotherapy at home, in contrast to those in a control group. At the end of the year, we assessed both the parents and their babies. When the children were 2 years old, we assessed them again and found that the intervention group had statistically significant higher scores in maternal empathy, maternal responsiveness, and maternal involvement with the baby. In turn, the babies had significantly less avoidance, less anger, and less conflict with their mothers than did those in the control group. Thus, this approach is promising from a statistical standpoint. We took 1 year to do it and it worked, but these were mothers who were eager for treatment. Many times parents do not want help, so it takes a long time just to persuade them to engage in treatment. Also, some parents have tremendous characterological disorders that are much more complex than the difficulties in the groups we treated. In such a case, the length of treatment becomes of special importance for the parents.

In many of these most difficult cases, helping the parents to understand how they are influencing what the baby is experiencing does not really help them change. Even when we use every modality available in our repertoire—crisis intervention, emotional support, didactic developmental psychotherapy, linking of past and present—it takes forever to see their behavior change. Even when parents can remember horrific scenes from their own past and can retrieve and relive the concomitant emotions, the key is their retaining the memory of those emotions. It is not sufficient just to remember intellectually. Such remembrance and the associated feelings must lead to a reorganization of the sense of self in relation to attachment; just remembering and reliving the emotions will not do that. One can say that even when the ghosts come to the exorcism ceremony, they do not easily relinquish their malevolent powers and have to be re-exorcised again, and again, and again. One case will illustrate this point—that of the mother of the 2-year-old toddler, Oscar, who was referred for severe and prolonged tantrums and biting episodes:

> This mother called her son a monster, and he dutifully enacted the monster role, acting like a wild, desperate, out-of-control creature. In home

visits and at the office, the mother screamed obscenities at Oscar, cursed him, told him she would leave him, hit him in a rage, and threw things at him. Oscar's father and mother had violent fights in front of him. The father was more loving toward Oscar, but he also spanked him routinely as a form of discipline. Treatment took many forms at different times to address different configurations of Oscar's problems. Most sessions were with mother and child, but there were also entire months of individual sessions with the mother; triadic sessions with mother, father, and child; and couples work. We also fielded numerous crisis telephone calls.

In this process, it emerged that the mother had been raised by a psychotic mother who force-fed her, made her eat her vomit when she threw up, locked her in her bedroom for hours, beat her with a broom, and cursed her with long, blood-curdling curses in her native Italian dialect. Although there was eventual improvement in Oscar's family, it took 2½ years for Oscar's symptoms to abate. During this period, the mother vividly remembered what had happened to her during her childhood: her hatred of her mother and her rage and contempt toward her father for not defending her.

We eventually understood that Oscar had come to represent his grandmother, that is, the mother's mother. He (she) was a monster on the loose who could not be controlled or contained. Oscar's mother could even identify ways in which she had provoked the child to be like her mother. On occasion, she cried bitterly, with guilt and remorse. But she also tended to dismiss Oscar's need for empathy from her by saying, "I treat him much better than my mother treated me." Similarly, she and her husband often dismissed Oscar's terror at their fights by saying, "Ah, there was so much worse stuff with our parents. He can take it." It took a very long time for them to feel that a replication of their own childhood was not what they wanted for their child.

CONCLUSION

I go into some length in this description because, as a society, we are seized by the fantasy that dismal situations can be resolved quickly, cheaply, and painlessly. Those of us in the public sector are constantly pressured to cure people quickly, both to save money and to make room for the large number of other people who go untreated because there is not enough money to treat them all at the same time. Those in private practice are pressured by insurance company policies and managed care firms. Those of us with theoretical predilections are also pressured internally by the beauty of a model prediction that if we can interpret malevolent parental fantasies, then we can make them go away.

We need to fight all these pressures, both internal and external. In addition, we must fight the pressure to feel bad about ourselves when we cannot work miracles and then are told, or tell ourselves, that we must be doing something wrong and surely must be ineffective therapists.

Indeed, we must fight all these pressures, particularly when long-standing psychological clinical experience tells us that we are not dealing with simple matters but with severe, long-standing, deeply structural problems. Unless we speak up for the urgent need for adequate time, human availability, and therapeutic continuity as essential healing agents; unless we speak up to our funding sources, of whatever kind; and unless we protest actively against the push for ever-briefer services, we will be colluding in a social course that dehumanizes not only the families we serve but all of us as well.

REFERENCES

Ainsworth MDS, Blehar MC, Waters E, et al: Patterns of Attachment: A Psychological Study of the Strange Situation. Hillsdale, NJ, Erlbaum, 1978

Albus KE, Dozier M: Indiscriminate friendliness and terror of strangers in infancy: contributions from the study of infants in foster care. Infant Mental Health Journal 10:30–41, 1999

American Psychiatric Association: Diagnostic and Statistical Manual of Mental Disorders, 4th Edition, Text Revision. Washington, DC, American Psychiatric Association, 2000

Boris NW, Zeanah CH: Disturbances and disorders of attachment in infancy: an overview. Infant Mental Health Journal 20:1–9, 1999

Fraiberg S: Pathological defenses in infancy, in Selected Writings of Selma Fraiberg. Edited by Fraiberg L. Columbus, Ohio State University Press, 1987, pp 183–204

Fraiberg S, Adelson E, Shapiro V: Ghosts in the nursery: a psychoanalytic approach to the problems of impaired infant-mother relationships. Journal of the American Academy of Child Psychiatry 14:387–421, 1975

Freud S: An outline of psycho-analysis (1940), in The Standard Edition of the Complete Psychological Works of Sigmund Freud, Vol 23. Translated and edited by Strachey J. London, Hogarth Press, 1964, pp 139–207

Greenspan S, Wieder S: Regulatory disorders, in Handbook of Infant Mental Health. Edited by Zeanah CH. New York, Guilford, 1993, pp 280–290

Lieberman AF, Van Horn P: Attachment, trauma, and domestic violence: implications for child custody. Child Adolesc Psychiatr Clin N Am 7:423–443, 1998

Lieberman AF, Zeanah CH: Disorders of attachment in infancy. Child Adolesc Psychiatr Clin N Am 4:571–587, 1995

Lieberman AF, Weston DR, Pawl JH: Preventive intervention and outcome with anxiously attached dyads. Child Dev 52:199–209, 1991

Main M, Kaplan N, Cassidy J: Security in infancy, childhood and adulthood: a move to the level of representation, in Growing Points of Attachment: Theory and Research (Monographs of the Society for Research in Child Development, Vol 50). Edited by Bretherton I, Waters E. Chicago, IL, University of Chicago Press, 1985, pp 66–106

Ortega y Gasset J: El hombre y la gente (1957). México City, Editorial Porrúa, 1994

Reik T: Listening With the Third Ear: The Inner Experience of a Psychoanalyst. New York, Farrar, Straus, Giroux, 1948

Thomas A, Chess S: Temperament and Development. New York, Brunner/Mazel, 1977

Winnicott DW: Collected Papers: Through Paediatrics to Psycho-Analysis. New York, Basic Books, 1958

World Health Organization: The ICD-10 Classification of Mental and Behavioural Disorders: Clinical Descriptions and Diagnostic Guidelines. Geneva, World Health Organization, 1992

Zeanah CH, Mammen O, Lieberman A: Disorders of attachment, in Handbook of Infant Mental Health. Edited by Zeanah CH. New York, Guilford, 1993, pp 332–349

Zero to Three, National Center for Infants, Toddlers, and Families: Diagnostic Classification of Mental Health and Developmental Disorders of Infancy and Early Childhood (DC: 0-3). Arlington, VA, Zero to Three, 1994

6

Multimodal Parent-Infant Psychotherapy

J. Martín Maldonado-Durán, M.D.
Teresa Lartigue, Ph.D.

Lascia parlare il tuo cuore, interroga i volti, non ascoltare le lingue . . .

Let your heart talk, interrogate the faces, do not listen to their tongues . . .

Umberto Eco, *Il nomme della rosa [The Name of the Rose]*

In this chapter, we describe a model of therapeutic intervention with infants and families that incorporates diverse modes of understanding and various therapeutic approaches. This way of intervening seems most applicable to the needs of families with many concurrent problems. Dealing with these situations in the infant mental health clinic requires maximum flexibility, sensitivity to the unique needs of patients, and an ability to comprehend the various problems in order of importance and severity.

This model relies on a process of intervention that involves the parents and the infant as primary partners with the clinician in understanding the problem and in attempting its resolution. The therapist changes roles and techniques depending on the initial problem and how the situation evolves. The presenting problem may be simple in itself but may become complex and difficult given the family context. Or it may be only one of many problems the family faces, including other stressors and adverse social and economic circumstances (see Figure 6–1).

Parent-infant psychotherapy can be described as the interaction of the family and infant system with the system of the therapist or therapeutic team. Optimally, the transactions between these two systems are mutually

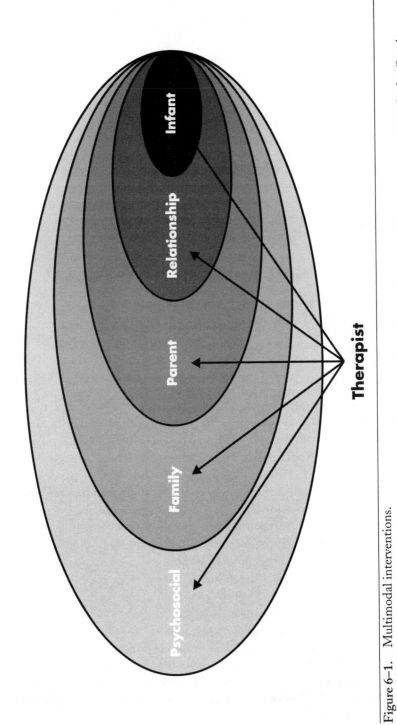

Figure 6–1.   Multimodal interventions.

The multimodal approach to therapy can help clinicians recognize and prioritize problems so that interventions can be more appropriately tailored.

informative, satisfying, and constructive and result in a positive outcome—or at least the problem situation improves. In these exchanges, the therapist is ready to modify interventions, depending on changes and shifts within the family-infant system. However, if the therapeutic interaction does not lead to a mutually adaptive response to the family's unique set of problems, therapy may prove unsuccessful.

Our therapeutic proposal demands the therapist be highly flexible and able to use a variety of techniques. Using only one method to address all problems is not likely to fit the realities of a particular family, child, or parent-child relationship. When therapists are trained to use different interventions, they can apply various strategies to specific clinical challenges, taking into account factors such as the family's motivation to change, the infant's particular problem, and realistic constraints of the situation (e.g., traveling distance to see the therapist, financial limitations). Some recommended techniques are useful when the family has limited motivation or resources for prolonged treatment or when there is a need for rapid change.

In addition, different "theoretical lenses" (e.g., family systems therapy, developmental psychopathology, behavior therapy, psychoanalysis) can be used at various moments in the therapeutic transaction to gain a better understanding of the nature of the problems. These perspectives will inform and guide the interventions. The available literature on parent-infant psychotherapy tends to emphasize a psychodynamic perspective and interventions that provide a broad framework for understanding infant mental health problems (Cramer 1995; Lebovici 1983; Lieberman 1992; Stern 1995; Stoleru and Morales-Huet 1989). This framework guides most other interventions. There is comparatively little information available on less interpretive but more immediate and practical techniques.

There is little empirical evidence for the effectiveness of psychotherapeutic interventions, including those during infancy, except for studies on the models of brief parent-infant psychotherapy at the Geneva school (Cramer 1995; Cramer and Palacio-Espasa 1993) and the interactive guidance model described by McDonough (1995). To address the question of effectiveness, we are currently conducting a follow-up study of our multimodal approach.

In this chapter, we describe the impact of using diverse theoretical perspectives in our technical interventions with infants and families. It will become apparent that many techniques commonly used in family therapy are incorporated into these different maneuvers. We also address some indications and contraindications of the models and illustrate several points with brief clinical vignettes from an infant mental health clinic in a community setting.

MULTIMODAL INTERVENTIONS

Not all families respond the same way to certain models of therapy. For instance, some parents with an infant who cries "almost all day" may come to the clinic asking for immediate advice on what they can do to help their child. They may feel quite disappointed if the clinician does not give them suggestions for how to help their baby cry less. Therapists who notice the parents' desperation may focus their inquiry, even from the first session, on what could make the infant cry so much and then recommend ways to alleviate this severe challenge (e.g., carrying the child more, reducing auditory stimulation, using a pacifier). Once the most troublesome symptom is alleviated somewhat or ameliorated altogether, the focus could shift to discovering other factors contributing to the baby's difficulty. Then the therapist may learn about an array of issues, such as the parents' feelings of anger and rejection toward the child or severe stressors they are experiencing. To help the baby, these problems must ultimately be addressed. Alternatively, the process may terminate once the parents notice their infant does not cry so much after they implement the therapist's initial recommendations.

In contrast, another family with a baby who cries excessively may not welcome the clinician's advice. Parents who have major difficulties with self-esteem or trust toward others, and whose own families have accused them of not taking good care of their baby, may feel resentful if the therapist initially suggests any concrete interventions. In such a situation, the therapist may find more useful a reflective model that emphasizes aspects of empathy toward the parents primarily and toward the infant secondarily. The therapist should try to establish a trusting relationship with the parents so that they do not feel suspicious of treatment recommendations. Conceivably, after these initial therapeutic moves, the parents may become receptive to techniques they can use to calm or comfort the baby and preempt further crying episodes.

A multidisciplinary team (including, e.g., family therapist, occupational therapist, language therapist, physician, developmental psychologist, and psychiatrist) can most readily design multimodal strategies. (Or one clinician may simply consult with colleagues from other disciplines.) When there is a team, clinicians with different backgrounds contribute their unique expertise to the understanding of the clinical problems. (In some cases, the use of a one-way mirror or videotaped sessions may be helpful. Of course, these methods require informed consent from the parents.)

Through case discussion, members of each discipline participate in designing a solution while also learning from each other and expanding their own therapeutic repertoire. This approach can be illustrated with the following case.

David

> Ms. G, an 18-year-old mother, brought David, her 11-month-old son, to the clinic with the complaint that the baby was extremely aggressive and frequently threw temper tantrums at the slightest frustration. According to her, David is rarely content for any length of time and seems very unhappy. When angry, the baby hits and also tries to bite her. Indeed, he has bitten her many times. Ms. G shows several small bruises on her arms. David also hits others who take care of him, including his maternal grandmother and aunts.

At this point, the clinician can explore in several directions, depending on his or her theoretical point of view and professional background. A family therapist may be interested in the systemic framework and meaning of these complaints and in the infant's and mother's behavior.

> Ms. G says while she is working, her mother looks after David. She regrets having to rely on her mother but chalks it up to multiple stressors in her life. She not only works in a fast-food restaurant but also attends college. She takes care of the baby the rest of the time. Later, when asked about her relationship with her mother, she mentions they have had many physical fights in the past. She would even bite her mother during those fights. Some recent confrontations were set off when her mother found out Ms. G was pregnant and kicked her out of the house.

The therapist could then examine the transgenerational aspects of the situation and try to explore with Ms. G how the aggression (biting) seems to traverse at least three generations. The therapy might proceed by focusing on that point of view. The therapist could also explore the multiple stressors Ms. G faces: poverty, the care of her baby while attending school, conflicts with her mother, and problems with access to the health care system.

In contrast, a clinician with a more child-focused, developmental point of view might focus on how the child has developed these problem behaviors. During the session, the therapist might explore and observe how the child plays, moves around, and speaks; how the child's emotions fluctuate; and how the child eats, sleeps, and reacts during transitions. The therapist could try to get an idea of the baby's cognitive status, sensitivities, and emotions.

> The therapist learns David has a long history of crying for extended periods and is highly sensitive and fussy. If things do not go his way, he immediately loses control and cries or attacks those around him. In the

session, the therapist observes David accidentally bump his head on a table. He then becomes angry, walks toward his mother several feet away, hits her, and tries to bite her, as if she were the one who caused his pain and he wanted to punish her. The therapist then suggests David is struggling because he does not know how to express his anger in a more adaptive way. The therapist recommends several interventions. One intervention is to diminish the intensity and array of stimuli in his milieu; another is to ease the transitions during his daily routine. The therapist also suggests Ms. G empathize with her son's pain by expressing her own concern when the baby is upset. Later on, in front of Ms. G, the therapist "teaches" David not to hit or bite and shows him with a doll what happens when someone bites another person. The therapist illustrates biting a doll and "marks" (Gergely and Watson 1996) the doll's ensuing pain by exaggerating the emotional expression associated with the pain. He then suggests an alternative and demonstrates it by asking David to touch the doll gently so as not to hurt it. David appears surprised. The clinician asks David (and his mother, who will also model for her son) to give the doll a kiss instead of biting it. David does so, and the therapist applauds. He advises Ms. G to practice this new emotion at home. He also recommends she name the negative feelings David displays when he appears so frustrated as being "mad," empathize with David, and soothe him, instead of chastising him and giving him a time-out.

This intervention is a more cognitive-behavioral approach to the same clinical situation and was the first level of intervention with this family. A clinician with more psychiatric orientation might be interested in the fact that Ms. G's mother suffers from bipolar disorder. The clinician would then attempt to explore symptoms of mood disturbance in Ms. G and the infant.

Ms. G says she is sad and angry most of the time because her hopes of going to medical school were shattered by the baby's arrival. If Ms. G endorses more symptoms of major depression, the first suggestion might be for her to engage in a trial of antidepressant medication. She mentions she is very irritable and tired and has little energy for dealing with the infant. She often feels like not getting out of bed in the morning and is pessimistic about her future.

A more psychodynamically oriented professional might explore the number of consciously mixed feelings that Ms. G expresses about David and his birth. Ms. G says she tried to have an abortion when she learned she was pregnant. When she went to a clinic, she was told it was "too late." She realized she would have to continue the pregnancy but had decided to give up the baby for adoption. When Ms. G's mother found out about this plan, she became enraged and pressured Ms. G to "keep the baby," saying it was a disgrace to the family that she could even think of giving the baby up for adoption. She offered to help Ms. G care for David.

The psychoanalytically oriented therapist may conclude Ms. G has not made space (Hoffmann 1995) for David in her life and her mind. The baby feels like an intrusion or even a punishment; he has spoiled her plans and now she must pay the consequences for her mistake. The therapist may begin the clinical work by talking about Ms. G's feeling that the child came at the wrong time in her life and that she did not really want him. This realization may help Ms. G start thinking about making room for her son in her life.

A child therapist may be more inclined to speak for the baby and thereby promote the development of empathy in Ms. G for her son. Observing the child in action with his episodes of aggression and biting, the clinician could reflect on the question of how David might feel when he is trying to bite his mother and how he may have chaotic feelings when he is throwing a tantrum. The therapist may also discuss how the infant could express his intense feelings differently. This possibility of change in the baby's expression of feelings may help Ms. G understand the intentionality in the child's actions and teach her to predict and perhaps preempt future explosions. These realizations could at least help her to contain David and accept his feelings, without reprimanding him and giving him a time-out.

These are only a few suggested points of view to use in approaching this situation. We suggest a clinician or therapeutic team could hold several of these models in mind and consider the clinical scene through different lenses. Then one or two strategies could be used to approach the problem. The decision of which strategies to use also depends on the therapist's intuition and his or her perception of the infant and family; it also depends on what the family wants and which therapeutic goals the family can achieve. The therapist and the family would then negotiate a therapeutic contract, understanding that both parties should be open to adjusting their focus according to the progress made in therapy.

DIFFERENT PERSPECTIVES AND TECHNIQUES FOR VARIOUS THERAPEUTIC GOALS

Factors in Therapeutic Goal Setting

At the beginning of clinical work with a family and child, several factors, as listed below, must be understood in order to arrive at a realistic therapeutic agreement or "contract":

- The infant's problems as well as his or her strengths and attributes
- The family's perception of the child's problems and what they wish to change

- The therapist's recommendations about what the problems are and what could be done to change them
- Real-life factors, cultural factors, limitations, and factors that operate in favor of and against therapy and change

Infant's Problems, Strengths, and Attributes

A patient profile can be made as a result of a hands-on assessment of the baby. Each line of development should be assessed in its own right: language, motor skills and coordination, sensory integration abilities, reciprocity and relatedness, emotional status, expressiveness and emotional regulation, play, attention span, and so forth. With this profile in hand, the clinician would know both the child's relative strengths and the child's most challenging areas.

Family's Perceptions and Wishes

The therapist clarifies what the family sees as the problem; what their theories are about its nature, cause, and maintaining factors; what they think should change; and their motivation for change and investment in change. The therapist also determines the family's systemic resources for making such change possible.

Therapist's Recommendations

By integrating the observation and assessment of the infant, the family as a whole, and the caregiver-infant relationship, the clinician develops a priority list of what needs to change and what should be addressed first. This list would constitute the therapist's "wishes," not necessarily what would be worked on.

Real-Life Factors and Limitations

The real-life factors and limitations would include the ability to come to sessions, work demands, economic difficulties, and family stressors (e.g., a mother with chronic fatigue syndrome, a father with diabetes). The therapist could also take into consideration what the family perceives as dysfunction and the parents' preferred remedy for the situation.

The Therapeutic Contract

The therapeutic contract should be the result of a mutual exchange, a negotiation, so to speak; it should not be decided by only the family or the therapist. Ideally, it would be a cooperative approach to the problem and would include the priorities for addressing it. The contract should be fairly explicit, but at times it can be left implicit. In many of the most difficult families, a contract can be most useful for focusing initially on the problems presented by the infant, that is, the problems that initially bring the family to the clinic. The clinician deals explicitly with these areas while also starting a therapeutic process on other aspects, such as the parent-infant relationship, the spousal relationship, or, if present, the parents' malignant projections toward their child.

Two extreme points of view illustrate the benefits of a negotiated therapeutic contract. At one extreme, therapy is dictated by "the expert" (the therapist). After exploring the situation, the therapist arrives at a conclusion about the problem and its solution. He or she then gives a "prescription" of what the family should do. This approach used to be the traditional medical model. At the other extreme, some family therapy involves having the therapist work only on what the family perceives as the problem. Logically, once that problem is resolved, therapy is terminated. Even at the other extreme, however, the parents must agree at least on a working definition of the problem and what should be attempted to solve it.

Both these extremes (and even more balanced approaches in between) sometimes forget the infant also has a contribution to make to the therapeutic contract. For example, the nature of the child's difficulties, development, temperament, and unique characteristics should inform the family's perception and the therapist's recommendations.

We suggest that in most situations it is optimal to seek an intermediate point between the two extremes. Neither the vertically designated prescription from the expert nor the unmodified and unquestioned view of the family and its definition of the problem is the best therapeutic approach. From our point of view, the clinician can make valuable contributions to the definition of the problem and its possible solution, which should not be ignored or set aside. The family also plays a major role in deciding what the problem is and what the therapy should be. Parents, however, vary in their knowledge of child development, child psychopathology, and other aspects of human relationships. Thus, their view of the problem may be either quite accurate or quite inaccurate. The knowledgeable therapist can help the family redefine the problem and inform them of possible interventions. Many parents welcome "expert" opinions and are eager to implement suggestions. In short, the family and the therapist should seek to arrive at a mutually agreed-upon area where clinical work can take place, that is, where the therapist, family, and infant can collaborate to reach a common goal.

DIFFERENT INTERVENTIONS AND TECHNIQUES

Apparently simple and practical interventions, such as giving advice or offering practical help to parents, do have a psychodynamic meaning that may or may not be discussed openly in the therapeutic relationship. All the interventions we describe here have a psychodynamic impact, but this aspect is usually not emphasized in the context of multimodal interventions (Figure 6–2).

Practical Help

Parents of young children, by the very nature of the demands of this stage of life, experience significant stress during pregnancy, delivery (or cesarean section), the neonatal period, and later on. Many of these stressful situations are usual, but families may go through additional adverse circumstances. Stress factors have not only a cumulative but also a multiplying effect, putting the family and infant at more risk. People are able to tolerate only a certain amount of stress, after which their homeostasis and ability to cope are likely to collapse.

When the therapist sets practical help in motion, at least one stressor may be eliminated. In some cases, the alleviation of some stress can make the difference between a positive and a negative course. Relieving some immediate concern may also enable a parent to face the challenges presented by the baby, be more emotionally available or patient, or even enjoy the child more.

In their model of infant-parent psychotherapy, Lieberman and Pawl (1993) described the use of practical help. This often preliminary step promotes the development of trust between the parents and the therapist and moves them closer to the ultimate goal of a corrective attachment experience.

Here we refer simply to the implementation of practical actions to alleviate the stress felt by parents. This provision of services may indeed be perceived as helpful by parents who are on the verge of succumbing to overwhelming psychosocial circumstances or are socially isolated, as is the case with many inner-city families.

Ms. B

During a house visit with a social worker (Mr. Jack Moseley, whose spontaneous help to the family was most useful), one of the authors consulted with Ms. B, a 20-year-old single mother of two children. One child was 2 years old, and the other was 9 months old. Ms. B's inner-city apartment was very old and quite dark. It consisted mostly of one big room with a stove in the middle.

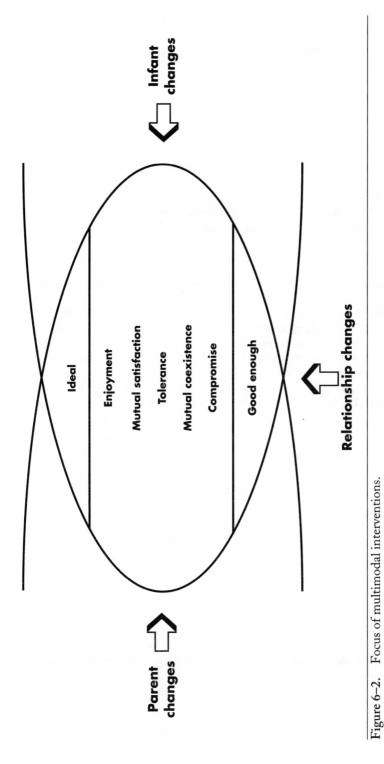

Figure 6–2. Focus of multimodal interventions.

The focus of multimodal interventions can be on the parent or the child, or on their interactions, so they can be helped to work toward developing a better relationship.

The consultation concerned the 9-month-old baby, who was not eating well and, consequently, not gaining weight. Ms. B appeared very hesitant and burdened, looking much older than her 20 years. Because the baby was not thriving, the pediatrician had called child protective services, suspecting the mother was neglecting the child. The social worker, on the other hand, thought Ms. B was quite devoted to her two children but felt overwhelmed and lacked the energy to try new strategies to feed her baby.

Ms. B said she did not know how to get her child to eat. He only wanted to drink milk and juices, which did not provide enough calories and protein to grow. The therapist suggested Ms. B give the baby puréed foods to play with and explore. He asked her whether she had a high chair for the infant. Ms. B said she did, but it was still in the box. Some relatives had given it to her as a gift several months before, but she had never opened the box and assembled the high chair. While the therapist was explaining to Ms. B about experimenting with food, the textures of different foods, and the critical periods for introducing consistent foods, the social worker unpacked the high chair and put it together. Ms. B then put her baby in it and placed some puréed food on the tray in front of him. The infant immediately proceeded to touch the food, pick it up, and put it in his mouth. In a follow-up visit several weeks later, the baby was found to be eating a variety of puréed and even "lumpy" foods. It appeared that assembling the high chair for Ms. B was the "jump-start" she needed to set in motion the process of working with her problem in feeding her child.

Practical help may be necessary, or a first step in therapy, for parents who have a sick baby and do not have a telephone, who have had their water disconnected, or who lack heating. At times, several social services can be drawn on with the intervention of the therapist, who is often more knowledgeable about such resources. The goal is to create a more favorable set of circumstances for the family and the infant.

Practical help should be offered with a clear goal in mind. The therapist should differentiate among adequate interventions; excessive, inappropriate, and unnecessary interventions; and those based on the therapist's sense of guilt. The therapist should also avoid interventions that the family may view as an intrusion or an indication that the therapist thinks the family is ineffective.

Information

Families in the United States and other developed countries are becoming increasingly nuclear, and many are quite isolated from a support network. As a result, parents often do not have any role models from whom to learn about child rearing, nor do they have anyone to ask about common infant problems. In the past, shared cultural values and practices made it easier to know what to do and how to manage child rearing. Some parents may turn to books, but in many circumstances they just do the best they can, creating novel interventions that may be quite useful sometimes but detrimental to the child at other times. It is well known that one major risk factor for child maltreatment is social isolation, especially for single mothers (Olds et al. 1997).

The therapist may give parents information about a number of issues, including child development, common and transient alterations in infant behavior and organization, and the emotional needs of young children. There are multiple situations in which the therapist can reassure the baby's caregivers with simple developmental information or help them with recommendations that experienced parents might find commonplace and unremarkable. For novice, isolated parents, such information may make a significant difference in their ability to care for their babies.

Although much of this knowledge can be gained from videotapes and pamphlets, the parents most in need tend not to avail themselves of such knowledge through those channels. They may also be more likely to welcome specific information suitable for their particular child—that takes into account the uniqueness of their situation—rather than material meant for a wide audience. To illustrate this principle, the following list gives examples of information that may be helpful to parents:

- The competencies of newborns and infants, including their ability to see and hear, their need for touching and holding, and the ways parents can promote a reciprocal relationship between themselves and their child (Maldonado-Durán 1996).
- Preparation of baby formula and monitoring of infant nutrition. For example, parents may dilute the formula too much or not notice situations in which the child does not gain weight because he or she drinks juices, which satiate the appetite but have relatively poor nutritional value.
- The transient nature of many infant behaviors. For example, children need to be held, but the need usually will not persist with that intensity after walking starts. Each stage represents different needs. The same is true with struggles over autonomy during the tenth month of life. Exploratory biting by the infant at 9 or 10 months of age can be misconstrued by others as attacks. Similarly, the child's insistence on dropping things on the floor to repeat an interesting spectacle can be interpreted as stubbornness.
- The importance of routines to help support the young child's efforts at self-regulation.

- The need for cognitive stimulation of the infant's developing brain and the importance of language, speech, and play. The stimulation for the baby may include face-to-face contact to support the development of reciprocity.
- The development and changes in the baby's emotional life, for example, the emergence of separation anxiety and consequent clinginess. Talking about the emotions of young children may foster in the parents an attitude favorable toward "mind-reading" the child, which is a crucial element of sensitive parenting (Fonagy 1998).
- Normal patterns in the development of eating abilities, sleep routines, crying, motor functioning, and sensory processing.
- Common health concerns and childproofing strategies for the home.
- Individual differences between children and the uniqueness of the individual child. For example, parents may need information about specific sensitivities, temperament, and the different "types" of children (Greenspan 1991). Parents may have preconceived expectations about how the child should be, while being less aware of healthy variations.
- Cultural variations in child-rearing practices, particularly for migrant parents or those from different cultures. For example, if the parents do not have a cultural perspective, they may practice co-sleeping with their baby or prolong breast-feeding and find themselves questioning their intuition about what to do (Moro 1994). In industrialized cultures, parents from nonindustrialized cultures often are perceived as not fostering their child's independence, yet being independent is not an important cultural value for these parents.

This information may alleviate many of the parents' concerns and help them solve problems and answer questions about what to do when faced with the unique demands or challenges of their child. The therapist, however, may encounter contraindications to providing such information. Some parents may feel annoyed or even insulted by the clinician's "lectures," notwithstanding the quality of the information or the obvious need for it. Except in situations in which the primary needs and safety of the baby are at stake, the therapist should respect the parents' defenses. Caregivers with conflicts originating from dealing with their own authoritarian parents may not be responsive to further information. The therapist also has to exercise "mind-reading" skills to ascertain how the initial pieces of information are received. It may be more strategically sound to offer no information until a trusting relationship is established, which may take a long time for some families.

Julia

The importance of establishing a trusting relationship can be seen in the case of the D family. Julia was a 4-week-old infant at the time of the first consultation. A social worker referred the family because Ms. D repeatedly alluded to the surprising capacities of her daughter. Ms. D was certain the baby knew all of her mother's emotional states, could make decisions about her clothing, and had specific tastes about the decorations in her room. As time went on, the mother attributed more capacities to her daughter. At 2 months of age, Julia was seen as having clear preferences for television programs and clothing, and her parents were making arrangements to have her learn Spanish, German, French, Iroquois, and Potawatomie (the last two are Native American languages). Initially, the clinician attempted to provide information about the cognitive development of children—how it would be hard for an infant to make choices in clothing and TV programs. Such statements went mostly unheard by Julia's parents until their reasons for perceiving Julia as a super child could be addressed. The therapist discovered that Ms. D had lost a previous child from sudden infant death syndrome, and she was afraid that Julia would also die. She saw Julia almost as a reincarnation of the previous child, whose attributes compounded Julia's. Ms. D felt as if life had compensated her for her previous loss with an extremely gifted and special child. When the therapist addressed the mother's need to mourn the loss of her first baby, Ms. D's excessive attributions toward Julia diminished.

Emotional Support

When a baby is born, a parent is also "born" (Lebovici 1995). The adult who did not have children has to be born into a new identity as a parent (parentification)—a challenging and demanding task. The perinatal period is one of great vulnerability and usually requires much support from other adults who are emotionally close to the new parent. This period of adjustment seems true even of gorillas; when a gorilla baby is born, other females tend to support and help the new mother (Bard 1995).

The therapeutic stance of providing emotional support means, among other things, "being with" the parents and the infant. Sharing in their experiences, concerns, anxieties, and emotional pain, as well as in their happiness and hope, can be helpful and sustaining. Such an intervention may be more necessary or meaningful when parents cannot rely on relatives or close friends to participate with them, especially when difficulties develop. When a baby with a malformation or major disease is born, the distraught parents need an opportunity to discuss the situation, including their feelings, uncertainty, and pain; such contact may help them cope not only in the here and now but also in the future. Processing their experience and feelings may prevent difficulties down the road.

The therapist can encourage the parents to express their feelings, even negative ones toward the baby, and can help the parents to process them.

One aspect of emotional support is the therapist's function as a "container" for the feelings and experiences of parents and infant (Maldonado-Durán 1997). This support involves helping the parents cope with a difficult or potentially devastating situation involving great uncertainty and tension. At times, therapists underestimate their role as a listener and container. Many parents benefit from and find relief in "telling their story" to someone who is attentive and interested in hearing it. Often the therapist just has to be available; he or she does not have to say anything or interpret the meaning of the experience. The narration of the story and the reexperiencing of contained emotions associated with the story can have a strong therapeutic impact on adults who have gone through difficult or traumatic events.

Emotional support may also be necessary to mark, amplify, or simply acknowledge the feelings parents have around certain developmental achievements in their child. Particularly when parents are isolated and lack social support, the therapist may function as a "mirroring" figure for their efforts at parenting. Mirroring involves affirming the joy felt by the parents when the baby achieves developmental milestones, such as growing a tooth, saying "Mama" for the first time, or taking the first few steps. Parents enjoy these celebrations and sometimes actively engage the clinician by pointing out milestones, anniversaries, and accomplishments. Emotional support may be particularly helpful a) when the baby is born with some malformation or known dysmorphic syndrome, b) when the infant develops a major chronic medical illness, or c) when the newborn must be sent to a neonatal intensive care unit.

Many young parents, in particular, need to be reassured that they are doing a good job. Praising their devotion, skills, and attunement to the infant may help them continue to carry out these difficult tasks. All parents need gratification and social feedback. When the baby is less competent to reward the parents, the support of others can substitute to some extent.

Most parents are willing to speak about their feelings and share them with an interested person. This self-revelation is sometimes not possible, however, with more suspicious or emotionally injured adults, who may fear any sense of vulnerability or emotional closeness with someone else. The therapist should recognize the need for distance and defenses (e.g., denial, intellectualization, and rationalization) when parents are not in a position to explore other reactions. These defenses sometimes aid parental adjustment when parents must cope with their baby in difficult circumstances.

Advice From the Therapist

Winnicott used to say that the most difficult aspect of his work with patients was imparting advice (Newman 1995). Imparting advice is, indeed, a very difficult aspect of any therapist's work, but one that may be necessary. In some circumstances, it may be helpful for the therapist to assume the position of an "expert" on issues of child development, behavioral and emotional problems, and interpersonal relationships. The giving of advice seems very distant from the work of interpretation and reflection more typical of psychoanalytically oriented therapy. However, advice may be the most indicated clinical intervention in certain situations.

In some clinical cases, not giving advice can be counterproductive. Giving advice may help to engage the family in therapy and preserve their interest in seeking help or their hope for some benefit from it. Parents may even feel quite disappointed when a therapist does not offer suggestions about how to deal with their baby's problem. For instance, a therapist may be asked to consult with parents about a youngster who frequently hits or bites other children and is on the verge of being expelled from his third day-care center. Such parents may feel desperate to deal with a problem that represents many complications for them. They may feel frustrated if the therapist takes a stance of exploration and prolonged reflection about the problem without offering alternatives that the parents or the day-care staff can implement immediately. If no suggestions are made despite their requests, the family may decide that seeing a therapist is not helpful.

One function of the clinician may be to alleviate psychological pain, as in the case of the parent who feels helpless or incompetent. Another therapeutic task is to foster the hope that the situation will improve. After the parent implements some of the therapist's advice, a problem situation may become much easier to manage. Once the major tensions and the sense of urgency have abated, the parent may feel better able to reflect and examine fantasies.

Many situations call for advice, including those in which the parents need to be taught techniques to soothe and promote the infant's self-regulation. Optimally, this advice should be grounded in a careful examination of the child. Concrete suggestions also can be given about how to help a child settle to sleep or how to attempt to feed an infant with a minor disturbance (e.g., frequent vomiting, falling asleep at feeding time, pervasively diminished appetite).

Alex

Alex R, a 2-week-old infant, was referred for consultation by the lactation consultant from the hospital where he was born. His mother is a young married woman who recently immigrated to the United States with the baby's father. A number of relatives live with the couple in their home and share in taking care of the baby. Ms. R's first pregnancy ended in a stillbirth.

Ms. R was quite apprehensive and worried because Alex "cries all the time," particularly at night. She was referred because she had lost her patience and had spanked the baby. In her mind, there was no reason for Alex to cry, but she could not console him. She regretted her outburst and wanted help to learn how to soothe her baby.

On examination, Alex appeared to be a very sensitive infant. He squirmed constantly and was quite restless and fussy. He quickly built up to active crying. Once he started crying, it was difficult to console him. Ms. R said this behavior was exactly what happened many times—day and night. The baby had very tremulous movements and was easily startled. He was hypersensitive to touch and did not accommodate being held in his mother's arms.

After examining the baby, the therapist recommended using a pacifier to give oral stimulation (i.e., nonnutritive sucking) to the baby as a soothing technique. It had been observed that the baby could better self-regulate while he was sucking. At first, Ms. R was surprised with this recommendation. She explained that her own parents did not like pacifiers, which were frowned on in their native country. But she said it would be fine to try using one. Then, infant massage was discussed and demonstrated, particularly the difference between superficial and deep touch. Finally, it was suggested she reduce surrounding stimuli (e.g., loud voices, television) for Alex.

In a follow-up interview, Ms. R reported she was enjoying her baby more than before. She appeared much more relaxed, and she felt the recommended techniques had proven effective. Her relief seemed helpful later on, when she was able to discuss her fears about losing Alex in light of the loss of her previous child.

Advice can be a "behavioral prescription" to try to alleviate a problem at hand. In several areas of infant functioning or symptoms, parents may not intuitively know what to do. For example, many parents may be surprised to be told that their baby naturally reacts cautiously and anxiously to new stimuli and that, therefore, such stimuli should be presented gradually, giving the baby time to get acquainted with them. In other words, each baby is unique. The clinician, who may have a fund of knowledge and experience about strategies for helping a baby cope with a changing environment and stimuli, can suggest two or three techniques that have been useful with other infants. Similarly, in dealing with a number of sensory integration difficulties (DeGangi 1991), some parents show great inventiveness and imagination to help their baby cope, and they modify their caregiving practices accordingly. However, many parents feel baffled and frustrated when what they do is not helpful to their baby. The clinician's experience may be necessary as a resource to deal with those situations (Zeitlin and Williamson 1994).

A common situation that requires advice from an "expert" is how to deal with an infant who shows little response to surrounding stimuli or interactions with caregivers. The baby can be hyporeactive or self-absorbed. If the parents do not persist in trying to engage the child, the child may eventually have delays in language, motor development, and the ability to engage in circles of reciprocal communication. Parents may require suggestions for techniques to prolong interactions and "seduce" the child into longer interactions. Left to their own devices, parents sometimes give up and let the child withdraw for significant periods. Letting the child withdraw extensively without any attempt to engage him or her is undesirable because in the first 2 years of life there may be more plasticity in the brain for the development of more refined pathways.

Parents often welcome such advice. However, as with the previously described interventions, advice may be contraindicated when parents feel vulnerable, criticized, or even "attacked" by the clinician's expertise. It may also prematurely close an issue that needs to be explored. In many situations, however, advice can open the door to further work once the parents' sense of immediacy and helplessness with the infant's symptoms has abated.

Translation of Infant Signals From a Developmental Point of View

In this intervention, the clinician may "speak for the infant" (Carter et al. 1991). A therapist who is experienced in evaluating children's problems can assess the baby's "symptoms" and then communicate to the parent some of the infant's needs and unique features. It is preferable to frame these needs as preferences and challenges rather than as difficulties or deficits. Here the therapist is a translator or an intermediary in the space between caregiver and infant. This translation frames the child's behavior from a new point of view that helps the parent understand the child's messages or states. As a result, the parent's perception of the baby may change, enabling the parent to invent strategies, develop new patience and empathy, and find new motivation for helping the baby overcome roadblocks. This situation is often the case with the infant who struggles with autonomy and tries to do everything on his or her own, which is developmentally appropriate. When the therapist points out that it is healthy for a baby to struggle to achieve autonomy, the behavior that the parent may have perceived as defiance or stubbornness can be seen in a new light. Something similar can be said about temper tantrums at 2 years of age. At times, parents will experience the toddler's territoriality and unwillingness to allow others to play with his or her toys as selfishness and greed. They may expect the toddler to understand the concept of "taking turns" or "sharing toys." However, they might revise their view after learning more about the normal development of prosocial behavior.

As described by Carter et al. (1991) and Fraiberg et al. (1989), the therapist can be a conduit for signals from the child to the parents, helping to promote sensitivity and empathy. The parents may have difficulties with their perception of the baby's communications, or they may even misattribute meaning. When the clinician notices that the parents' attribution involves distortions and actual misattribution of meaning, suggesting an alternative meaning may promote a more benign reading of the child.

A therapist who is well versed in infants' language can help parents understand the child's communication. For instance, in the first few months of life, turning the head to one side, yawning, or hiccuping may be signs of overstimulation and a need to take a break from interactions. This information may help parents adjust the amount of interaction with their baby. In addition, parents who learn to recognize states of quiet alertness in the newborn may be able to take advantage of them as a time for interacting better with their baby. It is also useful to recognize other states, such as somnolence and active alertness, in which such interaction is not possible. Smiling, trying to grasp the parent's face, and cooing vocalizations all may be noted by the therapist as the infant's attempts to say something positive to the caregiver. As the infant develops, such behaviors may be interpreted as reflective of the toddler's emotional life.

Pearl

Ms. M and her boyfriend were recently advised to have some conversations with a mental health clinician. Ms. M is 17 years old, and her boyfriend is 18. They brought in Pearl, their 10-day-old infant. Ms. M appeared highly stressed and uncertain about how to look after the baby. When Pearl started fussing and appeared uncomfortable, the therapist asked Ms. M why she thought the baby was upset. In a quite serious tone of voice, Ms. M responded that Pearl was just "being mean" and that she enjoyed bothering her mother. As the therapist and the parents explored this idea, other possibilities were suggested, such as the fact that, for example, the baby might feel sleepy or hungry. Ms. M proved sensitive to these alternative possibilities and began trying to remedy the possible causes of Pearl's discomfort. In this case, the misattribution of meaning was due more to a lack of awareness of the child's neediness and dependence than to a lack of empathy. Ms. M was sensitive to the child's discomfort once alternative interpretations were contemplated during the session.

Parents who have had difficult experiences in their own childhood may not find it easy to develop a repertoire of sensitive responses to their child. But with the assistance of another person, they may be able to learn the possibilities and nuances of their child's behavior. The therapist's knowledge of infant development and psychopathology can guide them not only in characterizing a problem but also in designing a strategy for its solution by means of a "developmental map" of what to suggest to parents.

Knowing about the normal development of feeding abilities, for example, can help a therapist design interventions for a child with a feeding disturbance. This process may involve deciding precisely where the child is having problems and then recommending the next developmental step the child can try to master, depending on when the disturbance began. For instance, the therapist may suggest that the child begin eating puréed foods rather than only liquids (Maldonado-Durán and Sauceda-Garcia 1998; Ramsay 1995).

A similar approach can be used to address diverse aspects of a child's development, including fostering the infant's ability to self-feed and explore new solid foods after he or she manages to tolerate semisolid textures and new flavors. This model also applies to an infant's difficulties with gross motor development, coordination, and fine motor skills. In addition, anxiety problems can be approached with this developmental frame of mind. The therapist can design interventions to help the child cope with each stage in the mastery of fears and anxieties, such as moving gradually from constant closeness to the mother to using transitional objects and playing games that involve separations and reunions. Another example of an intervention would be going from engaging in mutual attention and gaze to playing in a reciprocal way in simple interactive games (e.g., tossing a ball back and forth) to playing games involving a verbal exchange. This framework helps start treatment by meeting the child at the point at which he or she is developmentally and then going on to the next step, in what has been construed as a "Vygotskian" approach (Wertsch and Tulviste 1994).

PARENTS AS THERAPISTS

To deal with several problems, a behavioral modification approach may be indicated. The principles of behavior therapy include conducting a detailed analysis of parent-child interactions and examining the sequence of those interactions. The behavioral analysis helps obtain a picture of the transactions between parent and child and determine where an alternative sequence might be introduced. A common situation is that of the toddler with intense and frequent temper outbursts and difficulty calming down. A behavioral analysis could help the parent identify precipitating or at-risk moments, early signs of frustration, and ways to preempt those outbursts.

In the clinic, we frequently see parents who have a limited behavioral repertoire for denying their child what he or she wants. For instance, they may say, "No!" but then fail to provide any further engagement, alternatives, or interactions to help the child cope with the ensuing frustration. We suggest strategies for empathizing with the child and initiating other activities that may help prevent the temper tantrum.

Behavioral interventions often use measurements that involve keeping a record of some behaviors and then assessing progress. Merely asking parents to record their child's behavior can have a powerful impact on changing some behavioral sequences.

Implementing changes, particularly in negative interactions, encourages both the parent and the child. When a positive space for engagement is created along the lines of positive parenting (Howard 1991) and the child is rewarded (mostly emotionally) for adaptive or flexible behaviors, other aspects of the relationship may also improve.

Behavioral and Cognitive Interventions

Behavioral and cognitive techniques vary, depending on the child's age, but often can be used with quite young children of about 10 months and older. One can use these interventions with the child while the caregivers are also in the consulting room. In this manner, the therapist "trains" or models to parents some of the therapeutic interventions. The parents can then operate as co-therapists at home, where some techniques can be implemented more frequently than is possible in the therapist's office.

These techniques can be employed to help infants with sleeping and feeding problems, those with very short attention spans, or those who are less responsive to reciprocal interactions or who exhibit hyperactivity. These methods can also help expand the behavioral repertoire of children who express frustration in mostly physically aggressive ways, such as biting, kicking, hitting, or pinching. In addition, these techniques can benefit children with intense anxiety about brief separations who become "paralyzed" when they are exposed to some feared stimulus.

These cognitive and behavioral interventions are more visual and representational, with limited use of language, particularly with younger infants. A behavioral sequence can be represented either with people or with dolls, puppets, or stuffed animals (Lillard 1993). Using these objects in a way that the child can easily see, the therapist represents the challenging situation and suggests a direct message, for instance, by substituting one behavior for another. This teaches the child to substitute a new strategy for a maladaptive way of dealing with challenges.

The goal of these interventions is learning. The therapist (or the parent coached by the therapist) will help the child learn things that he or she has not mastered, such as self-control, response inhibition, delay in response, or attention to a scene for longer spans of time. Even a child with biological vulnerabilities can often benefit from learning new behaviors. For example, with an infant who often bites when he is angry, a disagreement or frustration could be depicted with two dolls, one representing the young child and the other an adult. In this theatrical display, the infant doll "hits" and "bites" while demonstrating anger at the adult doll. The play scene can be repeated with different interactions and outcomes and with different actors. If capable, the child could participate in the scene and in this way, in play, express or represent his own anger and reactions. Then an alternative scene might be suggested, for instance, in which the child does not bite, because biting hurts the other person, or does not hit and instead says, "I am mad at you." When the youngster substitutes an alternative, more adaptive behavior for biting in play, he is praised, and the more adaptive sequence is celebrated. Children can also be taught how to use soft touch to express tender feelings, elicit closeness, or receive reassurance from parents when they are afraid.

Children who are inattentive and distractible can be "trained," through repeated attempts and interesting sequences, to engage in longer periods of looking, playing, or interacting. The therapist will require skills to create funny, interesting, or engaging scenes that elicit the child's interest. For instance, the therapist may use somewhat exaggerated facial expressions or verbalizations, noises, or unexpected turns in the play sequences. The therapist may also be training the parents to do these things at home. This practice extends the parents' repertoire of strategies to engage their child. One uses different means to achieve this end, depending in part on the sensory preferences of the child: the representations may be more auditory (singing or making animated noises) or more visual, kinesthetic, proprioceptive, and so on. Whatever representation is used, the purpose is to capture the infant's imagination.

Through trial and error, the clinician can design an intervention suited to a particular child. For example, an infant may require that the caregiver or therapist play only in the corner of a room with one or two toys, lest the child become distracted and quickly disinterested. The clinician searches for a strategy that achieves the goal while the parent observes what the child seems to prefer or what is successful in eliciting interest or engagement. They can then recognize early signs of overstimulation, frustration, or the child's need to disengage and do his or her "own thing." These observations may help the parents and the child in their everyday interactions at home.

The child may need behavioral support to cope with a challenging situation (DeGangi 1991; Zeitlin and Williamson 1994). Engaging and helping the child maintain a state of alertness or contentment may require deep pressure or massage to the trunk and limbs, vestibular stimulation, or oral activity (sucking or, in the older child, chewing). Older children (perhaps above 2½ years of age) can use some biofeedback techniques to help control anger and cope with overstimulation or anxiety. Abdominal breathing, muscle contraction and relaxation, and hand warming can all be taught in the context of playing a game. The infant with intense anxiety or traumatic stress responses can be helped to master difficult situations by gradually bringing him or her closer to feared objects. As a behavior changes slightly, it can be "chained" to another new coping behavior.

Promotion of Positive
Parent-Child Relationships

For some parents, the prescription of play with their child can help them engage in a new, mutually gratifying space where the tension and strain of a relationship can be set aside. In this area, they can just have fun together and enjoy the moment. For the child, this relaxing play can create new memories of a positive exchange with the caregiver. In some cases, the therapist seems to give the parents permission to enjoy their child. At times, the clinician may have to subtly teach a parent by gradually including him or her in playful interactions with the young child. Without creating a sense of inadequacy in the parent, the therapist also needs the ability to play, using a sense of humor, laughter, and creativity. The therapist should convey that this interaction is not just a teaching moment but rather a true moment of relaxation and pleasure. At times, such reinforcement enables the parent to experience closeness and warmth toward the child and allows the creation of a no-conflict zone.

With the toddler, play can give a sense of effectiveness and of being in control. In the "floor time" technique (Greenspan 1991), the child takes the lead in play and the parent follows, so that the child can feel like an effective agent whose initiatives make a difference.

Psychodynamic Interventions

At times, psychodynamic approaches (more fully described in other chapters in this book) offer the only possibility for improvement or resolution of infant problems deeply entangled in relationship difficulties between parent and child. Addressing parental perceptions of the child and understanding and interpreting them (Vives-Rocabert and Lartigue 1995) can help release the child from ghosts of the past.

With many parents (particularly those with a history of previous losses, psychological trauma, problems with trust, and relationship difficulties), the more "naïve" interventions we have described are not effective or therapeutic. In these circumstances, the approaches described by Lieberman (1992), Lieberman and Pawl (1993), Cramer (1995), Cramer and Palacio-Espasa (1993), Lebovici (1983, 1995), and McDonough (1995) may be the only hope for helping an infant and parent.

Systemic Family Interventions

In clinical work with infants, it is useful to maintain a systemic point of view. The infant is seen as a member of a larger interactive system, encompassing not only the mother but also the father, siblings, and others in close relationship with the parents. These others have a profound impact, including transgenerational influences, on the mother-child relationship. Throughout this chapter, we have described interventions guided by these principles. Here we emphasize only two additional points: how to prioritize interventions and how to address other dysfunctional subsystems within the family.

The clinician often is faced with the question of what came first: the child's symptoms or the parent's way of dealing with the child. The systemic approach does not tackle the question from a linear point of view. Instead, it assumes simultaneous influences and multidirectionality. The intervention is directed to all members of the system at the same time, assuming that interventions with one member will have an impact on the whole.

Working With the Marriage

At times, the functioning of the marital relational system is crucial for understanding and addressing infant symptoms. When spouses have major differences in their approach to parenting, which may be part of broader marital disagreement, the differences can lead to confrontations on how to handle various aspects of caring for the child: discipline, limit-setting, feeding, sleeping, and so on. On occasion, the infant's problem should initially be addressed from the point of view of the marital system.

Julian

Julian K, 15 months old, was brought to the clinic because of a sleeping difficulty. He woke up during the night, and the parents disagreed on how the problem should be handled. Ms. K has tried the "ignoring approach," which her husband supports, and found it unsuccessful; the baby still continues to cry for periods of more than an hour. She has decided to change her method and soothe the baby whenever he wakes up and cries. She wants advice from the therapist about how to help Julian sleep through the night.

Ms. K has discovered that if Julian sleeps in his parents' bed, he doesn't wake up. When the issue of where the baby should sleep (in his room or with his parents) is brought up, a major disagreement surfaces between Mr. and Ms. K. The marriage was the first for Ms. K and the second for Mr. K. Crying, Ms. K says she does not like to sleep in the marital bed because it is where her husband slept with his first wife. Ms. K wants to buy another bed, but her husband argues repeatedly that they cannot afford it. Ms. K immediately and angrily points out that her husband had just bought a Mercedes-Benz. He quickly responds that he bought the car only because it was necessary for his business as a realtor. This initial issue is only one in a long list of marital disagreements.

The point here is that Ms. K apparently welcomed the baby's sleeping difficulty because it often compelled her to go to sleep beside his baby bed, which helped her express her own resentment about the marital bed. When this matter was addressed directly, the parents were able to agree on a number of issues about the baby's routine and about their involvement in parenting. In a few weeks, the child's sleeping problem disappeared.

Focusing on Strengths

Family therapists are interested not only in what the symptoms of dysfunction are but also in what aspects are functioning well. In therapy, the clinician often has to draw on the strengths of the child, the parents, and the family. At times, parents lose perspective about their basic strengths (e.g., the feelings they have for each other, their mutual commitment, their cohesiveness and love for each other) and get caught up in day-to-day conflicts. To help the parents regain perspective and to instill hope, the therapist may actively point out these strengths, which can become the point of departure for positive changes.

The technique of reframing can sometimes help change the parents' perspective about their baby. A child perceived as hyperactive and inattentive can also be perceived as very intelligent, curious, and actively engaged in exploring the world. These semantic maneuvers also allow a shift in the parents' point of view. "Defiance" in a child has positive elements (e.g., persistence, autonomy, and desire to develop one's own project) that parents can learn to appreciate. Thinking about these aspects of defiance may help parents allow their child more space to pursue personal projects. It may also help them engage in fewer face-to-face confrontations as they begin to appreciate their child's drive to succeed individually. In addition, differences of opinion on parenting, instead of necessarily leading to conflict, may give parents an opportunity to expand their views and consider alternatives.

Thinking of a family system as a whole helps the therapist be aware of where the interventions are focused. They could be focused on the child, on the parents, or on the parent-child relationship: Modifications in any one of these areas may bring about changes in other areas. Often the therapist must focus initially on the child because that is what the parents want. The child may have to be helped to take the "first step" in changing so that the parents can then also change their view of the child. At other times, parents are willing to change their own approach; their willingness, in turn, helps the child modify his or her responses or behavior. The perinatal period often seems uniquely suited to making changes and developing flexibility as members of the new family get to know each other in their new roles (Figure 6–3).

PSYCHIATRIC INTERVENTIONS: RECOGNITION OF A MENTAL DISORDER

With awareness of psychopathology, the clinician can at times notice behaviors and symptoms in parents that may lead the clinician to suspect a mental disorder in a family member. For the general population, the risk of having one condition is approximately 15% or somewhat higher. Particularly when the condition is not severe, it may go unrecognized by the family and the clinician. The main disorders to consider with new mothers are mood problems, depression (postpartum variety has been estimated at a 10%–15% prevalence in women in this period of life), posttraumatic stress disorder, or another major anxiety problem, such as panic disorder or a dissociative condition. Even attention-deficit disorder in a parent can lead to major difficulties in caregiving for a baby.

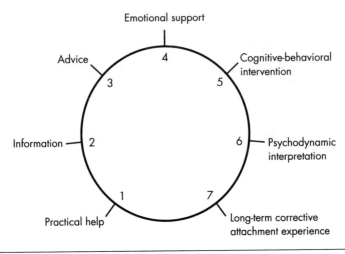

Emotional support

Advice

Cognitive-behavioral
intervention

Information

Psychodynamic
interpretation

Practical help

Long-term corrective
attachment experience

Figure 6–3. Continuum of interventions.

The continuum of multimodal interventions contains a range of practical approaches with psychodynamic overtones. They may be used either one by one or concurrently, as well as with one or more relationship problems.

Mary

Ms. A, a 16-year-old single mother, was referred for a consultation because her 4-month-old daughter, Mary, was highly irritable. As we observed parent-child interactions, the young mother clearly seemed to be doing her best. However, she often came to sessions without a bottle and diapers or would forget to give the child the medication for "colic" that had been prescribed by her pediatrician. Ms. A was herself in the custody of child protective services because of concern that she would neglect her baby. The clinicians suspected that Ms. A might have attention-deficit disorder and asked both Ms. A and her mother about her previous history. Ms. A's "being scattered" had been a major problem for a long time, not only during the perinatal period. When she was informed of the clinicians' impression, she seemed to feel relieved. Among other suggestions made to help her organize was a therapeutic trial of psycho-stimulant medication. She agreed. Ms. A was then able to think more clearly about future events, such as the fact that the baby might need a clean diaper or require feeding. She was also able to pay attention to several variables at one time, whereas before she had been able to focus on only one at a time. In addition, she could remember her child's needs, which before had seemed too overwhelming to handle.

Sometimes an adequate appraisal of the situation from the psychiatric point of view may mean the difference between success and failure in helping the infant. Problematic situations may include situations in which a young mother or father uses street drugs as a way to "treat" psychiatric symptoms. Also, a parent with marked irritability and mood lability may suffer from an undiagnosed mood disorder; treating this disorder might markedly improve a situation.

Anxiety disorders (e.g., severe social phobia, panic, generalized anxiety disorder, and posttraumatic conditions) can have a severe effect not only on the parent-child relationship but also on the family as a whole. A parent may live in constant fear that the baby will die and experience multiple somatic symptoms (e.g., lump in throat, palpitations, constant tension, sweating, diarrhea, shortness of breath) or may have unpredictable episodes of panic. When these symptoms are alleviated, parenting and family life become easier. The gamut of severe psychopathology can occur in the perinatal period as well, and the clinician can help by recognizing the problem and treating it or referring the patient.

At times, postpartum psychosis is very obvious, but often it is not. Only careful inquiry can uncover it. For example, a young woman recently said that she felt constantly nervous around her baby. When specific questions were asked, she alluded to the fact that she would hear her baby cry when, in reality, the baby was sleep. She would also visualize the infant covered in blood and hurt. She felt so frightened by these experiences that she had not told anyone. Adequate pharmacological treatment alleviated these symptoms of postpartum psychosis.

We suggest that the therapist who can reflect on several points of view when faced with a clinical situation can better take all of them into account. This diversity may lead to a more comprehensive understanding of the situation from several points of view. Then, based on what seem to be the clinical priorities, the therapist should decide on some formulations to present to the family and on what therapeutic interventions seem the most suitable for the problem, the child, the parent-child relationship, and the caregivers.

References

Bard KA: Parenting in primates, in Handbook of Parenting, Vol 2: Biology and Ecology of Parenting. Edited by Bornstein MH. Mahwah, NJ, Erlbaum, 1995, pp 27–58

Carter S, Osofsky JD, Hann DM: Speaking for the baby: a therapeutic intervention with adolescent mothers and their infants. Infant Mental Health Journal 12:291–301, 1991

Cramer B: Short-term dynamic psychotherapy for infants and their parents. Child Adolesc Psychiatr Clin N Am 4:649–660, 1995

Cramer B, Palacio-Espasa F: La pratique des psychothérapies meres-bébés: Études cliniques et techniques [The Practice of Mother-Infant Psychotherapy: Studies in Clinical Techniques]. Paris, Presses Universitaires de France, 1993

DeGangi GA: Treatment of sensory, emotional and attentional problems in regulatory disordered infants. Infants Young Child 3:9–19, 1991

Fonagy P: Mind reading as an element of sensitive parenting. Paper presented at the International Conference on Infant Studies, Atlanta, GA, April 1998

Fraiberg S, Shapiro V, Spitz Cherniss D: Treatment modalities, in Assessment and Therapy of Disturbances in Infancy. Edited by Fraiberg S. Northvale, NJ, Jason Aronson, 1989, pp 49–77

Gergely G, Watson JS: The social biofeedback model of parental affect-mirroring. Int J Psychoanal 77:1181–1212, 1996

Greenspan SL: Floor time: different types of children (shy, withdrawn, angry, distractible, negative, concrete, clinging), in Infancy and Early Childhood: The Practice of Clinical Assessment and Intervention With Emotional and Developmental Challenges. New York, International Universities Press, 1991, pp 501–542

Hoffmann JM: Making space. Infant Mental Health Journal 16:46–51, 1995

Howard BJ: Discipline in early childhood. Pediatr Clin North Am 38:1351–1369, 1991

Lebovici S: Le Nourrisson, la Mere et le Psychanaliste: Les Interactions Précoces [The Infant, the Mother and the Psychoanalyst: Early Interactions]. Paris, Paidos-Le Centurion, 1983

Lebovici S: L'homme dans le bébé [Within the person, the baby]. Revue Francaise de Psychanalyse 58:661–680, 1995

Lieberman A: Infant-parent psychotherapy with toddlers. Dev Psychopathol 4: 559–574, 1992

Lieberman A, Pawl J: Infant-parent psychotherapy, in Handbook of Infant Mental Health. Edited by Zeanah CH Jr. New York, Guilford, 1993, pp 427–442

Lillard AS: Pretend play skills and the child's theory of mind. Child Dev 64:348–371, 1993

Maldonado-Durán JM: La conducta del recién nacido normal [The behavior of the normal newborn], in Neonatologia [Neonatology]. Edited by Jasso-Gutierrez L. Mexico City, Interamericana-McGraw Hill, 1996, pp 49–59

Maldonado-Durán JM: Adjustment disorder, in Casebook of Infant Mental Health: Behavioral and Developmental Disorders. Edited by Lieberman A, Wieder S, Fenichel E. Washington, DC, Zero to Three, 1997, pp 181–194

Maldonado-Durán JM, Sauceda-Garcia JM: Evaluación clínica y tratamiento de los problemas de alimentación [Clinical assessment and treatment of feeding disturbances], in La Alimentación en la Primera Infancia y Sus Efectos en el Desarrollo [Feeding in Early Childhood and Its Effects on Development]. Edited by Lartigue T, Maldonado-Durán JM, Avila H. Mexico City, Plaza y Valdes, 1998, pp 363–390

McDonough SC: Promoting positive early parent-infant relationships through interaction guidance. Child Adolesc Psychiatr Clin N Am 4:661–672, 1995

Moro MR: Parents en exile: psychopathologie et migrations [Parents in Exile: Psychopathology and Migrations]. Paris, Presses Universitaires de France, 1994

Newman A: Noncompliance in Winnicott's Words. New York, New York University Press, 1995, pp 26–27

Olds DL, Eckenrode J, Henderson CR, et al: Long-term effects of home visitation on maternal life course and child abuse and neglect. JAMA 278:637–643, 1997

Ramsay M: Feeding disorder and failure to thrive. Child Adolesc Psychiatr Clin N Am 4:605–616, 1995

Stern DN: The Motherhood Constellation: A Unified View of Parent-Infant Psychotherapy. New York, Basic Books, 1995

Stoleru S, Morales-Huet M: Psychothérapies Mere-nourrison dans les Familles a Problemes Multiples [Mother-Infant Psychotherapies With Multi-Problem Families]. Paris, Presses Universitaires de France, 1989, pp 37–88

Vives-Rocabert J, Lartigue T: Apego y Vínculo Materno-Infantil [Attachment and Mother-Infant Bonding]. Guadalajara, Universidad de Guadalajara, Asociación Psicoanalítica Jaliscience, 1995

Wertsch JV, Tulviste P: Lev Semyonovich Vygotsky and contemporary developmental psychology, in A Century of Developmental Psychology. Edited by Parke RD, Ornstein PA, Rieser JJ, et al. Washington, DC, American Psychological Association, 1994, pp 331–356

Zeitlin S, Williamson GG: Coping in Young Children: Early Intervention Practices to Enhance Adaptive Behavior and Resilience. Baltimore, MD, Paul H Brookes, 1994

7

The Therapeutic Consultation

Serge Lebovici, M.D.
J. Armando Barriguete, M.D.
J. Luis Salinas, M.D.

Pour aller plus loin dans l'approche du terme empathie, il nous faut rappeller qu'il s'oppose à celui d'insight, équivalent de l'allemand Einsicht (voir en dedans) . . . le mot empathie en français est traduit du terme allemand Einfühlung. Autrement dit, il s'agit d'opposser "voir ou comprendre" à "sentir au-dedans."

To go further in our approach to the term empathy, we should remember that it is opposed to the term insight, which is equivalent to the German word *Einsicht* (to see inside) . . . the word empathy in French is a translation of the German word *Einfühlung*. In other words, one is trying to contrast "to see or to understand" to "feel from inside."

Serge Lebovici (1994a)

The term *therapeutic consultation* was used originally by Donald W. Winnicott in a brief paper he wrote in 1965 (Winnicott 1965/1989) and later in a book on the subject (Winnicott 1971). In the paper, Winnicott referred to a therapeutic approach designed for brief psychotherapy and oriented to the symptomatic management of a baby or child. This approach is in contrast to the traditional process of gradual opening common in the psychoanalytic technique.

The term was taken up by the senior author (Lebovici 1998a) and expanded to designate a therapeutic modality specifically for the infant (newborn to 3 years old) and his or her family. This technique also has

161

been elaborated by Mazet and Stoleru (1996) and others (Barriguete 1997; Barriguete et al. 1998). In France, the term has been used by many authors who wish to indicate that clinical work with young children should involve the parents, and that the therapist should not remain passive, imitating the psychoanalyst of adults who maintains an attitude of listening in relative silence and abstinence.

A therapeutic consultation is not psychoanalysis in the strict sense of the term. However, it is a clinical intervention undertaken by psychoanalysts or professionals in behavioral health with a vast knowledge of analytic technique and psychodynamics as described by Freud and others.

At the Centre Alfred Binet in Paris, where I (S.L.) worked for more than 20 years, I was in the habit of meeting with the parents and the child together. After having gained an understanding of the family genogram (genealogy) and the predicament (transgenerational mandate) of the child, I would see the parents by themselves. At the same time, I asked the child to make a drawing while waiting. I would then see the child without the parents. We customarily worked on the drawing as if it were a dream. Then we used some toys, such as wild or domesticated animals, that were representative of certain themes. Later, before asking the parents to reenter the office, I would ask the child whether we should show the drawing to the parents or just keep it between us. Along these technical lines, the intervention had a mutative character for the child—that is, it changed some dynamics and behaviors. Parents were always involved in the process.

The term *therapeutic consultation* has been applied differently in various centers. For instance, at the Centre Alfred Binet, Michel Ody has adopted the term, but with a very different meaning. The consultations of Ody's group may last many months. They also involve the parents in the treatment. But the original meaning of the term may be lost when it is also used to describe lengthy clinical work.

It is important to clarify that we understand the term to apply to the clinical approach to a symptomatic baby in the company of parents or caregivers. It is readily understandable why a therapeutic consultation is not a classical psychoanalysis: the subject that motivates the consultation is an infant in the literal sense of the word. Nevertheless, this therapeutic work demands a good deal of experience in the classical psychoanalysis of adults and children complemented by adequate training in the treatment of families and couples in conflict. Indeed, as practiced in some countries, the therapeutic consultation is a modality of psychodynamic family therapy. In Mexico, for example, it is the "family within the baby" that is studied and treated (Barriguete and Salinas 1999; Salinas et al. 2000).

CENTRAL CONCEPTS IN THERAPEUTIC WORK WITH INFANTS

Before we describe some of the main techniques used in therapeutic consultation, we will explain the concepts we have developed, which may be less familiar to English-speaking clinicians: a) transgenerational transmission, b) fantasmatic interactions, c) the tree of life or "psychic genogram," d) the earliest interactions, e) parentification, f) holding, and g) filiation and affiliation. These concepts are central to our therapeutic work; they form the basis for understanding what is happening with the baby and the family in their interrelationships. These concepts also direct the therapeutic intervention.

Transgenerational Transmission

The concept of transgenerational transmission involves the repetition of themes, perceptions, or behavioral patterns from one generation to the next (Lebovici 1992). We have even used the term *pathology of destiny* to denote extreme cases of such transgenerational transmission. Pathology of destiny refers to the idea that an infant may come into the world with a predetermined role or mission in life—for example, to save a marriage, to replace a lost child, to alleviate the loneliness of a woman, or to realize dreams and expectations unfulfilled by previous generations. If the pressure from these expectations is severe, one could say that the baby has come into the world with a destiny already charted. In less severe situations, there is no transgenerational mandate as such, but there is a tendency for the parents to perceive and interact with the child in a certain way that may represent themes from the life of the parents as children, or even from the life of the grandparents.

Even in the first interview, we may introduce the theme of transgenerational transmission. In this area of our clinical work, we have found a rich source of conflicts in the parents, many of which they are not aware of. These issues may become obstacles to the free and spontaneous participation of caregivers in interactions with the baby. Because of such unconscious conflicts, the parents' thoughts and feelings and their ability to care for the baby are clouded by what we call *fantasmatic interactions* (Kreisler and Cramer 1981; Lebovici 1983), discussed in the following subsection.

The transgenerational component of our work, therefore, addresses these kinds of "knots" that may exist in the mind of the parents or even the grandparents. The conflicts contribute to a deposit of unconscious psychic contents (metaphorically called "ghosts") in the parents' mind that will influence the formation of the infant's psychic structure, perhaps even shaping the child's self-concept as "bad." In this context, the work of Selma Fraiberg regarding "ghosts in the nursery" (Fraiberg et al. 1975, p. 387) is relevant to the idea of "ghosts" or fantasies deposited in the baby. Winnicott (1989) also reflected on the topic of unconscious fantasies, indicating that motivation has very deep determinants.

Fantasmatic Interactions

Fantasmatic interactions are unconscious ways of seeing, perceiving, and reacting to the baby that are rooted in the parents' own early experiences as a child reawakened or reactivated by the baby. Once reawakened, these feelings, perceptions, or conflicts are projected or deposited in the baby, regardless of the "real" characteristics of the child. For instance, one parent may perceive the baby's eyes as being similar to those of the parent's father and find them accusatory or persecutory (e.g., suggesting that the parent is not a good father or mother). Such accusations—a sense of not being good enough—are the reactivation of the parent's experience as a child with his or her own father. This distortion of the baby's eyes will influence future interactions between the parent and the baby.

The distortions occur to a greater or lesser degree in all parents. One cannot really be objective when it comes to one's children. Nevertheless, the distortions are a powerful influence on the parent's perception of the baby, which may be quite different from what an observer might see. For example, the clinician may see a happy baby, while the parent may see "a monster" or "a cross to be carried."

Tree of Life or "Psychic Genogram"

A corollary of transgenerational transmission, the concept of the tree of life or "psychic genogram," proposes to keep in mind a transgenerational and developmental perspective. Lebovici (1998b) suggested this idea to highlight a sort of "transgenerational saga" whose overture is the arrival of the newborn and that continues with a narrative of the history of how the family came to be. Ever since the pregnancy, the main actor in the scene has been the new generation, the future baby, who represents a re-generation, the new way of doing things. One could say that the tree of life grows and is modified with the birth of the baby. At this point, the ancestors make themselves present and are welcomed—or perhaps not. The parents may try to ward them off, to make them stay away from this occasion. With the modification of the family at the moment the baby

arrives, there is a new design to this tree of life. From a dialectical perspective, one could say that it is not only the past that determines the
present but also the present that allows the past to exist.

The fruit of the tree of life is the baby. In the conceptualization of the
so-called Bobigny (a section of Paris) school of earliest interactions
(directed by S.L.), four different aspects of every baby are crucial to take
into account. These representations are in the mind of every parent:

1. *The "real" baby.* The "real" baby is the actual baby in front of us, with
   his or her abilities, capacity to relate to and reinforce the parents, and
   so on.
2. *The imagined baby.* The imagined baby is a preconscious construction.
   It is an image of the baby produced during the pregnancy. It is formed
   during the states of reverie (daydreaming) of the mother or of the
   future mother and father. The selection of the name for the future
   baby usually takes place in this state.
3. *The fantasmatic baby.* The fantasmatic baby is essentially unconscious.
   It harks back to the mother's or father's wish as a child to have a baby.
   In the girl, it is close to her wish to have a baby with her own father,
   and in the boy, it is close to his wish to have a baby with his mother.
   These conflicts, when not elaborated, will influence the interaction
   between the parent and the baby in the present. What is not resolved
   comes back with intensified energy.
4. *The cultural (or mythic) baby.* The cultural (or mythic) baby is also the
   carrier of a cultural shadow of the past of the parents, mother and
   father. The concept was introduced by Marie Rose Moro (Moro
   and Barriguete 1998; Moro and Nathan 1995). The baby represents
   something or has a meaning or a mission depending on the cultural
   context. The infant also represents cultural images relevant to that
   social group as he or she is initiated into the traditions of a certain culture.

Earliest Interactions

The earliest interactions between mother and child make up a very rich
topic. We highlight here only what is particularly useful to consider during therapeutic work with parents and babies.

More is known every day about the incredible capacities in the baby
designed to interact with others. The neonate recognizes the mother's
voice from the first day of life and recognizes the odor of the mother in
the third day of life. In fact, as research with nonnutritive suction in utero
has shown, the fetus recognizes the mother's voice during the seventh

month of intrauterine life. Ethological observations (Montagner 1988) have suggested that the initial bonding between mother and child may determine the baby's ability to develop further capacities in a normal way. An adequate bonding may also help the mother to be more sensitive to her infant and to have a more positive relationship with the child months later (Kennel and Klaus 1998).

Our group has described what we have called the "affective bath" as a crucial aspect of the interaction between caregivers and the baby. In this process, the parents "wrap" the child through their different actions (e.g., stroking, talking, looking, holding). It starts with the first encounter between the parent and the baby and has many manifestations. Some are readily observable: touching the baby's fingers, smelling the child, exploring the baby's body. Some are perceived only intuitively, as in the tenderness the parent manifests while holding and talking to the baby. Indeed, to thrive emotionally, the infant needs a "bath" of affects as much as food.

Moving from ethological to clinical observations, we find that Montagner (1988) has multiple examples of the rich social life of even very young babies. According to him, the classic developmental sequence, point–touch–grasp, will evolve to the next sequence in motor, cognitive, and social development, which would be the sequence point–grasp–touch, all eminently social activities.

Winnicott (1970) proposed a metaphor: the baby moves forward in development in front of the mirror that is the mother and the family. The baby sees the mother who, in turn, is looking at the baby. By the age of 4 months, the baby is aware that the person he or she regularly sees is a mother—that is, there is a more exclusive and uniquely intimate relationship between two. (Winnicott emphasized that this exclusive relationship develops regardless of whether the mother is ugly or beautiful.)

At the same time, the mother looks at her baby who looks at her. There is, indeed, this effect of mutual mirroring through which the baby recognizes the mother and feels alive in her arms. Perhaps it is one of the first instances of the baby's feeling alive in a continuous way and that he or she is a functioning being. Sandler (1993) pointed out that this same gaze exchange occurs in psychoanalysis and is an important therapeutic element. In some cultures (e.g., some groups in Africa), mutual gaze exchange is forbidden and other ways of maintaining contact, such as touch, are preferred.

The baby in the mother's arms will usually cuddle and may direct the mouth toward her breast. Later on, this reflex will disappear, but it may be reactivated if the mother shows an animated facial expression. The animated face may be the first representation of maternal care. Bowlby

(1969/1978) has suggested that this precocious form of attachment tends to be replaced by other forms of interaction. In any case, the very young baby who sleeps in the arms of his or her mother does not need to find any other relationships outside the primary attachment.

The mother always tries to be reassured that her baby is all right. When she puts the baby in the crib, the infant may reach toward her. (The human baby cannot yet—as the baby chimpanzee can—run toward the mother.) At this point, she rejoices and says, "You are great, my baby, you recognize my voice." Within 2 weeks after the baby learns to extend his or her arms toward the mother when she comes into sight, he or she is able to reach out after just hearing her voice, without even seeing her.

If there is a disruption at this time (e.g., when a baby loses his or her mother), the maternal representations are damaged and the baby remains confused and frustrated. A reparation is possible when the mother returns after a separation. When the separation is too long and no specific person looks after the baby, the baby falls into a depressive state that may resemble autistic regression. In the very young infant, physiology and psychology in the strict sense are not really differentiated. The baby reacts to emotions with his or her whole being. This reaction is also true of adults, but it is more readily observable in infants.

As these interactions evolve, we can distinguish two major realms of development: one in the baby and the other in the parents. In the first realm, the child goes through a process that begins in a state of absolute dependency, moves into relative dependency, and, it is hoped, arrives at a state of psychological autonomy. (By autonomy, we mean a state of rational interdependence, which is a social and relational dimension. Without relationships, there is no autonomy.) In traditional terms, the process moves from the pleasure principle toward the reality principle, and from autoerotic satisfaction to object-relatedness. The other realm, discussed immediately below, is best described as the process of parentification.

Parentification

In addition to the baby's development, we have the parents' own development as caregivers and as participants in a new group. Lebovici (1992) suggested that as the baby is born, so too is the mother born. Of course, this "rebirth" would also be true of the father and the grandparents, particularly with the first child. The ability of the parents to take care of the baby and to meet his or her challenges and needs will either give satisfaction and self-confidence to the mother and father or lead to frustration. We call the process *parentification*. It is the psychological task of becoming a parent. The mother's "self-of-rearing" (Barriguete et al. 2000)—that is, her own upbringing—will influence her ability or capacity to become a mother. This self-of-rearing is rooted in what the caregiver experienced vis-à-vis her or his own caregiver during infancy and childhood.

There is also another subsystem: the marital couple vis-à-vis the baby. There are shared fantasies, perceptions, and wishes as the two families of origin in the mind of each parent interact during the process of having a child. The quality of the marital relationship will allow for the satisfaction of intimacy and dependency needs, for the needs of the parents to be looked after, and for the toleration of the baby's enormous dependency. Or, to the contrary, the marital relationship may drain energy and make the task of caregiving more difficult.

Indeed, during the perinatal period, there is an activation of what we call "the self-of-rearing" or "self-of-upbringing," which takes a temporal preeminence when the parents are called on to look after a dependent human being whose survival hinges on their ability and disposition to meet his or her needs.

We concur with the view of Stern (1995) that it is crucial to observe three interrelated levels of discourse in the interactions between a mother and her infant (this discourse is internal, but its content can be inferred): a) the mother's discourse or dialogue with her own mother, particularly when the mother was a child; b) the mother's discourse with herself as a mother (a new identity); and c) the mother's discourse with her baby. If the clinician keeps these three dimensions in mind, the themes that preoccupy the mother and that may cause disharmony vis-à-vis the baby usually become more apparent.

Holding

Holding refers to the emotional behavior of the mother and father with the baby. It involves the physical act of holding the child, but it does not stop there. Holding also involves providing support for the emotional development of the child and for the integration of the self. This ability to hold, a product of the primary maternal preoccupation, works as an auxiliary ego to the baby. The child's development of a true or false self will depend on the success or failure of this emotional support. A false self is the acquisition of behaviors that give the appearance of security but hide profound anxieties and insecurity in the child. The holding or containing of the baby buffers the interactions of the child with the environment and provides manageable experiences, helping the baby to avoid any overwhelming or traumatic ones as much as possible.

The self of the young infant is an incipient one; there are no organized functions of the ego, self representations, or representations of the other (object). However, an emerging self exists and continues to develop, conditioned by the "relational dominions"(Stern 1985). These interactions with others determine both the infant's self-experience and the experience of other people (to-be-with). As these relationships evolve, an identity is being generated; so, too, is awareness of the body, sensations, feelings, and perceptions. All of this development generates protorepresentations that evolve with time. The "prenarrative" experience (Stern 1993) will give way to narratives, actual recollections, memories, explanations of previous experiences, accounts of events, and so forth.

Winnicott (1965) was interested in the mother-infant interaction. Psychoanalysis has emphasized what happens in the mother's mind regarding this relationship. Winnicott, however, paid attention to the actual interaction between baby and mother. The mother creates a space in her mind in which she is able to comprehend and process the anxieties and concerns of her child using her intellect, intuition, and emotions. This process, in turn, contains the baby and helps the infant deal with anxiety.

Winnicott (1965) also looked at the interpersonal space. What he called the "sustaining environment," an actual activity of the caregiver, allows the infant to create an internal sustaining environment, so to speak. The caregiver helps the baby metabolize anxieties. Similarly, the mental health professional in the therapeutic consultation aims to create a sustaining environment where spontaneity and hope can emerge and where the drama of the baby and the family can be represented in the presence of the clinician.

Filiation and Affiliation

The senior author (Lebovici 1993) has proposed two additional terms that belong to the notion of the tree of life: filiation and affiliation. Filiation (from the Latin *filius*, son, and *filia*, daughter) is the psychological work in the baby, and later on in the child, of considering himself or herself to be a child of the parents or the child of a certain family and thus a part of that family. Affiliation makes a more complex psychic demand on the child, and later on the adult, to consider himself or herself a part of multiple generations, a social group, and a culture. This social group represents a number of things: how babies are looked after, how we play with them, what we want for them, and how we seek help when they have problems.

A developmental line runs from filiation to affiliation, from considering oneself as a child of one's parents to being a child of one's extended family and social and cultural group. The larger group represents models of relating, of psychic life, and of representing the world. The development of filiation and affiliation may proceed in a healthy manner. On the other hand, difficulties may arise when the person does not feel inclined to embrace the family or group, or when the belonging is denied, disavowed, or escaped from as if the person had originated de novo.

TECHNIQUE OF THERAPEUTIC CONSULTATION

When Winnicott (1965/1989) wrote, "I would not say that a full-scale psychoanalysis is always better for the patient than a psychotherapeutic interview" (p. 318), he was referring to clinical work with children and their parents. Of course, work with an infant does not mean that the parents of a symptomatic child cannot receive a recommendation to undertake psychoanalysis themselves. Winnicott continued: "It is well known that the first interview in an analysis can contain material that will come forward for analysis for months and even years. . . . That which I am calling the psychotherapeutic interview makes the fullest possible use of this relatively undefended material"(p. 319).

This relative lack of defenses is even more obvious in clinical interventions with babies under 1 year of age. The "motherhood constellation" (Stern 1995) provides extremely fertile psychological terrain. The parents of the infant, understandably worried and anxious about their baby's symptoms, show very few defenses and do whatever they can to help the therapist understand the situation.

In our work, we create a clinical setting with a global ambiance of trust and exploration. The sessions are intense and the interventions of the clinician are much more active—compared with the attitude of abstinence in the traditional psychoanalytic interview. Paraphrasing Winnicott (1971), we note a difference between the technique of therapeutic consultation and that of psychoanalysis. In the latter, the transference neurosis unfolds little by little and is used for interpretation. In the therapeutic interview, the therapist has a preestablished role based on the expectations of the parent, namely, that the therapist will be helpful, there is hope for the baby, and the situation will improve after the intervention of the clinician. In short, there is very active participation by the therapist. Such participation is informed by the therapist's understanding of the psychodynamics of the interactions and of the situation. It does not involve giving quick advice simply to satisfy the wishes of the parents.

Referring to therapeutic interviews, Winnicott (1965/1989) said that there was an inherent danger: the possibility of doing nothing. Such inactivity stems from excessive cautiousness or ignorance on the part of the therapist. In our clinical work, we suggest ideas or constructions that are also addressed to one or both parents. We are not averse to making an intervention that is appropriate in the context of individual psychotherapy or in couples therapy, although the parents or couple may not consciously realize that their relationship is a focus of intervention.

Following Fraiberg's method (Fraiberg and Fraiberg 1980) but adding the presence of the father, we proceed in the following manner in the early childhood clinic. The mother takes the baby in her arms while a psychotherapist observes the participants in this interaction. The psychotherapist also listens to the mother and father talking about their predicament. In the parents' discourse, the clinician discovers the imaginary baby who is the carrier of their latent wishes. These wishes, or desires, are a part of the transgenerational transmission of themes and hopes. A still deeper dimension of the parents' perception of the baby is unconscious, the fantasmatic baby. In a therapeutic consultation, bringing these unconscious fantasies to the surface in a fairly direct manner or early in the therapeutic work may have considerable therapeutic effect (Lebovici 1998a).

The therapist will pay particularly close attention to various dimensions such as all nonverbal interactions. In the earliest parent-child transactions, nonverbal exchanges are crucial. The clinician then reflects on, works with, and conceptualizes this relational dimension. He or she is a participant-observer. If the clinician is able to remain in the position of observer of relationships and nonverbal interactions, a number of intrapsychic processes will start becoming clear. These intrapsychic processes will throw light on what is happening now in the baby and in parent-infant interactions.

We pay special attention to the actual choreography that unfolds in the presence of the clinician—the movements, gestures, and communications between the baby and parents. Our colleagues from Lausanne, Switzerland (Fivaz-Depeursinge et al. 1996), have formalized this procedure in their observations of "triadic interactions" (baby-mother-father exchanges). We carefully note the parents' way of holding the baby and particularly their spontaneous gestures and verbalizations that take place without thinking, in a free response to the baby's movements or initiatives. We illustrate these points with a brief vignette:

> The first case of therapeutic consultation that I (S.L.) treated deserves to be recalled: It dealt with a "modern couple" who brought me their baby, a little boy named Pierre, less than 1 year old, who virtually did not sleep. He had been conceived after his parents had been lost in the Sahara Desert and had accepted the idea of dying together. The parents said that Pierre had been conceived in the mountains, in the open air.

They felt it was almost a miracle that they had not died, and that later on Pierre had been born from such circumstances. Drama surrounded the origins of this little boy.

At night, Pierre slept (or was expected to sleep) in a room far from his parents. His mother attempted to be very modern, free, and independent by working outside the home. But she also felt guilty leaving her son in the care of strangers during the day. She would often come home from work early and was eager to show Pierre that she was interested in him. She wanted to use the latest techniques to take care of him. She had read that she should provide the baby skin-to-skin contact, and she used to take the baby in her arms after removing or lifting up her bra and other clothing.

At the time of the consultation, I heard the baby crying in the waiting room where he was being held in his paternal grandmother's arms. The mother offered me a cigarette, which I declined. I asked that the baby be brought in. The mother took him and came into the consulting room. The baby was there, taking refuge in his mother's arms, but with a hyperextended torso. She provided skin-to-skin contact, but I noticed that Pierre did not look at her at all. On her part, the mother appeared tense and restless, and she could hardly keep from walking around. She crooned a vague song to her baby. It appeared as though she was trying to make contact with her "almost lost" baby but could not manage to connect. My immediate feeling was one of sadness at seeing that neither the mother nor the child could find each other, and that perhaps the mother felt she did not deserve to have a baby or that the baby was so fragile that he could die anytime.

I then remarked that she had a beautiful baby and that it would be all right to look at him. She covered herself and gazed at her baby. At that moment, a deep and long exchange of gazes took place between mother and baby. After a while, this mutual gazing appeared to allow Pierre to go to sleep. From then on, he had no more insomnia.

My impression was that during this brief exchange, a representation of her father (i.e., the therapist) had given permission to Pierre's mother not only to "have the baby" but also to enjoy him. The benign comment "The baby is beautiful and it is all right to look at him" seemed to produce a great sense of relief in the mother.

When I saw this family again several months later, the baby was now standing. About that time, I left the Centre Alfred Binet, where I had seen this family, to join the Faculty of Medicine at Bobigny. I wanted to follow up with this family. I was about to contact them, when I received a letter from them asking me for another consultation. The mother said that Pierre slept very well now but had become quite afraid when his father left to go on an airplane trip, which occurred frequently. Pierre's mother also thought he was afraid his father would be attacked by a lion.

Shortly after this, I visited with the parents about the intense phobia that had been reported in Pierre. The father asked to see the videotape we had made during the first consultation. When he saw his wife offer me a cigarette, he seemed unhappy and reproached her for having "come on" to me. She acknowledged that she had, indeed, tried to do so. She said she had been nervous and anxious and thought she acted this way in such situations. After some time, things settled down and the couple resumed their usual life together. When Pierre was 5 years old, he had a successful psychotherapy with me.

Fear of death was a persistent theme in this family, particularly in the mother. Later on, it manifested itself in the child's fear that the father would die. After the therapist spoke with them about the fear of death, the parents appeared to be less in conflict, and the phobia in the child abated. The mother's constant fear of loss also abated.

During consultation, we also try to observe the anticipatory responses of the parents toward the infant, as distinguished from their maneuvers to sustain and contain the baby. These anticipatory responses are actions, verbalizations, or gestures that occur not in response to the baby's cries or requests for food but in anticipation of the baby's actions and move-ments. It is particularly in these spontaneous and "guessing" reactions that we find the intensity and dramatic nature of fantasmatic interactions par excellence. This is so because the perceptions and desires to act in a certain way are not as clearly determined by obvious actions of the baby, but instead by perceptions of the meaning of what the infant is going to do, wants, or expects. The mother and father "guess" what the baby wants or needs, which is fertile terrain for enacting projections and distortions. In these moments, the "motherhood constellation," the family of origin, and the couple's relationship with each other are particularly influential.

The goals of the therapeutic consultation as practiced at the Bobigny School are

- To generate observations on the interactions between mother and baby, as well as on the interactions of other family members, particularly the father.
- To allow the parents to talk about themselves, their families, and their past, and perhaps about existing interactional patterns that might be repeating themselves in the present. This discussion allows for the evocation of possible fantasies projected onto the baby.
- To help the therapist understand, with the help of the parents and the baby, the unconscious meaning of observed behavior.
- To enable the therapist to identify intensely with the various members of the family: How would it feel to be the baby in this family? How would it feel to be, first, the mother and, then, the father?

For the parents, the therapeutic consultation provides a scenario in which words will surface to describe the turmoil of changing identifications they recently went through with the arrival of the baby. It includes experiences that are not yet named, representations that the therapist tries to help the parents put into words. A major purpose of the consultation is to help the parents unlock or disengage themselves from those primary identifications mentioned previously with regard to the baby and, instead, to be more themselves and, therefore, use the words "I" and "mine" with confidence.

Problem Areas

During the therapeutic consultation, a process of multidimensional observation is triggered (Lebovici 1983) that allows one to observe

- A narration or direct observation of the symptoms in the baby, as well as the infant's functioning in general.
- The details of the interaction and relationship between the baby and the mother and father or caregivers.
- Other factors surrounding motherhood and maternal care (stressors, adjustments, demands on the parents).
- The personality of the mother.
- The personality of the father.
- The family as a whole (Stierlin and Weber 1989).
- Any sociological and cultural issues (Moro and Nathan 1995).

This method of conducting the initial evaluation is similar to that proposed by Zero to Three (Lieberman et al. 1996). The clinician attempts to discover, rather quickly during the therapeutic consultation, the imaginary and fantasmatic images that the parents or caregivers have of their baby and any transgenerational issues impinging on the current situation. At least three generations are considered. The following areas are examined: a) the ordinal position of the child; b) the gender of the infant; c) the actual body of the baby, how the baby looks, or the phenotype, as well as any possible contributing genetic factors; and d) the degree of differentiation versus. fusion reached by the family. The fourth area is a crucial aspect that can determine the future differentiation of the child's self.

The cultural dimension is also explored because it dictates many of the early interactions. Knowledge of the cultural background allows us to understand what is conceived of as "the other" or the "not me" and how one deals with it—for instance, with the baby, with the family one has acquired (in-laws), and, in the case of immigrants, with caregiving practices that are different. The supplementation of the knowledge of psychodynamics with that provided by anthropology makes it possible to better understand the cultural issues involved in each family. This approach is practiced by clinicians who refer to their work as "perinatal ethnopsycho-analysis" (Moro and Barriguete 1998).

Our therapeutic work is the analysis of what we have named "the family within the baby," which is nothing other than the study of the family, taking the baby as the point of departure and the study of the parent-baby interaction into the transgenerational realm. We agree with Fraiberg et al. (1983) that "when a baby is at the center of a treatment, something happens that has no parallel in any other form of psychotherapy" (p. 56). It illustrates the positive role that the child's development can play in family change; the changes in the baby determine changes in the family system. The baby is thus an unconventional patient whose parents are collaborating in the treatment and are "talking patients." In turn, the therapist often "speaks for the baby" and takes into account the baby's affects, needs, and especially the response to the parents, who at times have difficulty noticing these cues.

The therapist becomes a bridge between parents and child and often has a sense of urgency to intervene on behalf of the baby, particularly when the baby shows a "failure to survive" (Fraiberg and Fraiberg 1980). This sense of urgency is a metaphor for what we describe as "enaction" (Lebovici 1994a), a particular modality of empathy (Lebovici 1998b) (see next subsection). In this sense, it is true that therapists often feel that "[n]o baby can wait for the resolution of the parental neurosis that is impeding his or her development. The baby also needs to get help" (Lebovici 1998c, p. 120).

By observing the parents' interactions, maneuvers, and ministrations and the baby's responses, as well as how accurately the parents "read" or interpret the infant, one can discern the unfolding of the parental representations of the baby, whether few or many. We have developed the concept of a "unity of the earliest interactions," meaning that the physiology and symptoms of the baby are closely linked with the mind/emotions/actions of the caregivers and their various expressions in multiple channels of interaction. What the caregivers do at this time has more impact on the physiology of the baby than on his or her psychology.

The Sacred Moment

Our group has placed special emphasis on the phenomenon of "the sacred moment" during the therapeutic consultation. This concept was originally advanced by Winnicott (1971). He thought that the first interview with any child and family was crucial and full of meaning. It had several opportunities for a therapeutic intervention, opportunities that could be used profitably by the consultant—or missed altogether. During the first session, there is the hope that the clinician-consultant can help. Parents deposit their magical expectations in the therapist and are prepared for the first interview, hoping that things will go better from then on.

The clinician-consultant has to create an environment where such trust and self-revelation are possible. Spontaneity and freedom in the consultant are essential ingredients, as well as an attitude of observing and listening to the situation of those who come to seek help or advice. In the first session, there is an element of surprise for all participants. The caregivers may find themselves surprised at what they are willing to reveal about themselves. The sacred moment is a genuine encounter between the mind of the therapist and the minds of the family members. The consultant "understands," while those who consult feel understood, held, and contained. This feeling of being understood is therapeutic in itself, providing hope and help for the family to continue therapeutic explorations and endeavors.

In the case of the infant mental health clinic, it is during the sacred moment that the consultant experiences a sense of surprise at understanding the predicaments faced by the infant, the family, or both. Pieces fall into place, so to speak, and there is a sense of "sudden understanding" of the forces that led to the present problem, fueling or maintaining it.

I (S.L.) have practiced therapeutic consultation for some 15 years as a variation of practicing brief psychotherapy with infants. In retrospect, I believe that since I began seeing babies for psychophysiological difficulties (e.g., sleeping, feeding, crying), I have been incorporating the notion of Winnicott's sacred moment in my work. In this moment, I am able to give the mother an interpretation that involves a metaphor (in French, *interpretation metaphorisante*, an interpretation that is expressed in a metaphor). In fact, during this sacred moment, I generate a metaphor based on a co-construction with the mother.

I once had the opportunity of presenting such a case to Anna Freud in which the sacred moment was a very salient feature. She told me (not without a certain disdain) that she already had heard about cases like mine from Winnicott. Be that as it may, I was quite impressed by Winnicott's attitude. During several consultations, in which Winnicott listened to our cases and presented his clinical work, he had shown a group of French analysts work in which he had acted in a very intuitive and novel fashion. He saw many families in his busy practice, and he gave them interpretations about their behavior. He assumed the role of the parents and probably imitated their behavior as he imagined it. It is well known that his interpretations were based on metaphor, which gave his theories their celebrated character. In a few words, one could say that he lived the object in its reality and that he made objects out of fantasies.

For example, a 9-month-old infant wanted to play with the mother, which suggested a metaphor to Winnicott (1947/1958) that he attributed to the baby: "Mom, I am too old to put your breast in my mouth, but I will play with you." At this point, the mother agrees to play. Her play quickly shows one side of her feelings toward her son: her anger toward him. In this instance, Winnicott reminds us of the multiple causes of a mother's anger at her baby. She has to wake up several times at night, feed the baby on demand, and tend to the baby whenever there is a call for attention. She may experience disgust at having to clean the baby's feces. Yet the mother accepts this role during this period of life because the baby needs her constantly. She, in turn, gives metaphors to her child necessary for the child's own emotional and cognitive development. In these metaphors, the mother presents the world to her baby in a manageable way, creating an illusion of more or less complete safety. Without these metaphors, the baby could become depressed or disorganized.

The anxieties or anguish that commonly develops in the baby at 8 months of age are compensated for by maternal reactions (e.g., protection, containment, reassurance, even the mother's mere presence). Research has shown that some babies are not able to arrive at the state of intersubjectivity described by Stern (1985). Even before this research, Winnicott (1953/1958) described the importance of the transitional object, a metaphor that helps the baby deal with anxieties and separations. If the anxieties and fears of this period in the baby's life are not adequately resolved, the baby may become fixated on objects later on.

Narcissism in the Therapeutic Consultation

It might seem surprising that we emphasize issues of narcissism in a description of this sort of therapeutic work. Through many years of experience, we have come to the realization that narcissism is a central topic in work with infants. The theme of narcissism is important when thinking about the following issues, which are present to some extent in all consultation:

- The dominant projections of the parents toward the infant
- The reactions of the baby to those projections
- The recent maladjustment or imbalance that led to the request for evaluation
- Elements in the baby and parents one could call pre-transferential (a transference relationship has not yet been established during the first consultation)

- Elements in the therapist one could call pre-countertransferential (initial feelings and reactions in the analyst toward the baby, the family, and the situation)

Concepts related to narcissism have been dealt with extensively by Palacio-Espasa and Manzano (Manzano et al. 1993). Their book is based on the idea of "narcissistic scenarios of parenthood." They show that although Freud studied child psychopathology and its future to some extent, he did not address the parental conflicts that may form the root of those difficulties. The authors suggest that the child essentially reacts or "gives in" to the fantasmatic pressure of the parents to behave and feel in a certain way because the child has needs for attachment and holding.

It should be recognized that in most situations the narcissistic elements of the parents, which lead them to pressure the child to assume certain attitudes and behaviors, are quite benign and ultimately produce normal and healthy situations. But in less fortunate circumstances, the infant is virtually "hit" with parental projections, which then become inscribed in the child's character. Manzano et al. (1993) describe in great detail a number of clinical constellations commonly observable in actions that lead to psychopathology.

A common situation occurs, for example, when the parents themselves were abandoned as children. They strive to achieve the identity and role of parents as if to establish their right to be good parents. This intention is also an indication of the guilt that the parents believe rests with the grandparents. However, the injured narcissism of the child is often not repaired or does not respond adequately to the hopes of the parents (injured children who are now adults) because the child may not act in a way suitable to reinforce or meet the parents' narcissistic needs. Instead, the child may not be ideal, that is, what the parents expected. Later, the child may behave in a way dictated by the Oedipus complex, perhaps demeaning the parents or competing with one of them and thereby failing to satisfy their narcissistic needs for reassurance, praise, and a feeling of having been "good parents." In such cases, the narcissistic wounds that the parents suffered as children reemerge or are reactivated.

The therapeutic work also can be complicated when these narcissistic issues are prominent but unresolved. This possibility is important because the therapist is often considered a parent, also perhaps within the narcissistic orbit of the parents of the baby. It is not infrequent for the analyst or therapist to react negatively to projections and expectations of this sort that originate in the parents. They can be considered under the general topic of countertransferential difficulties.

Finally, there is the issue of the narcissism of the therapist. Understanding one's narcissism may be an essential part of helping the family. I (S.L.) personally have found it very rewarding to reflect on these issues in my therapeutic work, something that is not common in the traditional psychoanalyst or clinician.

In the best-case scenario, the therapeutic consultation allows the parents to modify their fantasmatic projections on the baby and renounce their search for a narcissistic confirmation that they might otherwise impose on their baby. Through this work, the identificatory phenomena that occur with the succession of generations can be transformed. The baby will not be forced to stay in the assigned place, particularly in cases in which he or she is perceived negatively as an accuser, as a persecutor, or as a scapegoat. The following case vignette shows how a mother's perception of her baby revealed her view of her own self as a child:

> A mother and father came to the clinic with their 2½-year-old child, Andre. The mother had gone to the family doctor, who in turn called the psychiatrist because the mother was on the verge of "losing it" with her child. She was so distraught in the doctor's office that a consultation was arranged with the psychiatrist for later that day.
>
> Andre was a cute and very curious little boy. He wanted to explore everything within sight. Highly verbal and intelligent, he asked many questions. When his mother was asked what the problems were, she started sobbing. Andre's father also cried, but silently. The mother said that Andre was terrible and unmanageable and that he was an abuser.
>
> She said all these things in front of Andre. When the therapist asked Andre if he was a good boy, he said with conviction, "No." His mother proceeded with a number of "accusations" about how Andre had pinched her, kicked her, and called her names. She showed the therapist the places on her body where this had happened. As she cried with great feeling about her son, she kept saying, "He is an abuser. He is an abuser." The therapist had the fantasy that the mother was talking about an adult in her life as a child, someone who had treated her very badly, and the wounds were still raw. As the interview progressed, the mother revealed that she had, indeed, been very mistreated as a child.
>
> On seeing his mother crying, Andre asked why she was crying and appeared somewhat scared. His mother said she was not crying for any particular reason. Andre looked at the therapist, who suggested to the little boy that perhaps he could give his mother a hug. He did. At the end of the session, the therapist told Andre that it would be fine to give mother hugs if he wanted, hoping to reduce the tension between the "abuser" and the mother. In a follow-up session, the mother came with Andre. She said he was behaving much better and, smiling, that she "had gotten more hugs in a week from Andre than in the previous 2 years." It seemed that she needed a great deal of reassurance from her son that he loved her in order to allow herself to see him in a more benign fashion.

Requirements of the Therapist

We wish to emphasize one aspect of the therapist's work. Work with infants requires the expression of a new self in the therapist. The task at hand is to provide help to a baby within a family. The therapist has an analytic orientation and a family therapy dynamics (systemic) framework. The clinician must develop an analytic self, with the attributes of empathy, an ability to construct metaphors (*un self metaphorisante*) or to observe them, and the capacity to allow himself or herself to "become" (temporarily) the parent or the infant in order to experience—through ideation and somatic sensations—the "knot" in which the infant or family is tied up.

The therapist will use his or her own self-of-rearing to grasp the plight of the baby and the family. Through the self-experience of having been a child and having had a mother and a father, the therapist is capable of intervention that will promote the survival, maturation, and growth of the infant.

At present, I (S.L.) customarily see families in clinical practice two times over a 2-week period. The consultation involves constructing a story or narration that allows for an understanding of the parents' tree of life. It is not only a genogram but also an examination of the early relationship between the parents and their own parents, whether alive or not, so as to form an impression of this process of filiation.

Contrary to the opinion of some colleagues (e.g., Cramer and Palacio-Espasa) who believe that modifications take place only in the parents (e.g., in the identificatory projections of the mother toward the baby), we believe one can also have a direct therapeutic effect on the baby. Elsewhere, I (S.L.) have provided examples of situations in which one has a direct impact on the baby (Lebovici 1994b), as illustrated by the case of Matthew. This case also illustrates the process of using metaphors for a therapeutic purpose.

In the case of Matthew, I (S.L.) was able to interact with the baby and, through these pleasurable interactions, was able to elicit empathic feelings in the mother. These new feelings of empathy contradicted her previous negative feelings toward the infant. The child's positive response to me was the child's contribution toward making his situation better vis-à-vis his mother. After having carefully observed a videotape of these interactions between this baby and me many times, I have reached the conclusion that it was my interaction with the baby that had the most therapeutic value. While caressing his head, I told him, "You are beautiful." At that point, the baby became interested in me and responded even while he was in his mother's arms. It was as if, at this point, the baby had helped the mother recognize the importance of the father symbolically in me, the therapist. I introduced the father into the scene by telling him, "The baby dances with his mother like you have previously danced with your wife."

Incidentally, as will be explained in the next subsection, the enaction released in me by this family led me to experience a "metaphorizing emotion" leading to my decision to say to the baby "You are beautiful," and to show tenderness toward him. Perhaps it also gave permission to the mother to accept her baby and to reevaluate his attributes. It was a co-constructed moment of harmony (a sacred moment) between mother, baby, and me. This harmony allowed the mother to love her baby. She had previously been overcome by feelings of guilt and self-accusations that it was her negligence that had led to a daughter's death before Matthew's birth.

Enaction

I (S.L.) recently proposed the concept of "enaction" (Lebovici 1994a), an idea that deepens our clinical work with the transference from the parents and the baby to the therapist, as well as with the countertransference (the therapist's reactions to the parents and the baby or to the family). Enaction is rooted in the response of the therapist to motherhood and fatherhood (Barriguete 1997). One could say that it involves the therapist paying close attention to his or her own actions, verbalizations, and feelings vis-à-vis the family. Some of these feelings are an internal enactment of unconscious themes. The therapist may become critical, for instance, or may have a wish to criticize the parents or feel anger toward them, something perhaps out of character for the therapist or unrelated to what is being currently discussed. The feeling, the enactment in the therapist, would be used to inform him or her about the themes of anger and criticism in the parents as such. It might lead the consultant to explore this topic during the consultation. In other words, therapists use themselves in resonance with the family, analyzing their own feelings or wishes to act so they can understand the dilemma of the parents and the baby with whom they are consulting.

I (S.L.) have referred to enaction as a process of *mise en acte* (setting onstage). Anna Freud also used this phrase, but I was not really satisfied with that term. Rather than understanding enaction merely as a drama of the outward scene, I have concluded that enaction is what one *feels in one's body* during the consultation: what the therapist feels with his or her body in an empathic response. There is something felt but not acted on despite what the term might suggest. The therapist "feels" like doing something during the consultation. This reaction results from what is unfolding in the interaction between parents and baby: "My body responds, but the action is not externalized, it is an action inside my head . . . It goes a step beyond empathy" (Lebovici 1998b, p. 145).

In enaction, the consultant experiences an internal movement that may be initiated by countertransference, which is more verbal or language-based. Enaction is somatic; perhaps it is an agitation, something that stems from empathy. There is an internal *mise en scène* of the situation experienced by the baby and the parents. The therapist uses this bodily information to understand, to realize, to contain, and to interpret.

This important therapeutic tool requires the analyst to be comfortable being "taken over by the situation," perhaps even being overcome or temporarily swept along by it. It is an authentic internal movement in which the therapist is on the verge of losing control, thus allowing the experience to inform him or her of what is happening in this family. Only in this internal movement is it possible to know what is happening. The therapist is then guided by these experiences and emotions, registering but not acting on them. Perhaps it is a moment when, as an infant does from moment to moment, the therapist is able to experience with the body what belongs to other realms: emotions, words, visual and auditory messages being exchanged, and movements and actions taking place in the here and now.

CONCLUSION

We hope that this account of our clinical work and technique will elicit interest in the psychodynamic issues that we believe are important to consider when dealing with parents and children, particularly in the perinatal period. We find these concepts useful in working with many infants and families. As has perhaps become evident, our position gives less weight to the particular details of the "symptoms" presented by the baby, except as they may provide clues about the dynamics involved in the situation. In some families, addressing these psychodynamic elements proves extremely helpful in dispelling anxieties, distorted perceptions, and fears. These concepts also provide clues about the optimal development of the baby in the context of his or her caregiving environment.

REFERENCES

Barriguete JA: L'Enaction dans la Consultation Thérapeutique [Enaction during the therapeutic consultation]. Unpublished thesis for university diploma. Paris, University of Paris XIII, 1997

Barriguete JA, Salinas JL: La consulta terapéutica: la familia en el bebé [The therapeutic consultation: the family within the baby], in Violencia Social, Sexualidad y Creatividad [Social Violence, Sexuality and Creativity]. Edited by Vives J. México City, Plaza y Valdes, 1999, pp 215–226

Barriguete JA, Lebovici S, Salinas JL, et al: El papel del padre en la alimentación y sus dificultades [The role of the father in feeding and its difficulties], in La Alimentación en la Primera Infancia y Sus Efectos en el Desarrollo [Feeding in Early Infancy and Its Effects on Development]. Edited by Lartigue T, Maldonado-Durán JM, Avila H. México City. Plaza y Valdez, 1998, pp 252–272

Barriguete JA, Casamadrid J, Salinas JL: El self de crianza y la pareja parental [The self-of-rearing and the parental couple], in Observación de Bebés [Infant Observation]. Edited by Reyes N. México City, Plaza y Valdes, 2000, pp 179–188

Bowlby J: Attachement et Perte [Attachment and Loss], Vol 1 (1969). Paris, Presses Universitaires de France, 1978

Fivaz-Depeursinge E, Frascarolo F, Corboz-Warnery A: Assessing the triadic alliance between fathers, mothers, and infants at play. New Dir Child Dev 74:27–44, 1996

Fraiberg S, Fraiberg L (eds): Clinical Studies in Infant Mental Health: The First Year of Life. New York, Basic Books, 1980

Fraiberg S, Adelson E, Shapiro V: Ghosts in the nursery: a psychoanalytic approach to the problems of impaired infant-mother relationships. J Am Acad of Child Psychiatry 14(3):387–421, 1975

Fraiberg S, Shapiro V, Cherniss D: Treatment modalities, in Frontiers of Infant Psychiatry, Vol 1. Edited by Call JD, Galenson E, Tyson RL. New York, Basic Books, 1983, pp 56–73

Kennel JH, Klaus M: Bonding: recent observations that alter perinatal care. Pediatr Rev 19(1):4–12, 1998

Kreisler L, Cramer B: Sur les bases cliniques de la psychiatrie du nourrison [On the clinical bases of infant psychiatry]. Psychiatrie de l'Enfant 24:224–285, 1981

Lebovici S: Le Nourrison, la Mère et le Psychanalyste [The Infant, the Mother and the Psychoanalyst]. Paris, Centurión/Paidos, 1983, pp 145–160

Lebovici S: En l'Homme le Bebé [Within the Adult, the Baby]. Paris, Ed Eshel, 1992

Lebovici S: On intergenerational transmission: from filiation to affiliation. Infant Mental Health Journal 14:260–272, 1993

Lebovici S: Empathie et "enactment" dans le travail de contre-transfert [Empathy and "enactment" in the work on countertransference]. Revue Française de Psychanalyse 58:1551–1562, 1994a

Lebovici S: Le pratique des psychotherapies mères-bebés par Bertrand Cramer et Francisco Palacio-Espasa [The Bertrand Cramer and Francisco Palacio-Espasa method of mother-infant psychotherapy]. Psychiatrie de l'Enfant 37(2):415–427, 1994b

Lebovici S: La consultation thérapeutique [The therapeutic consultation], in L'Arbre de Vie: Eléments de la Psychopathologie du Bébé [The Tree of Life: The Basics of Infant Psychopathology] (Multimedia Collection "A l'Aube de la Vie" [At the Dawn of Life]). Edited by Lebovici S, Golse B. Ramonville, Saint-Agne, France, Éditions Erès, 1998a, pp 131–147

Lebovici S: L'empathie [Empathy], in L'Arbre de Vie: Eléments de la Psychopathologie du Bébé [The Tree of Life: The Basics of Infant Psychopathology] (Multimedia Collection "A l'Aube de la Vie" [At the Dawn of Life]). Edited by Lebovici S, Golse B. Ramonville, Saint-Agne, France, Éditions Erès, 1998b, pp 97–106

Lebovici S: Serge Lebovici: Psychanalystes d'Aujour d'Hui [Serge Lebovici: Psychoanalysts of Today]. Paris, Presses Universitaires de France, 1998c

Lieberman A, Wieder S, Fenichel E (eds): Casebook of Infant Mental Health: Behavioral and Developmental Disorders. Washington, DC, Zero to Three, 1996

Manzano J, Palacio-Espasa F, Zilkha N: Les Scénarios Narcissiques de la Parentalité: Clinique de la Consultation Thérapeutique [Narcissistic Scenarios of Parenthood: The Clinic of Therapeutic Consultations]. Paris, Presses Universitaires de France, 1993

Mazet P, Stoleru S: Psychopathologie du Nourrisson et du Jeune Enfant [Psychopathology of the Infant and Young Child]. Paris, Masson, 1996

Montagner H: L'attachment: Les Débuts de la Tendresse [Attachment: The Beginnings of Tenderness]. Paris, Éditions Odille Jacob, 1988

Moro MR, Barriguete JA: Aspectos transculturales de la alimentación del lactante [Transcultural issues in infant feeding], in La Alimentación en la Primera Infancia y Sus Efectos en el Desarrollo [Feeding in Early Infancy and Its Effects on Development]. Edited by Lartigue T, Maldonado-Durán JM, Avila H. México City, Plaza y Valdez, 1998, pp 337–362

Moro MR, Nathan T: Ethnopsychiatrie de l'enfant [Ethnopsychiatry of the child], in Nouveau Traité de Psychiatrie de l'Enfant et de l'Adolescent [New Textbook of Child and Adolescent Psychiatry]. Edited by Lebovici S, Diatkine R, Soule M. Paris, Presses Universitaires de France, 1995, pp 423–446

Salinas JL, Casamadrid J, Barriguete JA: Apego, self de crianza y ceguera [Attachment, self-of-rearing and blindness], in Observación de Bebés [Infant Observation]. Edited by Reyes N. México City, Plaza y Valdes, 2000, pp 139–150

Sandler J: On communication from patient to analyst: not everything is projective identification. Int J Psychoanal 74:1097–1107, 1993

Stern D: The Interpersonal World of the Infant: A View From Psychoanalysis and Developmental Psychology. New York, Basic Books, 1985

Stern D: L'enveloppe prénarrative [The pre-narrative wrap]. Journal de Psychanalse de l'Enfant 14:13–65, 1993

Stern D: The Motherhood Constellation. New York, Basic Books, 1995

Stierlin H, Weber G: Unlocking the Family Door: A Systemic Approach to the Understanding and Treatment of Anorexia Nervosa. New York, Brunner/Mazel, 1989

Winnicott DW: Hate in the countertransference (1947), in Collected Papers: Through Paediatrics to Psycho-Analysis. London, Tavistock, 1958, pp 194–203

Winnicott DW: Transitional objects and transitional phenomena (1953), in Collected Papers: Through Paediatrics to Psycho-Analysis. London, Tavistock, 1958, pp 204–218

Winnicott DW: The Maturational Processes and the Facilitating Environment: Studies in the Theory of Emotional Development. London, Hogarth Press, 1965

Winnicott DW: The value of the therapeutic consultation (1965), in Psycho-Analytic Explorations. Edited by Winnicott C, Shepherd R, Davis M. Cambridge, MA, Harvard University Press, 1989, pp 318–324

Winnicott DW: Therapeutic Consultations in Child Psychiatry. London, Hogarth Press, 1971

Winnicott DW: Psycho-Analytic Explorations. Edited by Winnicott C, Shepherd R, Davis M. Cambridge, MA, Harvard University Press, 1989

8

The Transgenerational Transmission of Abandonment

Hisako Watanabe, M.D., Ph.D.

Those who cannot remember the past are condemned to repeat it.

George Santayana (1863–1952), *The Life of Reason,*
inscribed over the entrance to the
Auschwitz Museum, Auschwitz, Poland

Studies in Western countries of the intergenerational transmission of trauma and psychopathology have yielded significant evidence of how unresolved parental conflicts can negatively affect the course of life and personality development of successive generations in diverse, invisible ways (Adelman 1995; Bacciagaluppi 1994; Fonagy et al. 1991; Kestenberg and Brenner 1986; Kogan 1998; Pines 1986; Pynoos 1996; Sorcher and Cohen 1997; Zeanah and Zeanah 1989). These findings alerted me to direct my attention to Japan. Here is where people continue to suffer from massive, unresolved conflicts related to World War II and the post-

Note. A brief version of this chapter was presented at the Sixth International Psycho-Analytical Association Conference on Psychoanalytical Research, London, March 1996. The cases presented here are part of the Keio Parent-Infant Project at Keio University in Japan. The author wishes to thank Bertrand Cramer for supervising the first case and Juliet Hopkins for her comments and advice. The author is grateful for support from the Japanese Ministry of Education Grant in Aid for Scientific Research and the Pharmacia Upjohn Growth and Development Fund.

war struggle to survive even while they remain bound by the cultural attitude expressed in such sayings as "Silence is golden" and "Just forget
and get on with life."

Seated in the renowned Nikko Shrine in Japan are three carved monkeys: Mi-zaru (See no evil), Iwa-zaru (Speak no evil), and Kika-zaru (Hear
no evil). They symbolize the traditional virtue of obedient self-inhibition
and denial for the sake of group harmony and *amae*, a unique Japanese
interpersonal relationship imbued with blissful interdependence. However, in more than two decades of clinical practice with families in Japan,
I have seen the ubiquitous dilemma of dysfunctional communication in
which wife and husband, or parent and child, cannot reach out to each
other to share feelings and mutual understanding (Watanabe 1987, 1992).
In many cases, these people experience years of silent suffering, whether
in hidden postnatal depression, unspoken intrafamilial deprivation, isolation, or covert abuse. This suffering culminates in manifest disruptive
symptoms and problems before family members learn for the first time
to confide from the heart in each other.

Because of this massive cultural repression of feelings, silent, unresolved conflicts tend to find expression most eloquently through nonverbal daily intimate communication (Ehrenberg 1992; Watanabe 1998).
These conflicts often take the form of particular patterns and characteristic interactive sequences in the family relationship. The sequences are
particularly active during the perinatal and neonatal periods, as well as
during early infancy. Throughout this time, there is a massive transmission of affect (Cramer and Stern 1988; Cramer et al. 1990). Selma
Fraiberg, pioneer of parent-infant psychotherapy, stated in 1975: "In
every nursery there are ghosts. They are the visitors from the unremembered past of the parents" (Fraiberg et al. 1975, p. 387). She noted that
behind every infant's symptoms are unresolved conflicts from the mother's
own deprived infancy that are evoked at the dawn of attachment. Fraiberg sought to free these mothers and infants from the cycle of abuse
and abandonment by home visits, carrying out her *kitchen psychotherapy*
with babies in their own homes.

This form of psychotherapy offers unique insight into the actual transmission of parental conflicts to the infant. By observing mother-infant
interactions (including, when possible, on videotape), one can study
infant psychopathology as it develops. By resolving early conflicts in
mothers, we can immediately prevent transmission of psychopathology
across generations. As Fraiberg stated in 1980: "When the baby is at the
center of therapy, something happens which has no parallel in any other
form of psychotherapy. Undo the impingements to forward movement
and the baby takes off. It is a little bit like having God on your side" (p. 56).

This same rapid, radical change occurs with mothers and infants in Japan, despite different cultural and traditional ways of child rearing.

What are the *ghosts* that alienate mothers and babies and the *god* that so dramatically retrieves secure, intimate relationships? Fraiberg suggests that they are early emotions powerfully evoked in a mother who is in touch with the strong organizational force of development in her infant. Cramer and Stern (Cramer and Stern 1988; Cramer et al. 1990) have studied how the infant's symptoms become the manifest expression of conflictual representations in the mother. Apparently, maternal projections or projective identifications often have an amazing power of penetration through subtle and repetitive interactional clues. By gaze, intonation of voice, emotional display, and physical exchanges, the mother precisely and compellingly conveys to her infant what she expects of the child whom the infant represents, what the mother wants the baby not to do, and what frightens or pleases the mother. The infant is exquisitely receptive to these clues and actively resonates to them. In a study of primary and secondary intersubjectivity, Trevarthan (1983) clarified understanding of the infant's early capacity to engage in nonverbal dialogue and concluded that babies are conversant from birth.

Winnicott (1987) said, "When the baby looks at its mother, it sees two things: its mother's eyes and its mother looking at it" (p. 100). The same statement applies to the mother: She sees the baby's eyes and the baby's state of mind in relation to her maternal care. It is this infinite mirroring of mutual states of mind that forms the basis for the development of self- and object-representations in baby and mother. This delicate mother-infant system is easily unsettled by influences on the infant's early life.

In his paper "Fantasmatic Interaction and Intergenerational Transmission," Lebovici (1988) proposed that three different images of the infant are activated when the mother looks at her baby (see Chapter 7, this volume). These images originate from different levels of the mother's psychic life: a) the real baby, whom she sees as a mature adult; b) the imaginary baby, which her girl-self has long wished for and conceived in her latent thought; and c) the *fantasmatic baby*, the representation of herself as a baby, with unfathomable memories deeply buried in unconscious memories now projected onto her baby.

In clinical work, it is useful to understand the multifaceted mirroring mechanism in the therapeutic relationship. When the therapist steps in to form the parent-infant-therapist triangle, he or she immediately becomes part of the process. This process entails three dimensions of parent-infant-therapist interaction: a) the real interaction (behavioral and affective), b) the imaginary interaction (semiconscious and wishful), and c) the fantasmatic interaction (unconscious and charged with primitive fantasies).

In the here and now of this parent-infant-therapist interaction, whether in the kitchen of the baby's home or in the therapist's consultation room, specific moments occur that open unexpected windows onto the intergenerational transmission of trauma. The therapist is alerted by a sudden subtle change, such as a heightened tone in the mother's voice or tension in a gesture or an affectively charged comment or anecdote. Most often, the change turns out to be an emergent moment in the mother's thematic conflict that can be explored in depth and unraveled on the spot.

The change usually takes place within the transference of the parent-infant-therapist triangle. In this triangle, the mother-infant duo spontaneously projects three dimensions of the object onto the therapist: a) the real therapist, a professional who has authority and can help; b) the imaginary therapist, an ideal, longed-for parent; and c) the omnipotent, fantasmatic therapist, who could harm the mother and infant just as the mother's parent harmed her in early life.

Especially at a time of crisis in the infant, when the therapist responds particularly to the mother's latent wish for an ideal helping figure, it is vital to be aware of the mother's urge to get rid of the unwanted aspects of her internal world by projecting them not only onto the infant but also onto the therapist. The mother will therefore construe the therapist as the perpetrator of her early trauma, the fantasmatic parent. By observing the mother's manipulation of the therapeutic situation and the manifest patterns in symptomatic interactive sequences, the therapist can better grasp the nature of the mother's unresolved conflicts and strive to prevent their transmission to the next generation.

PARENT-INFANT-THERAPIST INTERACTION

The following cases, which were videotaped, show how this interaction happens with a baby boy and a male fetus whose mothers had been abandoned by their fathers early in life. For these mothers, the infant and fetus initially stood for both the abandoning, alienating object and the angry, abandoned self whom the mothers had to fear and avoid. These cases also show how careful, understanding therapy and maternal care resolved the situations.

The first case features an abnormally regressed 19-month-old boy whose mother was brought up in an orphanage from the age of 8 months to 8 years after she and her own mother were abandoned by her father. The boy's mother acted out the abandonment by making the therapist leave the therapy room. The second case describes a male fetus and its anorexic-bulimic mother in a sadomasochistic conflict. To make up her mind to have the baby, this mother needed to accuse the therapist falsely of insisting on an abortion, thus making a rejecting object out of the therapist.

Nineteen-Month-Old Boy and His Mother

Bo, a 19-month-old boy, presented with autistic withdrawal and progressive physical and mental deterioration, suggesting possible organic brain disease. However, it took only three 1-hour mother-infant psychotherapy sessions over 8 days to resolve the baby's problems. This case is a poignant example of alienation and retrieval passed through three generations, from grandmother to mother to baby. Clearly, the mother's own unresolved feelings of abandonment in infancy were evoked by the baby and projected into him, eliciting his symptoms of avoidance and rejection. The major interactive themes of the mother's inner representations manifested both in her account and in her interaction with the baby in the therapy room, which, along with the hospital, formed a safe setting for her to reenact her past experience of abandonment. The video actually captured the very moment when the therapist's departure from the room made the mother tense and elicited mutual rejection in the mother-infant dyad. Bo, who is now 12 years old, portrays normal personality development.

How did this mother's inner representation affect the baby's development? How was it possible to prevent the intergenerational transmission of psychopathology, freeing the mother from past conflicts initially acted out in the current mother-infant relationship?

Bo was referred by a pediatrician. After a brief family trip to China 4 months earlier, he began to lose weight, his speech regressed, and he became withdrawn and difficult, with occasional outbreaks of hyperactivity and tantrums. His parents were middle-class; his father was a civil servant, his mother a housewife. After a normal birth, Bo had been an easy baby, saying "Daddy" and "bye-bye" by the age of 1, talking and walking at 15 months, and never showing any anxiety toward strangers or any separation anxiety.

This mother and baby posed a puzzling problem in the mother-infant unit where Bo was to undergo intensive investigation for possible organic brain disease. Bo's mother and grandmother both complained of episodes of upturned eyeballs. The pediatric neurologist suspected seizures, although neither the pediatrician nor the nurses ever witnessed them. Apparently the baby never sought his mother or cried aloud; she never hugged or caressed him. The pediatric neurologists were determined to find some rare disease that would entail endless tests. As the only child psychiatrist in the hospital, and with the mother's consent, I used a video camera to record and validate an urgent assessment of what was really wrong.

The first session. When Bo and his mother first entered the consulting room, Bo was solemn and tense, clearly avoiding eye contact with his mother. Not once in the first half-hour did he look, smile at, or even speak to her. The lack of reciprocity between them was pronounced. Oddly enough, their clothes were the same color, giving the impression that Bo was a part of his mother.

While Bo played with a toy animal, the mother concentrated wholly on telling me how strange and rejecting this boy was toward her. "It's so strange! Bo avoids me, ignores me. He does it on purpose. When Bo was 8 months old, we left him for an hour in a baby-care facility in a department store. When we came back, we called his name, "Bo-chan!" (Bo Darling), but he turned his head away, like this." She showed me exactly how he had turned his head, ignoring the child who was right in front of her as she spoke. She was so preoccupied with the strange baby inside her head that she was oblivious to the real baby before her.

Halfway through the session, she looked at her watch and said, "Daddy must be here by now. Please go and fetch him." I left the room, overwhelmed by the lack of normal attachment and referencing in this toddler. Perhaps he was showing the first signs of autism. But how strange it was that his mother could share her worries so fully with me so soon and yet not relate to the baby. The father had not yet arrived; intuitively, I realized that her real request was, "Please go and get my baby back." In fact, sending me out like that later proved to be an important reflection of the mother's central psychic conflict, which was repeated exactly in the third session.

I decided to intervene in the second half-hour, to explore with the mother the meaning of her baby's symptoms and behavior and to free her from the strong feeling of alienation that forced her to be so detached from Bo. Using a form of nonverbal dialogue, I asked the baby what he had to say about himself, testing his ability with gentle stimuli. I carefully included the mother all the while in an attempt to prompt the maternal preoccupation so essential for the baby's return to health.

Bo responded surprisingly well, first with fleeting interest, then coming up to me and showing affection. Acknowledging his mother's perception of his indifference, I showed her simple ways to improve the mutual interaction. I suggested that she not "miss small cues and demands from him; enjoyable repetition is also good." Once he accepted my overtures, I gradually added new ideas that expanded his responses. To his mother I said, "Make it simple and easy for him. Make it gentle and joyful for him."

I made them play peek-a-boo, with which Bo had no difficulty. The mother said this game was one of the few things he did. Then she noticed that Bo avoided her gaze and became tense again. "Look at me, Bo! Why don't you look at me?" She clearly felt rejected by him, and her demand made Bo avoid her all the more. So I said, "He has avoided you a bit. Maybe he remembered something unpleasant done to him. Maybe, in fact, he missed you when you left him alone." She agreed and cheered up, as if I had struck the right note. She added, "He did not cry at all. It puzzled me, but he may have stored it up for his current tantrums." I commented, "So he did have feelings." My suggestion had led the mother to see Bo's avoidance as a sign of his unvoiced separation anger and to link it with his symptoms. Behind the façade of an indifferent, avoidant baby, the mother began to see a lonely boy waiting for her to be in touch with his feelings. Because her way of being with Bo changed at this moment, I felt that she had been waiting for someone to allow her to be in touch with her baby's feelings.

Bo approached me, and I picked him up. I wanted to explore informally the extent of his responsiveness and his physical predisposition, including his muscle tone and reflexes. I explained, "Enjoyable repetition is good. See how he looks more intently at me? I think he is OK." The mother must have felt immensely relieved. In the following sequence, she elicited something I did not anticipate: Out of gleeful playfulness, she tickled him and made him burst into laughter for the first time in the session. Her mischievous face was turned toward him, ready to play and enjoy him.

I met the father that afternoon and told him to put all thoughts of some nasty disease behind him, as it was most unlikely. I also encouraged him to have fun with his son in every possible way, without any suggestion of discipline. In the latter part of the session, I had elicited mutual interaction between Bo and his mother. However, her preoccupation with the baby in her mind and her initial lack of emotional interaction were striking.

No enlightenment was forthcoming from the pediatrician's file, but at the end of the psychologist's report on Bo's development was a short comment: "This mother volunteered to talk about her infancy, which she spent in an orphanage from the age of 8 months to 8 years. Her father died suddenly in a building site accident, and her mother had to get a job to earn a living." I decided to take up this issue in the next session a week later, having also learned from the nurses that Bo's mother was 3 months pregnant.

The second session: unraveling the past. Three days later, Bo's maternal grandmother requested time with me during Bo's regular appointment. I took this opportunity to observe the interaction between grandmother and mother. They came together, with Bo in his mother's arms. A lumbar puncture had made Bo's leg sore and he was unable to walk, forcing him to cling to his mother. She began by saying that Bo had begun to respond to her and that he had started to get better. Yet she was worried about what would happen when the new baby arrived in June. She turned toward the grandmother, saying she wanted her to come and help her then. Bo's mother also described how the child loved and missed his grandmother whenever she returned to her own home. I felt she was talking about the infant inside herself, who had missed her mother in the orphanage.

I mentioned that I had heard about her history and appreciated that it must have been a tough thing to go through and that she might have been concerned about its effect on her role as a mother. I said it was not something irreversible or crucial, provided that she had stable support from her husband and mother. Because she had gone through such a long struggle on her own, she deserved extra mothering from both her husband and her mother so that they could make a good mother of her. Her strength in having survived the long separation from her mother was proof of her resilience.

The grandmother told me of the difficult circumstances that had led her to send her daughter to the orphanage. In those days, it was almost impossible for a woman to earn enough money to bring up a child, and it took more than she thought it would. The mother and infant listened solemnly, both with eyes downcast. Then the grandmother said something crucial to the discovery of the separation trauma: "Do you know, Doctor, my daughter insists on putting the baby alone at night in a room separate from his parents. The baby should sleep between his parents in the typical Japanese way, in the configuration of the Japanese letter *kawa*. (The word means "river" and is depicted by three vertical lines.) I have been telling her, but she won't listen to me."

I looked at the mother and, for the first time, saw silent rage and protest on her face. I immediately understood her feelings and said to her, "Maybe you thought it was best for him to sleep alone in a separate room because that was what you experienced and became familiar with in the orphanage. Maybe you thought your Mum chose this setting for you, and so you thought it was right to do the same for your baby." The mother cried out, "Yes, yes!" almost in tears. Then she looked into her mother's face.

The grandmother was dumbstruck and almost paralyzed with guilt. The room was filled with tense, negative emotions as a result of this remark. I instantly felt the need to modify the situation in order to safeguard the positive opening up of the mother's feelings toward her mother, probably for the first time. I told her what I thought could have supported her in her early ordeal. "Maybe you knew what it was to be alone. Maybe you could believe in your mother and had such a deep trust in her that you could endure the long days of separation and wait." "Yes, yes, Mother," the mother agreed. To the grandmother she said, "Oh, I never had a grudge. Oh, never! I knew it couldn't be helped. I knew you were striving hard for me." There was an intense emotional discharge between the two, resulting in great relief.

Later, I was told that it was the first time the two had been able to talk to each other about their painful past. The following day, the pediatrician in charge came to me with cheerful, inquisitive eyes and asked, "What did you say to them? I have never seen them chatting so happily to each other like that before." In the course of the session, I had helped Bo's mother recapture and relive her memories of the past and share them with her mother.

The third session: ghosts in the consulting room. The third session took place 1 week after the first session. Bo came in, closely followed by his mother, who sat down smiling at him. He turned toward her, looking more relaxed and natural. The mother said, "Bo has changed a lot! He now looks for me. He loves to be held and hugged. He giggles when tickled. He dribbles a lot, which he never did before." As I complimented her on all the splendid changes in Bo, she looked delighted and told me what a sensitive baby Bo was: "Do you know, even before Bo was a year old, he understood the situation when Grandma got carsick and had to push him to one side. He did not even cry but watched her anxiously and kept still without a whimper for a very unusual half-hour."

The mother spoke with such vivid emotion that I felt this episode must hold very special emotion for her. It seemed that she was unconsciously speaking about herself, recalling the highly sensitive baby suddenly thrown out of her mother's lap and forced to live in an orphanage because of an unavoidable situation. There was probably a distinct echo of all the mother's past for her in Bo's own sudden admission to the hospital.

Then the mother looked at her watch and said, "Daddy must have arrived by now." She sent me out to see. By chance, the video camera kept running, which enabled me to witness the reenactment of being abandoned in infancy. Immediately the mother became tense and quiet; unwillingly, I had dislodged her from the secure base of my psychological lap. The consulting room had become the institution where she had waited for years and years for her mother to earn her living and bring back her long-lost daddy.

The video camera recorded the following scene: Just like a small child stranded by its mother, the mother repeated the very words I said before leaving the room: "Speech and interaction!" she said with mock gaiety, as if to overcome her depression. Bo quickly sensed her tension. When she held out a toy in a rather pushy, unconvincing attempt to be playful with him, he hurled it aside. Let down, hurt, and scared by his aggressiveness, the mother withdrew from him and set two small dolls together, desperately singing to herself, "Kiss, kiss, kiss," in a thin little voice that dipped and faded. "Daddy is coming soon," she repeated, as if to soothe herself. Meanwhile, Bo came close and she inadvertently knocked him over. There they were, both of them, desolate, waiting for Daddy to come.

Clearly this reaction to my leaving was the reenactment of a lonely girl waiting for her father to come home while her mother went out to find him. The ghosts of the past were visiting the consulting room. Of course, when I returned, there was no sign that anything had happened. As the video later showed, in a matter of seconds both of them looked fine again. Bo was rather restless, and his mother said he was acting up. I assured her that his restlessness was a good sign and added, "How well you have done to have brought about all these changes in Bo! And how well you have done to have survived all those years of separation from your mother!" She smiled in reply and said in a sad, tender voice, "When I look at Bo, I feel as if I am confronting myself as a baby."

I asked about the orphanage. The mother responded: "The place was not good at all. I was a loner. I had no friends. I never managed to like it." While she was uttering these words, Bo came back from his exploration outside the room and begged her to come with him. She responded to his request while speaking to me at the same time, no longer oblivious of her son when talking to me. She seemed to be able to refuel Bo and, at the same time, also recharge the infant inside her (to use Mahler's terms). It was as if she had retrieved the good mother now available to her and understood and acknowledged her painful history (Mahler et al. 1975).

This change became all the more apparent when Bo, in his joyful exploration outside the room, fell, hit his head, and bellowed, something he had not done for a long time. His mother rushed to help him, and I followed with my videotape. She picked him up and soothed him tenderly. Bo pointed to the place where he had hit his head and began a long tale of woe: how he had stumbled, fallen, and hurt himself and how awful he felt. His mother, in her infancy, had not been able to cry out for her own mother's help, but now she was responding to Bo with all her emotion. I thought this interaction might afford a reparative experience for her, and that she might be dealing with her past wounds through Bo. I said, "Bravo, Bo! You cried and your Mum did hear it, didn't she? She did come to help you." I was addressing the mother just as much as Bo, indirectly encouraging her to unlock more and more of her unvoiced feelings. To the mother, I commented: "Do you see how Bo's voice grew louder after you rushed to save him? He now feels his voice is heard by Mum, and he is ready to communicate."

After this turn of events, the mother became very playful, inviting Bo to *onbu*, the traditional Japanese custom of carrying a baby on one's back. "Come, Bo, show Dr. W that you can do *onbu* now!" Bo went around the mother once and mounted her back. He then almost said "Giddyap" and egged her into running down the corridor. This the mother did with glee, mentioning Daddy again: "Daddy always does this to you, and you love it, don't you, Bo?" I said, "Daddy means a lot to both of you," referring to both their fathers.

We went into the room again, and Bo's father came in. Bo welcomed him with a radiant smile, and the mother looked wonderfully happy. The father brought in a good-smelling bag of food. Bo began to peek into it, and his father let him have some, also having a bite himself. Bo leaned against his father, who held him naturally, and all three family members sat close together with Bo in the middle, in the configuration of the Japanese letter *kawa*. The mother voiced her worries about her own mother: "I have long wanted her to live with us. After all these years of hard times, she must have a deep need to share with us. I now have this daddy to listen to me, but I wonder how she manages on her own." I said, "If this is how you feel, why not tell her? Call out and let her hear you." She said, "I will."

Follow-up. Thus the intervention ended, but I followed up with the family; the videotape section of the third session had alerted me to the problem of the mother's vulnerability concerning separation. In the first follow-up session 3 months later, Bo was completely recovered and had become a sensitive boy close to his mother. The mother gave birth to another boy just after Bo's birthday, and the grandmother helped her daughter to contain Bo's strong jealousy toward the newborn.

A year later, the grandmother came to tell me her story. A healthy, intelligent young woman when World War II broke out, Bo's grandmother was forced to marry a farmer's handicapped son. All healthy men were busy on active war service, and agricultural labor was badly needed. She was put to work like a slave, deprived of food and rest as her domineering mother took over the care of her two baby daughters. When she became too weak to work and was sent home, her own family rejected her out of shame. Then a stranger took her to a remote town where he made her pregnant. She resisted his demand to abort the baby, thinking it would be her sole blood tie. Thus Bo's mother was born. One morning 8 months later, the grandmother awoke to find her room empty. The stranger had deserted her, robbing her of her few possessions.

In shock and despair, she resolved to survive and defy the world. She put her daughter into the cheapest (and worst) orphanage and strove day and night for more than 7 years to work her way up in the world. She was eventually successful, setting up an au pair agency and buying her own house.

All this was too shameful for the grandmother to tell me during our initial encounter. She had lied to protect herself. However, as she observed and participated in her daughter's subsequent struggle to retrieve her lost childhood through caring for Bo and the new baby, the grandmother must have begun to come to terms with her own trauma of abandonment and alienation.

Bulimic-Anorexic Mother and Her Male Fetus

Mari, a 27-year-old woman with bulimia-anorexia, was referred to me because of her irrational fear of the "filthy, ominous male" in her womb and because of her sadomasochistic relationship (binge eating and dangerous vomiting) with her fetus. I slowly discovered that this woman's own mother had been abandoned after a promiscuous relationship. The patient had to suffer her mother's ensuing ambivalent feelings toward her, which ranged from hating her for causing the father's rejection to loving her as her only child. In order to decide to have the baby, the patient conjured up a story that the therapist was trying to force her to abort against her will, thereby acting out the very scenario of her own birth. The therapist represented, on the fantasmatic level, the patient's abandoning father and, on the imaginary level, the father she longed to have protect her.

Pregnant at age 27, Mari was referred by a psychiatrist for outpatient psychotherapy. She was in deep distress, even to the point of nervous breakdown, at the prospect of becoming a mother. She appeared slim and charming but immature. As soon as she opened her mouth, she vented all the ambivalence and anxiety she felt about the new relationship with a fetus:

> I am frightened about being pregnant. I don't know whether I really want this baby or not. It's a he, a male. I detest him. It makes me shudder to think a male is coming out between my thighs. I have been suffering from bulimia-anorexia ever since I was 18. I got married last year after having been treated for amenorrhea. Although at first I was overjoyed at becoming pregnant, my bingeing and vomiting have gotten worse. My husband does not know it. I dare not tell him. I binge and vomit in the bathroom many times a day. I vomit in an upside-down yoga posture and get terrible nosebleeds. Afterward I am so exhausted that I can barely crawl back to my bed. Oh, it's like torture! I dream every night and a demon appears in the dream demanding that I eat up a pool of vomitus, the very stuff I have vomited over the years. The demon says, "It's you who have vomited all this, so it's you who have to devour it."

Within 10 minutes after the consultation began, Mari had utterly revolted me with her grotesque story of bingeing. This consultation marked the beginning of a 9-month intensive involvement with her, during which she stuffed me with her undigested and indigestible feelings of abandonment and rejection from her early life. It was as if she had to make me taste the disgusting sickness and digest it for her, so that she could banish the ghosts and start afresh with hope.

Mari did indeed long for this pregnancy. Unfortunately it evoked a sense of danger and punishment, as if she were going to be killed or that she would kill the baby.

Why all this fuss and fear? What was invading her mind at the dawn of a new relationship? In our second and third interviews, Mari dwelt on her deep ambivalence toward the fetus. Apparently, she grew up like a "Siamese twin" with her mother, who died of massive esophageal bleeding from hepatic cirrhosis when Mari was 18. Mari had felt guilty and frightened ever since. She believed that she had killed her mother by going home instead of remaining with her on the night of her death despite the mother's plea to stay.

"I don't want this boy. He is filthy and ominous. I am going to terminate him," she declared, as if to see whether I took her seriously. When I suggested that she might be worried about something intruding into her intimate relationship with her husband, and that I might be more interested in the baby than she was, she said, "I become jealous when my husband talks happily about the baby. I feel murderously jealous." I concluded, "You seem to be telling me that one part of you wants the baby very much, but the other part feels that you cannot possibly accept the baby, who might push you out of your current intimate relationship." She urged me to comment on whether she should still give birth in the face of such fear and jealousy. In response, I conveyed the message that her feelings and security of body and mind mattered most.

Immediately after this session, she rushed to her obstetrician in another hospital and said that I told her to have an abortion against her will. This exchange prompted the obstetrician to phone me and ask what had actually transpired between us. I was flabbergasted by the way

Mari had twisted my words and the context of our interaction. I then reflected on how my touching on her intimate feelings had aroused fantasmatic levels of interaction between us. Mari had turned me into a fantasmatic object, the abandoning father; she identified with her mother, who had no choice but to give birth to survive, even though it might have been against her will. Mari decided to have the baby, having clearly gotten rid of her conflicts about giving birth by projecting them onto me.

Mari came to the fourth session with her husband, the first time they were there together. The way he followed Mari closely with a fearful, suspicious look alerted me to a paranoid transference: she had turned me into her fantasmatic object, the father who had threatened her mother with abandonment unless she aborted her baby. It was only through creating this bad object that Mari could feel safe enough to bring in her husband to share her fear of destructive bingeing and vomiting and her ambivalence toward the baby in the emerging new triangle of the mother-infant-father relationship.

I could fully appreciate the way she made me experience alienation by turning me into someone who could not be trusted in the patient-husband-therapist triangle, an experience similar to Mari's own sense of alienation in her original family triangle. It was then possible for Mari to tell her husband how much she needed him at this delicate time of transition to motherhood when she could well be expected to require warm maternal care from him. When he showed concern about her ability to be a good mother, I drew their attention to the way Mari had been gently stroking her belly even while she was talking about her ambivalence and hatred. "Look how Mari's body knows how to caress the baby even before it is born." I suggested to the husband, "If you want to help her, why not stroke her and hug her warmly and tightly each day before you go out to work."

The husband complied. In subsequent sessions, Mari reported that her bouts of bingeing and vomiting had dramatically decreased to once or twice a day. Her husband had volunteered to take control of her destructive impulses, limiting and taking part in her bingeing, vomiting, and obsessive bathroom cleaning. Interestingly, the husband was the second son of a priest of a Shinto shrine, a man from a family that exorcised devils and washed down sinks and toilets. The activity recalled a traditional Japanese saying, "Washing down the past in the water," which implies the cleansing of past sins. With such concrete and tangible support from him, Mari was able to confront her incessantly ambivalent, aggressive feelings toward the baby. She continued to be jealous of the baby, however, and insisted that her husband declare her a "good girl," enabling her to be more content. Nevertheless, as the time to give birth approached, she became frightened and besieged by feelings of abandonment and disorganization.

In the tenth interview, which included her husband, 2 weeks before delivery, Mari told me her traumatic family and life history. Prior to Mari's conception, her mother had had seven or eight abortions. When she was denied another abortion on medical grounds and subsequently abandoned by her lover, she gave birth to Mari out of wedlock. She refused to look at the baby for 3 days. Mari was brought up by her mother in her grandmother's poverty-stricken household, smothered by a symbiotic tie with her mother. As described earlier, they were as close as conjoined twins when Mari's mother was in a good mood, but Mari was physically and emotionally abused when her mother was in a bad frame of mind. Her mother would often beat and curse Mari, saying, "If you hadn't been born, I could have been happier."

When Mari was 8, her mother married the owner of a large hotel. Mari felt betrayed and abandoned by her mother, who urged her to behave perfectly in public to enhance her mother's status in the new household. To her mother's dismay, however, Mari was charged with shoplifting when she was about 16. Soon afterward, her mother developed and then succumbed to hepatic cirrhosis. Thereafter, Mari was haunted by dreams of her dead mother. The next year she left Japan to study in the United States for 6 years, during which time she developed anorexia nervosa, then full-blown bulimia-anorexia.

At the prospect of childbirth, Mari was haunted by nightmares about her baby breaking out of her abdomen hungry, emaciated, and damaged. Psychotropic drugs were required to dampen her excessive persecutory fears. She gave birth to a healthy baby weighing 2,540 grams (5 pounds, 8.9 ounces) early one morning the week she was due. She made a lot of fuss during labor and immediately after the birth declared: "There must be something wrong with it [the baby] because it was starved and abused during pregnancy." Later that day, she told me sadly, "I felt released after my baby was born, but I felt no feelings toward him. Since my mother rejected me for 3 days after I was born, I felt it would be a pity to repeat this rejection with my baby. So I plucked up my courage and went to see him. It is sad not to have my mother around. But I find my boy sweet. We have named him Ta, and I want to breast-feed him."

Arrangements were made for her to try her initial breast-feeding, and it was very noticeable how beautifully the baby attuned to Mari. We provided her with an extra week of careful nurturing on the ward. Yet 2 weeks after she returned home, she was in the emergency outpatient clinic frantically complaining, "My baby Ta has bulimia and is vomiting. He suffers from the same diseases I have. What shall I do?" Although there was nothing wrong with Ta, both mother and baby were admitted to the children's ward.

When I saw Mari breast-feeding on the ward, 1-month-old Ta was gazing into her eyes with keen, untiring interest for more than a minute at a time. Mari repeatedly said to him, "Yes, you are hungry and angry because you have been starved while you were inside the womb." The baby's gaze and the mother's repeated comment of how he must be feeling continued with powerful intensity. Mari described the baby's accusation of her: "Of course, you are angry. You must be angry." Mari seemed to be projecting onto the baby her own resentment and guilt toward her promiscuous mother who grudgingly gave birth to her and refused to see her after she was born.

Throughout pregnancy, this bulimic-anorexic mother had suffered from past memories, confusing the baby inside her womb with the baby inside her mind. I had to intervene by saying, "The baby moving and kicking inside you reminds you of your painful experience in the past. And because of that, you cannot eat properly for yourself and for the baby. And eating improperly makes you all the more guilty and convinced that the baby must be angry and hungry."

Over and over again, Mari reiterated her resentment toward her mother for refusing to see her after birth. In Ta, she saw her own deprived baby—self born in utter misery, only to be stranded in a sadomasochistic, symbiotic relationship with her mother. I repeatedly pointed out that she felt sorry and guilty toward Ta for neglecting him during pregnancy when she was struggling with her own fears.

What about the baby? The way he gazed intently at his mother revealed some aspects of his emergent mental representation. His eyes were fixed on his mother's face while she talked about her rejection. He highlighted elements in his mother that I would not have noted without his gaze. He was attracted by her rich milk, soft voice, and gentle way of holding and rocking him. The baby seemed to be eloquently saying to her, "Mum, you make me attach because you are nice." He showed his potential for positive object-representation. His way of relating to her eloquently declared, "Don't be misled by what my mother says. Can you really believe that she hates me while she gives me such gentle and ample motherly care?"

The infant's way of relating to the mother usually helps the therapist sense what is actually being experienced between the two. I told Mari, "The baby is looking into your eyes because he knows you well. Look at his excellent eye contact. He must be happy." She replied, "Oh, no. Oh, no. I am a bad mother. I neglected him, and I hated him while he was in my womb." I said, "Isn't it interesting that you tell me you are bad while your body clearly knows how to love your baby with such rich milk?" On another occasion, Mari repeated the same words, and I told her how during pregnancy, she caressed her abdomen with the palm of her hand while talking about her hatred. Her mouth may have expressed rejection, but her hands, arms, and body expressed love and concern.

Through the repeated interpretation of Mari's ambivalence, in which I accepted her resentment toward her parents as reasonable and acknowledged the positive elements in her as a mother, she gradually came to accept that she was also in love with her baby. It then became clear how carefully she fostered my concern, as if fearing that she would be forgotten by me as soon as she showed improvement. Fortunately, the clear understanding of Mari's conflicts, conveyed in a positive context of consistent maternal care, enabled her to look at the baby without projection. In this case, although the mother had enormous difficulty in her conscious attachment, the procedural, nonconscious attachment was almost intact. Without therapeutic support, there could have been serious transgenerational transmission of the mother's borderline psychopathology to the infant.

Discussion

The cases of Bo and his mother and of Mari and her fetus share the theme of alienation and retrieval transmitted through three generations. Both grandmothers grew up in poor, oppressed wartime Japan, were alienated from their partners, and had babies born out of wedlock. They both struggled to support themselves as poor single mothers and to raise their daughters in the face of cultural stigma. In their reactive depression and unavailability for maternal care, they were "dead mothers" (Green 1986/1998) in their babies' eyes, thus inflicting cumulative trauma of emotional abandonment. Bo's mother, despite her 7 years in an orphanage, somehow survived unscathed. Mari suffered because of the ambivalent sadomasochistic tie with her mother and developed bulimia-anorexia. Both women graduated from a university and married decent men, but eventually they became alienated, one from her baby boy, the other from a male fetus.

Parent-infant psychotherapy conducted in a hospital setting helped the mothers acknowledge their past abandonment, mourn the loss of their happy infancy and proper family life, and confirm and facilitate their mothering capacity through the reinforcement offered by their husbands' nurturing. Empathic understanding of the mothers' unvoiced conflicts was crucial because it promoted sufficient containment and the resolution of issues of motherhood, thus freeing the infants from their mothers' transference. It was at the level of both unconscious nonverbal and conscious verbal interactions in the therapy room that the central themes of the mothers' core conflicts of alienation and retrieval were played out (Ehrenberg 1992). Bo's mother spoke of her concern about her baby's avoidance while her body neglected and avoided him. Mari spoke of immense hatred and fear of her baby and indulged in self-destructive bingeing and vomiting while her hands and arms nevertheless consistently caressed first her fetus, then her infant.

Like a phrase in an orchestral piece, with various instruments playing their parts, concurrent components of the mothers' self- and object-representations were played out in different parts of the body. In his paper on the concept of the prenarrative envelope, Stern (1995) referred to a very young infant's ability to grasp a constellation of invariant features in the mother that forms a narrative-like shape, similar to a musical phrase, with a motive, goal, and high point laid out in temporal sequence. The infant can grasp the sequential pattern of the whole, which is internalized to form the basis of his or her emerging representational world.

Could the following particular patterns of interactive sequences in Bo's and Ta's cases be similarly identified? Bo's mother sent me out to get the father twice in exactly the same way: Looking at her watch, she said to me, "Daddy must be here by now. Please go and get him." She was unconsciously acting out her identification with a visiting mother, who caused repeated frustration by glancing at her watch and then ruthlessly departing the orphanage. Bo's mother made me experience what it was like to feel pushed out of a secure place. At the same time, she forced me to be the departing mother going out to work to retrieve her lost Daddy. Furthermore, perceiving me as a professional with authority, she projected onto me a representation of the imaginary father who could legitimize her birth and afford her a proper family.

In the third session with Bo's mother, the chance recording of her reaction to my absence eventually brought me in touch with her actual lived moments of abandonment. At the fantasmatic level of interaction, I apparently stood for the abandoning father, who had subjected the mother and infant to misery and deprivation. It is fascinating how sensitively Bo discerned the sudden change of mood in his mother from calm to tense anxiety. Instantly, he mirrored his mother's aggression by harshly rejecting her mock overture. The mother became frightened and withdrew further. Could this be the very moment when the transgenerational transmission of rejection and avoidance took place in the form of symptomatic interactive sequences? The fact that, a year later, both grandmother and mother came on their own to tell me what their pasts really entailed showed how much this therapeutic encounter had helped them to mourn and redeem the family's history of separation and loss.

Mari, whose biological father had abandoned her mother because she would not comply with his demand to have an abortion, was frightened by her own murderous rage, which she initially projected onto the male fetus. She turned it into a persecuting object that might destroy her tie with her husband. Gradually perceiving me as a trustworthy professional, Mari shifted her projection from the fetus onto me, making me a fantasmatic father who demanded an abortion. Thus, she secured the survival of her fetus in the face of her own aggression by unconsciously drawing on the scenario that had ensured her own survival as a baby.

Both cases show striking contrasts in terms of the mothers' personalities, the quality of transference and countertransference, and the provision of care required. Bo's mother was a mature, resilient, likable woman despite the cumulative trauma of her early infancy and childhood. In contrast, Mari was an immature, vulnerable person who unceasingly complained about her symptoms and sought my attention. The tone of transference in Bo's case was positive. The mother was ready to absorb and make full use of all I offered, and was able to openly share her worries with me and reflect on herself, although she was somewhat reserved in seeking attention. In my countertransference, I felt like a mother with a sensitive, autonomous, reserved daughter who appeared content with minimal maternal care, and for whom intimacy or closeness was a delicate issue requiring caution. Without the chance video recording of her sudden change into a depressive state during my fleeting absence from the therapy room, I could not have gained insight into her vulnerability regarding separation issues.

With Mari, the tone of the transference was markedly ambivalent and unstable. She filled the therapy room and the children's ward with relentless demands for attention and nauseating accounts of her symptoms. I felt like a mother with an angry, tearful, premature baby whose very existence depended on me and whose exhausting demands would overwhelm me and drain all my energy.

These two patients required markedly different help, highlighting distinct points in the spectrum of disturbed mother-infant relationships. This difference suggests the notion of a whole range of parent-infant psychotherapy, from prevention of deviant character development to treatment of severe psychopathology. To use Winnicott's (1958) metaphor of therapy as midwifery, Bo's case represents a natural delivery by mother-infant psychotherapy, while Mari's case represents a high-risk delivery requiring a psychological neonatal intensive care unit. For Mari, who had bulimia-anorexia, the past that she dwelt on was linked to the present with very real, vivid persecutory fear and rage directed toward her internal object. For such a mother, to be heard by the fearful baby inside her, words had to be made more convincing and comforting in a reliable setting with ample care and physical contact.

REFERENCES

Adelman A: Traumatic memory and the intergenerational transmission of Holocaust narratives. Psychoanal Study Child 50:343–367, 1995

Bacciagaluppi M: The relevance of attachment research to psychoanalysis and analytic social psychology. J Am Acad Psychoanal 22(3):465–479, 1994

Cramer B, Stern DN: Evaluation of changes in mother-infant brief psychotherapy: a single case study. Infant Mental Health Journal 9:20–45, 1988

Cramer B, Robert-Tissott C, Stern DN, et al: Outcome evaluation in brief mother-infant psychotherapy: a preliminary report. Infant Mental Health Journal 11:278–300, 1990

Ehrenberg DB: The Intimate Edge: Extending the Reach of Psychoanalytic Interaction. New York, WW Norton, 1992

Fonagy P, Steele M, Moran G, et al: Measuring the ghosts in the nursery: a summary of the main findings of the Anna Freud Centre-University College London Parent-Child Study. Bulletin of the Anna Freud Centre 14:115–131, 1991

Fraiberg S: Treatment modalities, in Frontiers of Infant Psychiatry, Vol 11. Edited by Call J, Galenson E, Tyson R. New York, Basic Books, 1980, pp 56–73

Fraiberg S, Adelson E, Shapiro V: Ghosts in the nursery: a psychoanalytic approach to the problems of impaired infant-mother relationships. J Am Acad Child Psychiatry 14(3):387–421, 1975

Green A: On Private Madness (1986). London, Hogarth Press and the Institute of Psychoanalysis, 1998

Kestenberg JS, Brenner I: Children who survived the Holocaust: the role of rules and routines in the development of the superego. Int J Psychoanal 67:309–316, 1986

Kogan I: The black hole of dread: the psychic reality of children of Holocaust survivors, in Even Paranoids Have Enemies. Edited by Berke J, Pierides S, Sabbadini A, et al. London, Routledge, 1998, pp 47–58

Lebovici S: Fantasmatic interaction and intergenerational transmission. Infant Mental Health Journal 9:10–19, 1988

Mahler MS, Pine F, Bergman A: The Psychological Birth of the Human Infant: Symbiosis and Individuation. New York, Basic Books, 1975

Pines D: Working with women survivors of the Holocaust: affective experiences in transference and countertransference. Int J Psychoanal 67:295–307, 1986

Pynoos R: The transgenerational repercussions of traumatic expectations. Paper presented at the Sixth International Psycho-Analytical Association Conference on Psychoanalytical Research, London, March 1996

Santayana G: Reason in Common Sense: Volume One of "The Life of Reason" (1905). New York, Dover, 1980

Sorcher N, Cohen LJ: Trauma in children of Holocaust survivors: transgenerational effects. Am J Orthopsychiatry 67:493–500, 1997

Stern DN: The Motherhood Constellation. New York, Basic Books, 1995

Trevarthan C: Interpersonal abilities of infants as generators for transmission of language and culture, in The Behaviour of Human Infants. Edited by Oliverio A, Zapella M. New York, Plenum, 1983, pp 145–176

Watanabe H: Establishing emotional mutuality not formed in infancy with Japanese families. Infant Mental Health Journal 8:398–408, 1987

Watanabe H: Difficulties in amae: a clinical perspective. Infant Mental Health Journal 13:26–33, 1992

Watanabe H: Paranoia and persecution in modern Japanese life, in Even Paranoids Have Enemies. Edited by Berke J, Pierides S, Sabbadini A, et al. London, Routledge, 1998, pp 189–202

Winnicott DW: Collected Papers: Through Paediatrics to Psycho-Analysis. New York, Basic Books, 1958

Winnicott DW: Babies and Their Mothers. Reading, MA, Addison-Wesley, 1987

Zeanah CH, Zeanah PD: Intergenerational transmission of maltreatment: insights from attachment theory and research. Psychiatry 52:177–196, 1989

9

The Challenge of
Multiple Caregivers

Alice Eberhart-Wright, M.A.

Throughout history, the relationship between mother and infant has been considered essential not only for the survival of the baby but also for healthy psychological growth. Many factors in current society, however, dictate that the baby be cared for by others. As a result, young children across the country are growing up with multiple caregivers. In this chapter, I explore caregiving situations, their impact on the young child, the complications that lead to various outcomes, and the implications for prevention, intervention, and research.

HISTORY

Beliefs about children and their needs undergo continual change, yet some ideas seem to withstand the vagaries of time (Cable 1972; Konner 1991). Judging from portrayals of mothers and babes that decorate gallery walls, the mother-infant relationship has been considered noteworthy from the days that artists first portrayed human life. In these portraits, one may observe all states of dress, the trappings of the age, and all manner of emotion, but the baby is almost always on its mother's lap. Depictions of the Nativity show a realm of admirers, but, again, the babe maintains the closest proximity to his mother.

Surprisingly, as far back as the sixteenth century B.C., a Mycenaean sculpture (*Three Deities*, 1500–1400 B.C.) raises the question of who is attending a small child—the mother or the grandmother? Just what is the relationship of the three (Janson 1963)? Likewise, the Ara Pacis commissioned by the Roman Senate in 13 B.C. depicts male figures (perhaps a father and brother) offering protection and guidance to a young child who clings to the toga of the man but seems to be listening to the older child behind him. And, of course, the famous Romulus and Remus bronze from 500 B.C. Rome depicts a she-wolf nurturing twin babies.

Someone must always be there to care for the helpless young. Moving from art into both fiction and nonfiction, we find that themes abound about the care of children. *Heracleidae,* a play written by Euripides sometime between 480 and 406 B.C., tells the story of two orphaned children who receive protection from their dead father's friend, who whisks them off to another country to try to protect them from prophesied death in their own land. In the Bible, the infant Moses is adopted by Pharoah's daughter after having been found floating down a stream, and Solomon threatens to cut an infant in half when two women fight for custody.

Many infants in Western civilization have been raised by wet nurses, mammies, nannies, stepmothers, and extended family. Before the advent of modern methods of birth control, infants and toddlers were cared for by a host of big brothers and sisters, enduring the deaths and replacements of mothers when illnesses and complications of childbirth were commonplace. Israel's noted social movement that produced the kibbutzim meant that whole societies of children basically grew up in groups with designated caregivers and visits from parents. Other cultures have unique caregiving practices, but generally there is a defined group of people who deliver consistent love and care for the baby.

The "Century of the Child" is the name sometimes given to the twentieth century by writers who acknowledged a mass turning toward the knowledge of child experts. Child-care books, psychoanalytic theories, developmental psychology, and behaviorism produced a steady stream of ideas that sometimes were diametrically opposed. Scientifically verifiable explanations were sought by researchers to explain both the failures and the successes in human lives. One of the most intriguing areas for exploration has been attachment and the consequences of broken attachments (Karen 1994).

Perhaps Rene Spitz should be credited for the first powerful documentary showing the dark despair of institutionalized infants. Removed from their mothers and placed in a Mexican foundling home, these infants showed the ordeals of being cared for in a group of 45 babies with one head nurse and five assistants (Spitz 1945, 1947). From Dorothy Burlingham and Anna Freud's (1942) studies of toddlers separated from their parents during World War II to Bowlby's (1944) famous paper on the 44 juvenile thieves taken at young ages from their parents and Robertson's (1953) film *A Two-Year-Old Goes to Hospital,* the data pointed to the importance of attachment and the trauma that ensued when critical relationships were broken. In psychoanalytic and behaviorist circles, bitter fights developed over what was happening in the minds of babies (Bowlby 1973, 1982). Were they fixated on the breast and the narcissistic injury that resulted from its loss? Was environment or subjective experience to blame? Would ethology be able to provide the answers? After all, with monkeys, Harlow (1958) showed that it was not just the food that was important but that something soft and cuddly was also needed. This questioned the belief that the baby was attached to the mother only because she provided milk.

Carefully observing the African mothers and babies, Ainsworth (1967, 1984) made the connection that the babies of absent or nonresponsive mothers exhibited different behaviors. These early studies led to the development of Ainsworth's Strange Situation (Ainsworth et al. 1978), which became a primary research tool to determine whether children were securely attached, avoidantly attached, or ambivalently attached. Through the use of a carefully constructed paradigm designed to observe toddlers' relationships to their mothers in comparison to relationships with a stranger and reactions to separation and reunion, researchers identified classifiable patterns. Securely attached toddlers enjoyed close proximity to their mother, searched for mother when she left the room, and were joyous and welcoming when she returned. Insecurely attached babies demonstrated a variety of behaviors that included avoidance, temper tantrums, and ambivalence.

Working under Sroufe (1977) at the University of Minnesota, Waters (1978) tested the stability of attachment patterns by assessing babies at 12 and 18 months of age. He found that 48 of 50 maintained their original classification. In a subsequent study, Sroufe and colleagues observed 2-year-olds confronting a series of tasks; the study reinforced the better functioning of children who had been designated securely attached at 12 and 18 months (cited in Karen 1994). Egeland, working with a poverty sample over two decades, conducted numerous studies with Sroufe (Egeland and Farber 1984; Egeland et al. 1988) to further reinforce early research studies showing that securely attached children did better over time in areas that included such major factors as ego resiliency and social skills.

While research on the mother-child relationship was being carried on across the United States, other people were continuing to look at the results of broken attachment and the impact of other caregivers. Robertson and Robertson (1971) produced a powerful series of films in the early 1970s about young children in foster care. In one film, 2-year-old Thomas, who seemed to have a secure, loving relationship with his mother, became anxious and avoidant when separated from his mother during her 10-day hospitalization.

Entering the realm of multiple caregivers from another angle, Belsky (1986) joined the cadre of researchers with a child-care study indicating that children who were placed in extensive day care during the first year presented more pictures of avoidant attachment and exhibited aggressive behavior in their preschool years. His findings ignited the world of infant researchers, infant mental health professionals, and child-care professionals. For years, Bowlby (1958) had insisted that babies belonged with their mothers, who could be supplemented with outside help if necessary. Scarr (1984) said that mothers deserved rewarding lives in the workplace and that quality day care was good for children. Kagan (1984) also studied and supported positive outcomes from preschoolers in child care, contending that labeling children as insecurely attached might be erroneous when, in fact, children could simply be demonstrating healthy independence. Belsky's (1986) landmark study unleashed a host of day-care research.

Four years later, studies by Howes et al. (1990) indicated that the quality of the parent-child relationship and the quality of the infant care could lead to different outcomes, both positive and negative. Critical factors included the empathic responsiveness of the caregiver and the size of the day-care group. Good external child care could even ameliorate the effects of problematic mother-child relationships; in fact, toddlers used the external care providers as models for their peer relationships. In an interview with Mary Ainsworth for *Becoming Attached*, Robert Karen (1994) learned that she was supportive of early day care, provided it was of high quality and not meant as a substitute for a mother who might be absent for up to 10 hours a day. Pianta (1992) also examined the relationships between children and nonparental adults as reported in research projects around the world. Recent research from a variety of sources has repeatedly indicated that young children can have secure attachments with the important people in their lives if those people are sensitive and consistent. In Zaire, for example, Morelli and Tronick (1991) found that babies less than a year old had multiple caregivers but slept with their mothers every night. The importance of the sleeping arrangement has also been documented in studies that examined home-based and communal-based kibbutzim (Sagi et al. 1995), which found the communal-based arrangement to be somewhat detrimental to attachment.

As we review the history of nonmaternal caregivers and examine our own images of such situations, we realize that, although there is a historical precedent for multiple caregivers, it is critical for infants and toddlers to have a limited number of enduring, important relationships with adults. But what, exactly, are the current issues in society that are creating the multiple-caregiver phenomenon?

MARCH INTO THE TWENTY-FIRST CENTURY

Multiple caregivers are on the increase because of major changes in society. These changes affect family composition, household wage earners, child-care providers, special-needs children, adolescent pregnancy, and social problems for a number of reasons:

- Nuclear families are becoming increasingly rare. Many children will experience attachments and losses repeatedly when parents marry, divorce, find new mates, and repeat the process.
- Most women work outside the home. Two-parent families feel that they need both incomes to survive or maintain a certain standard of living, and single-parent families have no choice. Although some women still choose to stay home and rear their children, and even some fathers become househusbands, the majority of parents spend considerable time in the outside workforce. Welfare reforms in the United States increasingly require low-income mothers to find outside employment within a designated period of time that varies from state to state. Thus, the demand for child care is escalating rapidly. In developing countries, economic necessity may force both parents to work, and child care may be left to relatives or siblings.
- Although demand for child care is increasing, the high cost of infant care, the low wages paid child-care providers, the American worker's increasingly nontraditional work hours, and our own lack of knowledge about the emotional needs of infants and toddlers make high-quality child care almost impossible to find. Staff turnover at child-care centers is great, and families must often paste together a hodgepodge of relatives and external care arrangements that change frequently.
- With the emphasis on identifying and diagnosing special-needs children before their third birthday, multidisciplinary treatment or intervention teams frequently require infants and toddlers to be moved around the community to access a variety of services. Programs tend to offer special services within traditional work hours, which poses additional problems for working parents.
- Adolescent pregnancy has been a major social problem since the sexual revolution. Caught in their parents' quest for identity, search for a mate, and confusion over life goals, babies of teen parents more fre-

quently experience an unusual number of lifestyles and caregiving experiences. Secondary schools generally focus first on the adolescent's needs to obtain a high school diploma or GED (general education diploma, roughly equivalent to a high school diploma), to find child care, and to learn parenting skills. The babies' needs come last as a host of people care for each baby every day in the infant-care laboratory.

- Social problems (e.g., substance abuse, character pathology, mental illness, poverty, child maltreatment, AIDS, and violence) have led to more out-of-home placements for young children. Some children are subjected to a progression of foster homes, while others are raised by an assortment of relatives, frequently grandparents, who may be worn out from experiences with preceding generations and pass the children along to someone else to continue caring for them whenever they become too overwhelmed. A number of these children also may have biological components that make them more difficult to care for, which makes them at even greater risk of experiencing a succession of caregivers.

The contemporary children's book *Bye Bye Baby* (Ahlberg and Ahlberg 1989) tells the story of a motherless baby who searches until he finds an empty-handed mother who wants him. For babies and toddlers who experience multiple caregivers, it may feel as though no one wants them. The book highlights the fact that too many people have priorities that do not include caring for a needy infant. And, in fact, attachment is hard work. First of all, babies need sufficient time and caring from a loving adult. If the attachment is disrupted, the baby experiences pain. The baby may dare to attach again, but another broken attachment increases the risk that the young child will turn away from subsequent attachments (Hodges and Tizard 1989).

WHEN PARENTS WORK

The multiple-caregiver situation is like a theme with variations. When a well-loved infant from a stable home encounters a variety of caregivers through daily child care, the results are less onerous for him or her than for children who do not have a safe, predictable haven. In fact, studies in Israel and Holland show that children benefit most by having relationships marked by three secure attachments—mother, father, and nonparental caregiver (van IJzendoorn et al. 1992). Infants and toddlers in group child care all must master the following tasks: They must experience separation, share the caregiver with other infants, and experience daily routines slightly different from those they experience at home. Caregivers who understand infant development and the importance of their caregiving to healthy development will communicate regularly with parents; learn about the babies' needs, cues, and expectations through them; and try to replicate as closely as possible the home culture. When parents understand the needs of their child, they will screen caregivers to select the one they like and trust, the one who practices their beliefs and reflects their culture. Depending on the age and temperament of the child, the adjustment may be smooth or difficult.

The following child-care scenarios may arise when parents work outside the home: a) family child-care homes; b) group care; c) au pairs, nannies, and other in-home providers; and d) extended family care. Although there can be positive outcomes in these scenarios, frequently there are problems. The following examples of each type of care illustrate both negative and positive situations.

Family Child-Care Homes

Family child-care homes abound in small communities, in metropolitan areas, and throughout the countryside. They are appealing because of their familial context. Scheduling is more flexible. There are fewer babies and mixed ages that resemble a typical family. When they are regulated, the safety, health, and numbers of children are controlled. Family-care providers have many opportunities to obtain training in child development, nutrition, appropriate developmental activities, health and safety precautions, communication with parents, children's special needs, management of a small business, and so forth.

Unfortunately, however, there are probably more nonregulated providers whose convenience—and often lower cost—appeals to parents. They may be less concerned about numbers and more likely to take in two or three siblings, adding to a group that is already too large. Parents may not realize the emotional and physical risks they are taking, and the child-care providers may not realize the impact of what they do or don't do. Frequently, this type of provider may take in children to bring in extra money for a short time or as a favor to a desperate parent. They may avoid licensure because of fears of government interference in their lives and because of the increased cost, both in time and in money, that accompanies quality programs. Yet the true cost is borne by the child who must try to cope when a child-care arrangement fails.

Unattached Parent, Unsupported Caregiver

Kerry brought her 3-month-old daughter to a parent support group offered by the community. As leader of the group, I was impressed with Kerry's attachment to her delightful baby. Tiny Christina engaged her mother by smiling and waving her arms. Kerry met her baby's gaze, returned her radiant smile, and danced with her as they talked, cooed, and engaged in playful touching games. Kerry shared with the group her joy in her child, predicting each new stage before it occurred, and reveling in sharing the latest tales of their adventures together. One day when Kerry came in with two babies, I thought that Tanya, the new baby, was indeed fortunate. After being home for 6 weeks, Tanya's mother, Tracey, had felt the need to return to work, and Kerry had agreed to provide child care.

Now Kerry had two babies to shower with her loving attention. She did a masterful job. Christina cruised the room on hands and knees, returning to her mother for refueling. She seemed not to mind the new baby cradled in her mother's arms, and Kerry seemed to be able to share her gifts of love.

As weeks passed, however, worrisome signs appeared. At first, they were subtle. Although Tanya laughed and smiled at Kerry, Kerry seemed more distant and not as responsive. Kerry talked about how Tanya's mother was not attached to her infant. Using her excellent observation skills, she related that Tracey never seemed eager to pick up Tanya. She had begun bringing her in earlier and picking her up later. Even when Kerry talked to her about the importance of respecting the hours they had agreed on, Tracey continued to ignore the rules. Kerry noted that Tracey was married for the second time and already had teenage children from her first marriage; Kerry speculated that Tracey may have had this baby only to please her new husband. Tracey complained that her older children spoiled Tanya by holding her too much. Kerry began to feel that Tracey was expecting her to be Tanya's attachment figure, and although Kerry fully understood the importance of attachment, she was not volunteering for that job. She was providing child care because she needed extra income, liked babies, and thought she did well as child-care provider, but she did not want to be the mother of someone else's child.

As Kerry distanced herself from Tanya, Tanya smiled less and slept more. She lost her bright-eyed interest in her surroundings and seemed to retreat into her protective shell. My efforts to support Kerry and coach her about how to communicate with Tracey fell on deaf ears. One day, Kerry came to the group with just one baby; she had decided to stop providing child care for Tanya. Tanya was headed down the risky path of multiple caregivers, where the lack of attachment at home coupled with rejection from an external caregiver would affect her fragile, beginning sense of identity. This succession of caregivers is, unfortunately, not so rare.

New Connections

Teddy had the chance to be the cherished baby in a family day-care home, where Karen, the day-care mother, cared for six children, including two of her own. She liked having a variety of ages, so she generally took infants through elementary school, one at a time, until they were ready to leave child care. Karen was active in the local association of family care providers, was registered as meeting state standards, and regularly attended meetings and annual workshops.

Before Teddy came into her home, Karen met with his parents to listen to what they wanted. She agreed with their ideas about holding the baby to feed him, rocking him before putting him down to sleep, taking him outside whenever the weather permitted, monitoring a limited amount of television for all the children, playing and talking with Teddy every day, encouraging the older children to interact with him, and taking him to events at the schools "the big kids" attended. They all agreed that it was important to allow time every morning and every evening for communication. Over a period of several weeks, Teddy's parents observed, spent time with the child at Karen's home, and built up to full day care. Health and safety factors were discussed and acknowledged from both the parents' and Karen's perspectives. Plans were made for the parents to take turns staying home from work with Teddy when he was sick, and both sides planned vacation times far in advance to minimize Karen's loss of income and ensure the most continuity for Teddy.

Teddy entered child care at the age of 3 months and continued it until age 12, when he entered the seventh grade. Karen and her family were like extended family for this child, whose own relatives were many miles away. In this case, the "substitute" caregivers become emotionally like the equivalent of an extended family and true attachment figures.

Group Care

Group-care centers come in all shapes and sizes. Because of the high cost associated with all child care, most are nonprofit. Sponsored by churches, businesses, and civic groups such as YWCAs and the United Way, they struggle to meet financial constraints and, at the same time, provide quality care (which means education as well as care). Chain child cares are new for-profit options that entice families to enroll by providing transportation, attractive buildings, and sleek brochures that promise a set of services. Through their large corporate structure, they are able to buy equipment and supplies in large quantity, promise bonuses to directors who operate within a tight budget, and use cost-saving business practices that have children sharing expensive equipment. Infant and toddler care, with its high staff ratio of one staff to three or four children, is so costly that few programs elect to offer these services. Also, states may fight licensing policies that stress the importance of small groups.

Two critical issues that plague group child care are 1) attachment and loss and 2) cultural synchrony and confusion.

Attachment and Loss

Although consistency is considered important, few families are fortunate enough to find child-care providers who will remain constant during the first few years of life. Whitebrook et al. (1989) reported that day-care staff turnover averaged more than 40% per year in the United States. Only now is there a major effort to keep children with the same provider during the first 3 years of group care (Lally et al. 1995). In many states, licensing requirements mandate that children be placed in age-segregated groups. As a result, group-care centers often move a baby to a new room and a new provider either when the child learns to walk or by by the time the child is 18 months of age. The video *Together in Care: Meeting the Intimacy Needs of Infants and Toddlers in Groups* (Lally et al. 1992) shows the grief of toddlers—and sometimes of caregivers—as children experience new situations where they must once again teach the adults to understand their cues. Children may lose a caregiver because of center policy, but regardless of policy, staff turnover is large. Most often, staff members leave because they desire better wages. To survive financially, even idealistic, well-trained early-childhood professionals often move into either administrative jobs, public education, or business and retail.

Time for Tears

Two-year-old Laura was well settled in her church-based child-care center. Her caring and devoted parents worked outside the home and chose the center because of its long history of providing good care for young children. Laura was part of a small group of 2-year-olds who spent their days in a bright, cheerful room with a stained glass window showing Jesus Christ tending lambs and children. Every day Laura could count on a predictable schedule, learning opportunities, nutritious food offered at just the right intervals, and developmentally appropriate activities both inside and outside on the attractive playground. Staff, however, did not recognize their own importance to the young lives that relied on them. After all, competent substitutes were always available when a regular caregiver had to be absent.

Laura's beloved "teacher" needed a vacation and notified the child-care director but did not think about what her absence would mean to her young charges. She left without talking about it either to the children or to their parents. Shortly thereafter, she decided it was time to move on, and she left altogether. Laura's parents noticed an immediate change in their daughter's behavior, especially an increased reluctance to go to school and sleep problems that persisted for 6 weeks. They wrote a poignant letter to the director and the board about the trauma Laura had experienced. Unable to talk about her loss in words, Laura showed everyone her distress through her behavior. Fortunately, she had sensitive parents who became her advocates and helped her acknowledge her feelings. They also alerted the child-care center so that teachers' departures and absences could be handled differently in the future.

Together for Three Important Years

Jill was enrolled in a child-care center as an infant assigned to Lizzie, a primary caregiver. Lizzie obviously understood her importance to children and was there to celebrate each new developmental accomplishment, nurse wounds, wipe away tears, listen, respond, and guide and teach. She learned to enjoy the challenges of each stage—valuing both Jill's dependency and her independence. Lizzie was able to change diapers, join parents in toilet training, and celebrate the newly toilet-trained child. By age 3, Jill was an empathic child who loved the world. With sensitivity and continuity both at school and at home, Jill seemed to have a strong, confident internal working model of self (Lally et al. 1992).

Cultural Synchrony or Confusion?

Frequently, child-care providers have taken courses focusing on child development and appropriate activities for their young charges. Although they know parents are important, they have experienced little training for communicating with parents, understanding their culture, and learning how to work out disagreements. Directors of child-care programs have not understood the importance of hiring staff who speak other languages and understand other cultures. They may not understand the importance of reading, acquiring training, or consulting with the parents about their particular culture. As a result, babies may be fed, talked to, put to sleep, and changed in unfamiliar ways. Without a parent-caregiver partnership, the baby experiences a world that is hard to understand and integrate. Out of frustration, the infant may develop behavior that is considered unacceptable. The following examples are taken from events that infants and toddlers from other cultures may experience every day.

Importance of Language

José comes from a Spanish-speaking home. Every night and weekend, he is surrounded by people who speak only Spanish. But at the child-care center, he hears only English for 8½ hours a day. At 20 months, both his receptive and expressive language scores lag behind the norm. Unless a bilingual parent is available to translate whenever his Spanish-speaking parents bring him in or pick him up, important communications between caregivers about his activities are lost.

Importance of Values

Antonia is the beloved little girl in a family of boys. Her family's cultural beliefs promote dependency, protection, beautiful frilly dresses, and cleanliness. At her child-care center, the teachers work to make Antonia more assertive, independent, and messy. She is beginning to exhibit tantrums, alternating with withdrawal, both at home and at school. She receives contradictory messages and has conflicting expectations due to the very different emotional fields with which she has to cope.

Survival Skills

Marcel is a 14-month-old from a neighborhood known for its danger and violence. From the time he could crawl, his adolescent mother encouraged him to hang on to his toys, fight, and "be a man." When Mommy went to work, Marcel began child care. Already he has been rejected by several child-care providers because of his "bad behavior." Again, there is a cultural dissonance between the two settings.

Right Fit

The new Early Head Start program was located in a rural area that had experienced an influx of families from Mexico who had moved first to follow the crops and then to immigrate. Having offered Head Start for many years, the community researched how best to serve children under age 3. Although the Early Head Start program already employed a number of Latino staff members, the Policy Council recognized the importance of hiring Spanish-speaking home visitors and child-care providers to help with the children's language acquisition and support identity formation that recognized family culture. As a result, 3-month-old Miguel entered a program that was a comfortable fit. The family advocate was able to listen to the family's goal to learn more English, while helping them share their wonderful sense of community, spiritual roots, and celebrations with other Early Head Start families.

Au Pairs, Nannies, and Other In-Home Providers

Higher-socioeconomic-status families generally have more child-care options, but if they do not understand the needs of their young children and the importance of quality and supervision, their children can suffer as much as children from economically deprived families. Au pairs or nannies are frequently used by families who want to provide more continuity, maintain more control, allow their children to stay within the context of a familiar home, and set more flexible working hours. To provide maximum availability to the family, au pairs or nannies frequently come from great distances to live with them. Unfortunately, tragic accidents have been in the news because young women enter the field for the wrong reasons or have inadequate supervision, training, and ongoing communication.

In some parts of the country, however, families hire in-home, daily child-care providers. Again, their success or failure depends on the family who hires them, their knowledge of young children's needs, and the support they receive in the home. Like all nonparental caregivers who become important supplementary attachment figures for children, the best child-care providers take on the job with a commitment that acknowledges their importance to the family over a period of time.

Tragic Scenario

Heidi came from Germany with high hopes of having wonderful adventures in the United States. She had attended an au pair school but had little supervised experience with young children. She took the job to learn whether she liked children, but her first experience was a disaster. There were more children than had been promised and no private room for Heidi. Objecting loudly to her agency, Heidi was moved to another state.

Her new family had two children—a 10-month-old and a 2-year-old—who had been through three au pairs since the birth of the older child. Heidi soon discovered why. The parents worked long hours, did nothing to make Heidi feel welcome, and gave her minimal instructions and support. In desperation, Heidi went to a community parent-infant group to make friends. The devoted, stay-at-home mothers had never met an au pair and didn't know how to relate to her. Heidi's lack of familiarity with the culture and her poorly developed social skills didn't help. The two young children sat quietly on her lap, soaking up the unfamiliar experience of a room full of active, joyous mothers and babies. Unlike other babies who attended the group for the first time, they had no secure base to either venture from or return to, so they sat doll-like for the entire hour. As group leader, I offered to visit the family and help with communication, but the situation was already hopeless. Heidi requested another placement, was turned down, and was soon on her way back to Germany. The children were in line for a fifth au pair—victims of both the parents and an agency that did not seem to understand attachment issues for young children.

Doing It Right

Several states away, another family searched for in-home help. Prioritizing the needs of everyone was important, and finances were not an issue. Because the parents knew the importance of the early years and put a high value on those years as well as on their own careers, they hired Jennifer, a teacher with early-childhood certification, as a caregiver. These parents were willing to offer considerable financial support and ensure that their child-care provider felt respected and valued. They were committed to sharing the job of parenting while handling their own demanding careers because they wanted their children, Jason and Joseph, to feel secure. Their house was always filled with the aroma of

Mommy's homemade cookies (frequently made late at night). The father read to his sons daily, making regular trips to the library to bring home the stacks of books that reflected the parents' devotion to education. Although these parents had heavy work demands, they also paid careful attention to Jennifer's needs, as well as to those of their children, thus ensuring that Jason and Joseph would grow to adulthood feeling competent, valued, and strongly versed in their family values.

Extended-Family Care

While parents work, many children are cared for by relatives. Sometimes grandmothers who were adolescents when their own children were born are now ready to devote real time to their grandchildren. At other times, the grandparents are still in the outside workforce, so other family members take over. Although it seems most acceptable to have one or two regular family members that the child can count on, some families have a tight network that works well with careful planning. For the children, it is most important that whoever cares for them understands and is sensitive to their needs and does the job out of love and caring rather than as a resented obligation. Because of the changes in our society, the new understanding of the importance of the early years, and the need for quality in every situation, intervention programs such as Early Head Start are broadening their training and support networks to reach out to extended family.

One More Time Around

Lavonia had raised four children under stressful conditions, but she did her best. She had no husband and lived in high-rise, urban, crime-ridden housing. She spent hours waiting in line for benefits from the welfare system and learning how to make the most out of the minuscule amount of money from the federal government. She had made her mistakes but was proud of her ability to get beyond them and nurture her children. Now, at 45, she was ready to begin doing a little living for herself. Through the community action program, she had gotten her GED and secretarial training and could finally become self-supporting.

What she hadn't counted on was a houseful of grandchildren. Despite her valiant efforts to teach her children different values, the power of the neighborhood and peer influences had made their mark. One son and one daughter had not been able to escape the tantalizing temptation to feel good by going the cocaine and heroin route. After providing short-term safe havens for five young children, Lavonia began to realize that she was committing her life to another 20 years of child rearing. She saw that the children were well fed, clothed, and immunized and had the basics, but she struggled with resentment because these children needed so much love, time, and attention. When would she ever have time for herself?

Lavonia put the children in child care during part of the day. At child care, the five young children vied for time on a teacher's lap, skirted ongoing relationships, and demanded attention from any adult who walked into the room. They showed through their peer interactions and play that life did not feel quite right. Caregivers worried about the neediness of these children. Some were eager to pass them along; others mourned their inability to provide the ongoing love that seemed lacking. All struggled with ways to support the grandmother while getting the children on the right path.

Circle of Love

When Joshua was a few months old, his mother needed to return to work. Her large extended family decided they did not want Joshua cared for by outsiders. They divided up the days when Joshua needed care, and various relatives took one or two consistent days each week—two days with Grandpa, one with Grandma, one with an aunt, one with another relative. As I talked with Joshua's aunt about the plan and its results, she glowed with pride. By the time he was ready for preschool, Joshua was outgoing, secure, competent, and developing well in every area. As we pondered why such a complex schedule would work for a young infant, the key words seemed to be family love, commitment, continuity, and communication. Joshua repeatedly saw his extended family together, celebrated important occasions with them, was with his parents every night, and felt completely wrapped up in a culture that believed that family togetherness and shared responsibility were important.

SPECIAL SERVICES AND THERAPEUTIC INTERVENTIONS

Although attachment and cultural synchrony are important, many authors and researchers have produced evidence that suggests there are exceptions to this rule. Thousands of children are born each year into homes where they will be maltreated. Thousands more are born with or develop special needs within the first few weeks and months of life. In these cases, babies require something other than a replication of their home experiences. There are mandates to report child abuse and requirements to assess, evaluate, and provide services for children with special needs. Professionals need training opportunities to learn how to recognize such needs and intervene early. Together, these requirements mean that increasing numbers of children under age 3 may spend significant time in a combination child-care and special-education facility or in a therapeutic center. In some cases, the child needs protection as well as rehabilitation. In other cases, there is no child maltreatment, just babies and families in need of special techniques to help children. Unfortunately, the vast array of services, appointments in various parts of town, and sometimes two half-day programs that carry the child by taxicab from one point to another may be overwhelming experiences to a child, who has no concept of time and cannot understand what is happening. Service providers may be too busy to send notes or maintain daily communication.

Caught in the System

Stephanie was happily enrolled in a therapeutic preschool program for 2-year-olds whose staff worked with her, her foster family, and her birth family. The program was jointly funded by the school district and a psychiatric clinic. Stephanie's life had been filled with tragedy, but she was finally in a place that provided integrated services. Her foster family had to give her up unexpectedly because of their own circumstances. With foster care homes at a premium, the only available home was located in another school district. Preschool staff breathed a sigh of relief when they were assured that the new foster home was within commuting distance. What they did not realize was that the new school district had a special-education, home-visiting program that refused to pay for Stephanie to attend another district's program, and her original school district had to have funds to be able to continue Stephanie in its program. Furthermore, school buses could not transport children out of a district, and the new foster parent could not transport her because of the other children's needs. In the new school district and in her new home, placid Stephanie's behavior became a problem.

Happy Ending

Billy was enrolled in a therapeutic child-development center when he was 11 months old. During his short life, he had experienced skull fractures, a broken leg, and numerous bruises. His 2-year-old sister sat quietly and passively on her teacher's lap, seeming more like a 3-month-old baby than a preschooler. The parents were required to bring their children to the daily program and begin the long process of changing their views that children were private possessions to be treated however the parents chose. There was no continuity between what happened at home and what happened at the child-care center. The nonparental caregivers were sensitive and responsive. The parents were insensitive and nonresponsive, the products of their own miserable childhoods. The road was long and rough, with babies needing to learn to trust and parents needing to learn what children are. Two years passed before these parents could begin to admit that they had made some major mistakes. Being able to give love and nurturing was such a difficult job for them. Learning to trust their autonomy and feel good about themselves was equally difficult for their children.

The program was center-based, with monthly home visits. While Billy was a baby, one or both parents attended the half-day program with him every day. When he moved to a preschool group, their participation dropped back to 1 day a week. Along with all the regular developmental experiences in their intervention program, both children had play therapy. Groups for the children were small, with a high adult-to-child ratio. Although trainees from a variety of disciplines did internships for a semester or a year, the family had consistent staff who maintained primary relationships over the course of the children's 3-year treatment program. Parents had family therapy and individual appointments and attended a parents' group and parent-child counseling sessions. The team worked closely to meet the family's needs, and regular social events at the center helped the family feel part of a positive, loving network.

Sixteen years after their initial referral, the family returned to see me with a minor family therapy issue. Billy, the beaten baby, and his sister, Susie, the "robot child," were bright, competent adolescents who had overcome their difficult pasts to succeed in school, form wonderful friendships, and approach adulthood with positive plans. In this case, multiple caregivers had been their salvation. Perhaps the most important aspect of this work, however, was that it included the entire family. Although the center did not replicate the caregiving that the children were receiving at home, staff members worked to change the parenting provided at home so that it gave the children what all children want: love, understanding, positive guidance, and responsiveness to their individual needs.

The program that Billy participated in started a number of years ago when there was more support for long-term programs to address long-term and very serious problems. Since then we have learned more about the importance of attachment, integration, and communication and the need to keep the child and parents in the center of the circle. Thus, there is more effort now to have a few key people in the driver's seat, focus more on family strengths than on family problems, and establish short-term, reasonable goals with the family. Because of welfare reform and the demand on families to become self-sufficient faster, it has become paramount to develop interagency teams, train parents to do specific activities with their babies, establish flexible hours, provide creative planning, and use volunteer and community groups. Programs such as Early Head Start (with its quality Performance Standards), Parents as Teachers, and Healthy Families America keep the baby in the center of the picture and may achieve positive outcomes by partnering with parents.

FOSTER CARE

According to Williams (1998) of the U.S. Children's Bureau, maltreatment of children under age 3 years quadrupled between 1988 and 1993 (U.S. Department of Health and Human Services 1998b). Only 50% of the children (ages 0–3) placed in foster care are able to remain in one home (U.S. Department of Health and Human Services 1998a). Nine percent have four or more homes, one after the other. Not only do the children sustain psychological damage from their own homes, but they also must deal with the system meant to protect them. Despite continuing efforts to correct and protect, the system is still in crisis.

Foster parents undertake the difficult job of caring for needy children for all sorts of reasons, many of which lead to failure. Not many emotionally injured children can provide the emotional rewards that foster parents anticipated, the money earned does not come close to compensating them for the difficult work, and the behavior problems can be overwhelming. Because there is always a tremendous need for homes, many agencies do not have the luxury of being particularly selective.

Once accepted into the foster-care network, foster parents have all too often been treated as second-class citizens. Although they have the challenging task of trying to rehabilitate children who are not ready to listen to anyone, the foster parents may find that, in turn, few people want to listen to them. Visitation schedules, reintegration plans, and therapeutic interventions may be planned without their input. Case managers may have too large a caseload to be able to give enough support to the foster parent when a child is having a difficult time. As a result, young children may be shifted from one home to another, frequently with little or no time for preparation. A 5-year-old who had experienced multiple moves during Christmas vacation once told me, "And God says it ain't over yet."

Just One More Chance

Angelina experienced nearly 20 moves between the ages of 2 and 4. Starting out as a sweet but neglected toddler, she developed into a child who believed she was bad. Acting out her magical thinking of controlling her own destiny, she repeatedly found a foster parent's vulnerable spot and triggered another rejection. During a 2-year period, Angelina had foster parents who became tired, case workers who thought she was becoming too attached and needed to be moved, supervisors who were concerned about preferential treatment in a home, and foster parents who had unrealistic expectations. Efforts were made to reunite Angelina with her birth mother between some of the foster home moves. Each time she experienced another trauma: no food to eat, domestic violence, and sexual abuse. Yet there was always the belief by caseworkers and the judge that her mother needed one more chance.

Angelina's most consistent adult was a therapist who was willing to stay with her through correspondence, telephone calls, and occasional visits over the course of her growing years. Parental rights were eventually severed, and Angelina was free to be adopted. The therapist was willing to stay involved as a telephone support to both Angelina and her new adoptive mother. The mother, however, decided that Angelina needed to make a clean break to forget the past—a fantasy that often leads to heartbreak in adoptive parents who want to make all the hurt go away.

My Cup Runneth Over With Despair

Christina had sustained multiple broken bones at the hands of her very disturbed, mentally handicapped parents. Removed from her home, she took months to begin to trust her foster parents. Intensive work with the birth parents produced no results, yet a judge returned her to a home where she was abused again. Her familiar foster parents could not take her back because their home was already filled with new children.

Agonies of Skin Color

Alexander was an African American toddler who was extremely attached to the European American foster parents who wanted to adopt him. However, the judge felt that it was not right for him to grow up with a white family and give up his ethnic roots. Alexander knew only that his foster mother had been there continuously to rock him through sleepless nights when he was tormented by the impact of his mother's heroin addiction. The foster parents had been given verbal assurance by the child protection agency that they could adopt him because his own mother had shown no interest in Alexander for the first 12 months. When he was 15 months old, she changed her mind and entered a drug rehabilitation program. The judge ordered reunification with an accelerated move back home. The pace was traumatic for both Alexander and his foster family. Overnight visits were increased every week, although Alexander became sick, began to bite, screamed hysterically, and threw the "other Mommy" doll away in play therapy sessions. The foster parents offered to invite Alexander's birth mother into their home to visit him. They wanted to communicate about how best to help him and were willing to put their own heartbreak aside for Alexander's best interests in meeting the court order for reunification. The birth mother could only feel jealous of Alexander's attachment to his foster parents; she was determined to get him away quickly and make him forget his past. The government agency's attorney advised the case worker not to alter plans because of Alexander's despair and to ignore the therapist's recommendation to slow down the process because of Alexander's desperate cues. On the day that his permanent return was to take place, there were still no signs of attachment to his birth mother. Alexander tried to throw his packed toys out of the bag while screaming, "No go." The foster mother entered counseling to recover from the loss and her disillusionment about the foster-care system.

HOPE FOR THE FUTURE

Our society at present is midstream in the process of allowing children to be adopted by people previously considered unsuitable matches. As a result, adoptive parents can now be single, homosexual, older than before, and from different ethnic backgrounds. Although it is still important to evaluate prospective parents carefully, there is increased recognition that love, understanding, and commitment are more important than color, age, and sexual preference. Only time will tell whether the new process is successful. Through it all, attention should be focused on attachment work with the young child and the new family, while grief work and support for new, constructive goals are offered to the birth parents, who may be inclined to start new pregnancies to replace lost children.

ADOLESCENT PARENTS

Adolescent parents frequently have babies to fill the emptiness in their lives. Abortions or adoptions that take place without processing the decision may lead to a repeat pregnancy within a short time. In the days of the scarlet A, pregnant girls generally aborted or gave up their babies; now they are much more inclined to keep them. Teenage pregnancy is particularly a problem when 13- and 14-year-olds, still children themselves, have babies (Osofsky et al. 1992). Because of the research that has defined and addressed the problems, prevention and intervention programs have sprung up across the nation. To ameliorate the poverty that frequently accompanies adolescent pregnancy, major efforts have been made to keep young parents in school through the twelfth grade or until they are able to acquire a GED. A major deterrent to finishing school has been the lack of affordable, readily available infant care. As a result, many alternative education programs have started group infant care within the school or within walking distance of the school. Quite often, the child-care program has doubled as a parenting laboratory for adolescent parents and occasionally for other students. The adolescents are able to learn about child development and good parenting practices. One important factor, however, gets short shrift. Rather than experiencing a protective environment with a few consistent, predictable caregivers, the babies in the laboratory school, which has only a few consistent staff members, may be cared for and handled by different people every hour of the school day. On the surface, the program looks good. From a baby's perspective, this daily world is a bit overwhelming.

On the Move

At first glance, Todd appeared to be a healthy, delightful 7-month-old. Having mastered crawling, he was on the go. The soft carpet, foam furniture, and developmentally appropriate toys offered a variety of interesting things to do in the infant laboratory of his mother's school. Todd never stopped. As mothers came and went from hour to hour, he crawled over laps and was picked up and fussed over by a succession of adolescents who spent their child-development hour in his room. Todd rarely cried. He also rarely made eye contact and practically never stopped to really explore a toy. At lunchtime, when his mother was scheduled to feed him, he looked so tired that he was barely able to eat. Although his mother was full of energy and ready to play, Todd was worn out. When Mommy played an animated game of moving her head back and forth a few inches from his face, Todd looked around her. To Todd, the world may have seemed like a daily amusement park, with little time and energy to establish meaningful relationships.

I Just Want You, Mommy

In the same infant laboratory, another 7-month-old boy handled his environment in just the opposite way. When Sammy's mother left, he cried. The busy but compassionate head teacher picked Sammy up, consoled him, and sat him in the lap of a foster grandfather who rocked him until he stopped crying. Not understanding the importance of individual relationships, the gray-haired man never spoke to Sammy or attempted to relate to him. Instead, he looked like a human rocking machine, and eventually the motion quieted the distraught baby. When he was put down on the carpet, Sammy cried again, with other people providing momentary comfort. When his mother arrived at lunchtime, Sammy was delighted to see her. As he ate his food, his one-tooth smile and comfortable sprawling over the side of his high chair told the world that he finally had what he wanted, but not for long.

Each girl who came into the nursery donned a smock and an attitude of professional caregiving. If her baby was awake, she spent some time with her baby but soon left to attend to others or play with one who was particularly cute and active. As soon as Sammy had swallowed his last bite, his mother saw another baby who was ready for lunch. She deposited Sammy on the floor across the room and turned her attention to the new baby now in Sammy's high chair. Sammy collapsed in grief. With tears rolling down his cheeks, he tried to pull himself across the floor to his mother, who blocked out his wails. Needing to get a washcloth for her new charge, she stepped over the crying Sammy, seemingly unaware of the depths of his despair.

WHEN PARENTS DIVORCE

According to divorce expert Monica McGoldrick (1997), 60% of all first marriages will end in divorce, and 75% of those who are divorced will remarry. Although much research has been done on children of divorce, little research has focused on the child under age 3. A study based in Boulder, Colorado, found that 20% of the divorcing couples in that town had children under 3 years of age (Hodges et al. 1991). Taking a strong stance that issues of time, perspective, object constancy, and attachment are important in determining visitation, the authors emphasized the importance of frequent short visits to ensure that babies maintain attachments to both parents while feeling secure in a consistent custodial home. The researchers found that frequency of visits increased the emotionality in the child, with some children responding more positively and some more negatively. In addition, early intensive contact led to more involvement with fathers as children became older.

Because of a belief in parental rights, the courts all too frequently treat children like pawns on a chessboard and disregard or minimize children's confusion and distress. Judges, lawyers, and parents with little knowledge of child development do not realize the trauma that children endure by being shifted from house to house when they have no concept of time, only fragile object constancy, and a need for ritual. Instead of attention being paid to the child's best interests, the focus is on fairness to both parents, with each having equal time. Children's emotional signals (withdrawal, tears, regressions, illnesses, or tantrums) are considered necessary transitional behaviors to be overcome by the passage of time. Despite the landmark book *Beyond the Best Interests of the Child* (Goldstein et al. 1979), courts continue to divide up children like property, except when compassionate judges have educated themselves about the far-reaching ramifications of their decisions.

Split in Two

Lucia's father moved to a neighboring state after his divorce from her mother, but he insisted on having his share of his child. Because of the distance involved, 2-year-old Lucia traveled 500 miles to spend 2 months with each parent on a revolving cycle. Following 2 months with her father, Lucia was brought for consultation because of tantrums, sleep problems, and regression in established toilet training. Her mother reported that after their long separation, they needed to become reacquainted all over again, a traumatic experience for both the child and her mother. Her father, on the other hand, refused to acknowledge that the visitation schedule might be beyond Lucia's coping ability and insisted that the court-ordered schedule be maintained.

Mommy and Daddy Both Love You

Matthew enjoyed an early infancy filled with wonderful regular time with his father, who bathed, fed, diapered, and rocked him almost as frequently as his mother did. Unfortunately, marital problems that had been building long before his birth were not magically resolved when he entered the world. Along with the love bestowed on him, he was exposed to violent anger between the two people he loved the most, depression in his mother, and, finally, separations and reunions that produced constant turmoil. Matthew reacted with an unusual amount of illness and insecurity and a facial expression that indicated he could not quite trust the world to be a safe haven. Through the counseling sessions ordered by the divorce court and services of a mediator trained to consider the needs of children under age 3, the parents were able to put aside their anger at each other long enough to plan for Matthew's future. Although they each wanted him half time, they became cognizant of the emotional price Matthew would pay for their own desires. Reluctantly, they made a pact to work out daily sharing in a way that would keep Matthew connected and secure.

Matthew's primary residence would be with his mother because she was still nursing him several times a day. Whenever his mother had evening classes or activities, his father had first choice to care for him at either his mother's or father's house. In addition, Daddy could pick him up from child care each day, play with him, feed him his evening solid food, and then take him home at the agreed-upon time. These parents decided to stay in close proximity during Matthew's preschool years. They also supported one another's relationship with Matthew, avoided angry outbursts in front of him, and renegotiated their shared relationship when he was 3, then 6, or whenever a developmental stage indicated it might be time for another arrangement. If the parents had trouble communicating, they would bring in a mediator or family therapist. Matthew's parents also recognized that acquiring new mates should be a time when they would also need to put forth more efforts to understand Matthew's needs and reactions and make sure that they and their new mates understood Matthew's best interests and their respective roles.

IMPLICATIONS FOR RESEARCH AND INTERVENTION

Everything we know about child development stresses the importance of relationships, yet we still seem to do things counterproductively in our current society. At the very point when children are most vulnerable, need to establish basic trust, and need to form the beginnings of their own identity, they are often placed in situations where there is little stability and where they are cared for by an overwhelming cadre of caregivers with different ways of doing things. We need longitudinal research to study the long-term impact of multiple caregivers while continuing to try to provide the kind of constancy and caring that has been effective in the past. Wherever we can, we need to promote education about the needs of infants and toddlers. We also need to encourage the best practices by being child-care advocates, providing good child care, offering therapeutic interventions, supporting those who provide foster and other out-of-home care, and developing teaching strategies for coping with adolescent pregnancy, divorce, and remarriage.

Advocacy

Mental health professionals must begin to sponsor and support legislation that provides for the care and nurturing of young children and their families. We must be willing to speak to community groups, using such materials as *Heart Start* (Zero to Three 1994), *Starting Points: Meeting the Needs of Our Youngest Children* (Carnegie Foundation 1994), and the latest magazines to educate the general public about infant development and community needs.

Child Care

Mental health professionals should educate parents about the needs of babies, support resource and referral agencies that maintain lists of licensed child-care facilities, and promote continuing education for child-care providers. They should also attract people to the caregiving field by fighting for higher salaries and professionalism, insisting on quality programming that specifically addresses the needs of infants, and encouraging business and child-care partnerships that support the needs of families. By helping communities develop multiple funding streams to support quality child care, we can ensure that families can afford to place their children in good programs. We can also work with universities and training providers to meet identified training needs through a variety of options. Finally, we can support efforts to build strong communication and partnering between parents and child-care providers, emphasizing understanding and supporting cultural factors.

Therapeutic Interventions

As much as possible, we should take our services into the child's home or the child-care center, training parents and primary caregivers to carry out special programming. Doing so would simplify and minimize ongoing appointments at numerous places with multiple providers. Although a multidisciplinary team may do an initial evaluation, creative strategies may produce interventions that are less overwhelming to a young child than to have multiple professionals in their offices meeting with their child. This would help maintain the infant's ability to remain in an inclusive program. We can also work with interagency special-education teams in the community to ensure that training and support are available to meet individual needs.

Foster and Out-of-Home Care

When it is absolutely necessary to remove a baby from the parents, we can support the alternative caregivers as they try to understand the baby and his or her needs. We can also provide consistency, appropriate care, and love as well as acknowledge the loss a baby may experience. We can support the supervising agency's knowledge of and advocacy for the best interests of the child, and we can treat the alternative caregivers as valuable partners. We can provide educational workshops for judges and encourage programs that not only work to preserve the family but also help the family understand the need to improve parenting ability within a limited time. In this way, a baby can have some permanency within a reasonable time. We can also encourage regular communication between adults providing care for the infant and be respectful of and responsive to the ideas of everyone working to ensure the best interests of the baby. We can see that mental health supports are there for the baby, the out-of-home provider, the family of origin, and the case manager. If and when the baby is released for adoption, we can plan carefully for a smooth transition by seeing to it that the adoptive family has a thorough understanding of the baby's past experiences and their implications for development.

Adolescent Pregnancy

Mental health professionals should understand that the needs of a baby and an adolescent parent are diametrically opposed. Thus, programs must be designed to meet the developmental needs of both. If child-care programs are used as parenting or child-development laboratories, we must design practices to give priority to the parent-infant relationship, reduce the number of daily caregivers, and keep the activity in the room at any given time from being overwhelming and overstimulating. We must help both father and mother relate to their baby appropriately while nevertheless supporting their own need for fun and for developing their identities and goals in life. We ought to help them find constructive support systems within their extended families, peer groups, and community services. We must also nurture those support systems and the young parents themselves. We have to support the efforts of adolescent parents to finish school and find work while maintaining their daily priority relationship with their baby. We should also find ways to help adolescent parents understand their impact on a child's life.

Divorce and Remarriage

Mental health professionals can play a unique role in divorce and remarriage. We can help attorneys, judges, and parents understand the unique needs of babies and toddlers under 3 years of age and can encourage them to make decisions concerning visitation and custody based on those needs. We can train family therapists and mental health practitioners to include babies and toddlers in consultations and therapy processes that provide healing therapeutic interventions for them, as well as for the older, more verbal members of the family.

SUMMARY

Infants and toddlers in today's society are experiencing rapidly changing lifestyles. Because of all the indicators that signify the importance of attachment to key caregivers, we, as mental health professionals, must constantly study, redesign, and observe the effects of circumstances that place babies with other caregivers. Families, service providers, and society as a whole must take off their blinders and look objectively at the results. If we are able to do so, multiple caregivers may be used in ways that enhance babies' lives rather than contribute to problems that lead to a society in distress.

For many years, both parents and children have loved the stories and poems about Christopher Robin and Pooh. A. A. Milne's understanding of the importance of primary caregivers in a young child's life is summarized in this excerpt from his poem "Vespers" (Milne 1924/1996). As we read of Christopher Robin saying his prayer, we recognize that it is up to us to be the protectors and advocates for young children—and their caregivers—everywhere.

> *God bless Mummy.* I know that's right.
> Wasn't it fun in the bath tonight?
> The cold's so cold, and the hot's so hot.
> Oh! *God bless Daddy*—I quite forgot.
> If I open my fingers a little bit more,
> I can see Nanny's dressing-gown on the door.
> It's a beautiful blue, but it hasn't a hood.
> Oh! *God bless Nanny and make her good.*

REFERENCES

Ahlberg J, Ahlberg L: Bye Bye Baby. New York, Little, Brown, 1989

Ainsworth MDS: Infancy in Uganda: Infant Care and the Growth of Love. Baltimore, MD, Johns Hopkins University Press, 1967

Ainsworth MDS: Attachment, in Personality and the Behavioral Disorders, Vol 1. Edited by Endler NS, Hunt JM. New York, Wiley, 1984, pp 559–602

Ainsworth MDS, Blehar MC, Waters E, et al: Patterns of Attachment: A Psychological Study of the Strange Situation. Hillsdale, NJ, Erlbaum, 1978

Belsky J: Infant day care: a cause for concern. Zero To Three 6 (September):1–7, 1986

Bowlby J: Forty-four juvenile thieves: their characters and home-life. Int J Psychoanal 25:19–52, 107–127, 1944

Bowlby J: The nature of the child's tie to his mother. Int J Psychoanal 39:350–373, 1958

Bowlby J: Attachment and Loss, Vol 2: Separation. New York, Basic Books, 1973

Bowlby J: Attachment and Loss, Vol 1: Attachment, Revised Edition. New York, Basic Books, 1982

Burlingham D, Freud A: Young Children in Wartime London. London, Allen & Unwin, 1942

Cable M: The Little Darlings: A History of Child Rearing in America, 3rd Edition. New York, Charles Scribner's Sons, 1972

Carnegie Foundation: Starting Points: Meeting the Needs of Our Youngest Children. New York, Charles Scribner's Sons, 1994

Egeland B, Farber E: Infant-mother attachment: factors related to its development and changes over time. Child Dev 55:753–771, 1984

Egeland B, Jacobvitz D, Sroufe LA: Breaking the cycle of abuse: relationship predictions. Child Dev 59:1080–1088, 1988

Goldstein J, Freud A, Solnit AJ: Beyond the Best Interests of the Child. New York, Free Press, 1979

Harlow H: The nature of love. Am Psychol 3:673–685, 1958

Hodges J, Tizard B: Social and family relationships of ex-institutional adolescents. J Child Psychol Psychiatry 30(1):77–97, 1989

Hodges WF, Landis T, Day E, et al: Infants and toddlers and post divorce parental access: an initial exploration. Journal of Divorce and Remarriage 16(3–4): 239–252, 1991

Howes C, Rodning C, Galluzzo D, et al.: Attachment and child care: relationships with mother and caregiver, in Infant Day Care: The Current Debate. Edited by Fox N, Fein G. Norwood, NJ, Ablex Publishing, 1990, pp 169–182

Janson HW: History of Art: A Survey of the Major Visual Arts From the Dawn of History to the Present Day. Englewood Cliffs, NJ, Prentice-Hall, 1963

Kagan J: The Nature of the Child. New York, Basic Books, 1984

Karen R: Becoming Attached: Unfolding the Mystery of the Infant-Mother Bond and Its Impact on Later Life. New York, Warner Books, 1994

Konner M: Childhood. Boston, Educational Broadcasting Corporation, 1991 [Companion book to nine-hour public television series of same name]

Lally RL, Mangione P, Signer S: Together in Care: Meeting the Intimacy Needs of Infants and Toddlers in Groups (videotape). Sacramento, Far West Laboratory for Educational Research and Development, Center for Child and Family Studies, and California Department of Education, Child Development Division, 1992

Lally RL, Griffin A, Fenichel E, et al: Caring for Infants and Toddlers in Groups: Developmentally Appropriate Practice. Washington, DC, Zero to Three, 1995

McGoldrick M: Remarried families. Presentation at Continuing Education Workshop at The Menninger Clinic, Topeka, KS, November 7–8, 1997

Milne AA: Vespers (1924), in When We Were Very Young: The Complete Tales and Poems of Winnie-the-Pooh. New York, Quality Paperback Book Club, 1996, pp 449–450

Morelli GA, Tronick EZ: Effective multiple caretaking and attachment, in Intersections With Attachment. Edited by Gewirtz JL, Kurtines WM. Hillsdale, NJ, Erlbaum, 1991, pp 41–51

Osofsky J, Eberhart-Wright A: Risk and protective factors for parents and infants, in Future Directions in Infant Development Research. Edited by Suci G, Robertson S. New York, Springer-Verlag, 1992, pp 25–42

Pianta R (ed): Beyond the parent: the role of other adults in children's lives. New Directions for Child Development, 57, 1992

Robertson J: A Two-Year-Old Goes to Hospital (film). University Park, PA, Penn State Audio Visual Services, 1953

Robertson J, Robertson J: Thomas, aged two years, four months, in Foster Care for Ten Days (videotape). Young Children in Brief Separation Film Series. University Park, PA, Penn State Audio Visual Services, 1971

Sagi A, van IJzendoorn MH, et al: Attachments in a multiple-caregiver and multiple-infant environment: the case of the Israeli kibbutzim. Monogr Soc Res Child Dev 60(2–3):71–91, 1995

Scarr S: Mother Care/Other Care. New York, Basic Books, 1984

Spitz R: Hospitalism: an inquiry into the genesis of psychiatric conditions in early childhood. Psychoanal Study Child 1:53–74, 1945

Spitz R: Grief: A Peril in Infancy (film). University Park, PA, Penn State Audio Visual Services, 1947

Sroufe LA, Waters E: Attachment as an organizational construct. Child Dev 48:1184–1189, 1977

U.S. Department of Health and Human Services: Adoption and Foster Care Reporting System, 1998a

U.S. Department of Health and Human Services: National Child Abuse and Neglect Data System, 1998b

van IJzendoorn M, Sagi A, Lambermon M: Beyond the parent: the role of other adults in children's lives. New Dir Child Dev 57:5–24, 1992

Waters E: The stability of individual differences in infant-mother attachment. Child Dev 49:483–494, 1978

Whitebrook M, Howes C, Phillips D: Who Cares? Child Care Teachers and the Quality of Care in America. Oakland, CA, Child Care Employee Project, 1989

Williams C: The role of Head Start in strengthening families, protecting children, and assuring permanence. Presentation at the Head Start Institute for Programs Serving Pregnant Women, Infants and Toddlers, and Their Families, Washington, DC, January 23, 1998

Zero to Three: Heart Start. National Center for Infants, Toddlers, and Families: Diagnostic Classification of Mental Health and Developmental Disorders of Infancy and Early Childhood (DC: 0–3). Arlington, VA, Zero to Three, 1994

III

Therapeutic Approaches to Psychophysiological Disturbances

10

Excessive and Persistent Crying

Characteristics, Differential Diagnosis, and Management

J. Martín Maldonado-Durán, M.D.
J. Manuel Sauceda-Garcia, M.D.

When a baby is born, everyone rejoices as the child announces the beginning of extrauterine life with a vigorous cry and the onset of breathing. Crying is a signal not only of the baby's hope but also of its need for comfort and assistance.

As time goes on, the crying, particularly when prolonged or difficult to soothe, is more difficult to listen to. The problems associated with prolonged episodes of crying are stressful not only for the infant but also for the caregivers. In the most extreme situations, unsoothable and excessive crying can precipitate maltreatment, such as shaking (Becker et al. 1998) or slapping (Van der Wal et al. 1998), of the infant (Mrazek 1993). To better understand excessive crying, it is important to understand normal crying and its normative progression in the first months of extrauterine

The authors wish to thank Jill Glinka, OT (USD 501 School District, Parkdale Preschool, Topeka, Kansas), and Winnie Dunn, OT (University of Kansas Medical Center, Kansas City, Kansas), for their help and teaching regarding sensory abilities and vulnerabilities.

life. Such knowledge establishes a better basis for understanding the possible causes and manifestations of excessive crying and possible interventions to alleviate it.

Crying has long concerned parents and clinicians. There is even an international society for the study of infant crying, whose aim is to share research results on the nature of crying and its disturbances. Yet much work remains to be done to fully understand the nature and consequences of crying in infants, and excessive crying in particular.

NORMAL CRYING

Crying is an adaptive response of infants (and, to some degree, of all children and adults) when they face stressful circumstances. It is usually associated with some unpleasant state, such as physical discomfort (e.g., pain, hunger) or emotion (e.g., anger, fear, boredom). In the older child and adult, crying can also occur during a state of joy or sadness or when the person is moved by some act of tenderness.

From an evolutionary point of view, crying may have a purpose and a survival value. It is a signaling mechanism par excellence that the newborn infant uses to communicate with caregivers (Eibl-Eibesfeldt 1987).

Crying has also been reported in primates, such as infant chimpanzees (Bard 1995) who cry in a manner similar to human infants during their first weeks of life. In other species, crying occurs in the form of distress calls to elicit rescue efforts by the parent. Bird chicks cry persistently to convey their need for food. In essence, these signals make the adult bird feed the chick and continue searching for nourishment.

In the human infant, crying can be seen as a communication device with two main purposes: to signal and to support the parent-infant relationship. As a signal, crying in a startled newborn can signal pain, discomfort, hunger, and fear. Later, at the end of the first and second years of life, crying can also originate from frustration, anger, boredom, and sadness. Crying is an immediate and peremptory stimulus to convey the internal state of the child to the parent (Bensel and Haug-Schnabel 1996). The second main purpose is to serve as an instrument to foster, maintain, and strengthen the parent-infant relationship. Bowlby considered crying part of the baby's behavioral repertoire, together with clinging, social smiling, and so forth, that promotes caregiving behavior and, eventually, attachment. As a "releaser" of caregiving behavior, crying can elicit empathic and tender responses that promote closeness and togetherness.

In the individual infant, crying occurs along a maturational curve. In terms of the amount of crying, its accumulated duration per day peaks around the sixth week of postnatal life for a baby born at term. This peak consists of about 2.5 hours of crying over a 24-hour period, a figure found to be fairly consistent in studies of crying that use audio recordings activated when the child cries (Barr 1998; St. James-Roberts and Halil 1991). In a study in Manchester in the United Kingdom, this duration was a little shorter than encountered in other studies (Baildam et al. 1995). The maturation process in the duration of crying has also been observed in premature infants, whose crying peaks in the sixth week of life (corrected age) (Barr et al. 1996).

In the months after their crying peaks, the majority of infants will cry less often. Not only does the total crying time decline, but the episodes also become less frequent, particularly at night. This reduction has been attributed to maturation in the child's ability to stop crying and become more settled and regulated, and thus more able to cope with the surrounding world. However, a proportion of infants will continue to cry intensely, more than 3 hours per day, during the whole first year of life. In a recent survey, about 40% of infants who cried excessively during the first 3 months continued to cry a lot during the whole first year (Wurmser et al. 2001).

In addition to changes in duration, this early crying changes in both quality and effect in the months after birth. In the first months of life, the cry of the baby has a tonic quality—that is, the episode starts and continues for some time—with unique acoustic features recognizable as the crying of a very young infant. In the second 6 months of life, crying becomes more phasic, and each episode is more discrete, briefer in duration, and acoustically different from the early cry (Papousek and Papousek 1995).

CRYING AS A TRANSACTIONAL PHENOMENON

Crying is also a form of communication aimed at eliciting a response from the person (e.g., the caregiver) who receives the signal. Many characteristics of crying, such as duration, depend not only on what elicits the signal in the first place but also on the response of the caregiver to the cry. Crying is therefore also a transaction between the baby and the caregiver (Acebo and Thomas 1995). To a considerable extent, the response of the caregiving environment determines features of the crying.

Mothers think they can distinguish somewhat between different types of crying and accurately ascribe the apparent causes of it. For instance, mothers can distinguish between crying caused by hunger and crying caused by pain (Gustafson and Harris 1990).

One of the ways crying promotes caregiving—up to a point—is by making parents feel distressed when their infant, or indeed any infant, cries (Corter and Fleming 1995). From an evolutionary or ethological point of view, humans appear to become distressed with the crying and try to make it stop, which normally would trigger soothing behaviors to alleviate the crying infant's distress.

To compound the situation, parents vary in their ability to cope with crying, not only because of their own personality, experience taking care of babies, and knowledge of infant development but also because of the amount of stress they experience at any given time. The perinatal period is full of normative stressors associated with the pregnancy, the birth of the baby, and the need for many adaptations after the birth of the child. In these circumstances, the more distressed a parent is or the more the parent experiences crying as difficult or intolerable (Crowe and Zeskind 1992; Gustafson and Harris 1990; Murray 1985), the greater the risk of a negative response toward the baby.

> Ms. P, the caregiver of an 8-week-old baby, Brent, called the emergency pediatric services at 10 P.M. one night asking for help. She said Brent was crying all the time and had done so for the past month. During a brief hospitalization of the baby, the pediatrician sought a mental health intervention after ruling out physical illness. Ms. P said Brent fussed or cried whenever she put him in his crib or did not hold him. He wanted to be held all the time and would not cry only when she did so. However, Ms. P said she had to do housework and tend to her older child. Ms. P spoke about her anger with the baby, with whom she had gotten very upset earlier. She had yelled at the baby to "shut up" because he had been fed and changed and was warm, so there was no reason for him to cry. Ms. P complained that this baby wanted to be "attached to her" physically all the time, and she could not stand it. Ms. P later cried and said she had very little support in her life because her husband would never talk about feelings. Also, she said that she herself had always "wanted a mama" but had never gotten one.

CRYING AS A SOCIAL AND CULTURAL PHENOMENON

Among the !Kung (Barr et al. 1991) and in Manali, India (St. James-Roberts et al. 1994), a crying peak was encountered, although children tended to cry for shorter periods per day. It has been proposed that the shorter duration of crying has to do with the amount of carrying the baby receives, its proximity to the mother's body, and the frequency of breast-feedings (on demand rather than according to a schedule). If one studies the normal progression of crying, socially and culturally determined caregiving practices become a crucial factor. For instance, Bensel studied the crying patterns in infants in Freiburg, Germany, and found a shorter duration of crying in that community within an industrialized country (Bensel and Haug-Schnabel 1997). The shorter duration was attributed to the caregiving practices recently adopted in that part of Germany. In Manali, India, and among the !Kung in Africa, the episodes of crying were of shorter duration compared with those in industrialized countries. Brazelton (1972) made a similar observation about the caregiving of babies in Yucatan, Mexico, among the population of Mayan descent.

As a communication, crying also has social and cultural dimensions. As noted earlier, cultural practices of soothing babies and taking care of them (i.e., the normative responses to crying) determine what babies do in this respect. In some cultures, babies are left to cry it out, while in others this technique is not considered adequate. Thus, the beliefs of parents and society about what is normal and how parents should respond determine the baby's behavior.

It could be argued that the culture, determined in large part by social and economic circumstances such as the practice of substitute infant care or maternal work, has superimposed its beliefs and practices on caregiver reactions to crying. The programmed responses from the ethological or evolutionary point of view can be overshadowed by social mandates, obscuring responses that might be considered intuitive (Papousek and Papousek 1995). These same factors operate in caregiving behaviors such as feeding, sleeping arrangements, and child rearing in general. A researcher in South Korea, Lee (1994), has attempted to replicate the studies carried out in other countries concerning the epidemiology of crying and colic. She discovered that in Korean culture and language, the phenomenon of colic is not known. Mothers do not report their babies having colic nor observe it in their infants, and there is not even a word to designate the condition. In the United States and other countries, many parents worry that if they respond to their child's cry consistently or promptly, the baby will be spoiled. Many health care professionals also advise parents not to respond too quickly so that the child will learn to self-soothe. This notion appears to be based on the social value of self-reliance and individuation.

EPIDEMIOLOGICAL ASPECTS OF NORMAL CRYING

Several researchers have studied the phenomenon of normal crying in nonreferred infants within the community in countries such as Canada, the United Kingdom, Germany, and Denmark as compared with those within the community in nonindustrialized countries (Alvarez and

St. James-Roberts 1996; Baildam et al. 1995; Barr et al. 1992; Bensel and Haug-Schnabel 1997; St. James-Roberts and Halil 1991). These studies seem to suggest a normative progression in the duration and quality of crying. Breast-fed infants seem to cry less than formula-fed infants (Van der Wal et al. 1998), perhaps because they are fed more frequently and more on demand than formula-fed infants. Mothers of higher socioeconomic status also tend to report a longer duration of crying.

PHENOMENA OF NORMAL CRYING

In this section, we describe two controversial concepts—difficult temperament and colic—generally accepted by the public and the professional community. We include them because these constructions are typically invoked to label some phenomena observed in the first few months of life.

Difficult Temperament

Several behavioral traits tend to co-occur during the first months of life of all very young infants, coloring the baby's behavioral responses. These traits form the temperament of the child. In the early conceptualizations of temperament, the traits were considered mostly constitutional (Hinde 1989). In later formulations, they were seen as the result of an innate predisposition in interactions with caregivers that influence behavioral manifestations (Prior 1992). One of the temperamental subtypes, called "difficult" by Chess and Thomas (1985), was thought to occur in approximately 10% of infants. Difficult temperament consists of the qualities of short attention span, difficulty focusing on a stimulus, irritability, and poor rhythmicity.

Although difficult temperament is considered a normal variant of infant characteristics (the others being easy temperament, slow-to-warm-up temperament, and undifferentiated temperament), it is not clear how much the difficult temperament overlaps with behavioral dysregulation. Such dysregulation would include feeding and sleeping disturbances, subtle neurophysiological alterations (Von Hofacker and Papousek 1998), and difficulties in regulating states, transitions, and changes. Of the children estimated to exhibit difficult temperament (Prior 1992), it is unclear how many of these children would, instead, have been characterized as having regulatory difficulties or diagnosed with having colic. It seems reasonable to assume that difficult temperament is a variation of normality when the child tends to experience more difficulties but falls within the realm of normality. Thus, perhaps other terms should be used to denote behavioral difficulties.

Colic

Colic is a traditional construct widely used by the public and health professionals in the Western world, despite its poor characterization and the many uncertainties about what it really is (Barr 1990; Maldonado-Durán and Sauceda-Garcia 1998a) and its causes and physiology (St. James-Roberts et al. 1995; Stifter and Braungart 1992). In addition, different clinicians and researchers use various definitions, making it difficult to interpret studies on how to define and treat it (Lucassen et al. 1998). It is commonly thought that colic affects 20%–30% of infants during the first 3 months of life. But it seems useful to differentiate colic from persistent and excessive crying that lasts after the sixth month. Colic could, therefore, be considered a relatively normative entity that typically appears in the second month of life and disappears spontaneously (maturationally) at around 4 months of age. When excessive crying persists after 6 months or so, it seems more useful not to call it colic anymore; colic typically is benign and self-limiting (Stifter and Braungart 1992).

It is not known what causes the crying: contractions in the intestines (as the word colic would imply), an interactional problem (Miller and Barr 1991), or even a normal variation in the amount of crying. Lehtonen (1994) identifies the level of stress and psychosocial problems in the family (e.g., marital conflict, a history of complications during delivery, a negative attitude toward the pregnancy) as contributing factors to colic, whereas others (Crowcroft and Strachan 1997) relate colic to higher socioeconomic status. Intense crying could have two main manifestations: one, a benign form of early excessive crying as it might present in colic; the other, more problematic and long-standing, occurring after the first 6 months of life.

In the typical description of colic, the crying episode often appears in the evening or at night. During this period, the baby cries intensely and does not respond well to being carried or to stimulating maneuvers by the caregiver. The baby retracts his or her legs, and the abdomen appears distended. Thus, colic could consist of intestinal contractions. Whether the noticeable abdominal distension has to do with excessive production of gas remains uncertain; it could be that the distension occurs as the result of, rather than being the cause of, the crying.

There is also uncertainty about the best way to treat an infant with colic. After ruling out major causes (e.g., illness, hunger, allergies), some clinicians simply reassure parents about the benign nature of colic and the fact that it will disappear (the reassurance is usually helpful) (Lucassen et al. 1998). Other clinicians commonly treat colic with anticholinergic medications (e.g., dicyclomine) or even opiate solutions. But these medications carry a risk for negative—even lethal—side effects and should be avoided whenever possible (Lucassen et al. 1998; Pickford et al. 1991). Common side effects are that the baby is too sedated, sleeps a lot, or appears "dopey." At times, parents may wrongly use a higher dose in their attempts to calm their child.

One of the best approaches seems to be to reassure parents about the benign nature of the condition, which should improve over time, and encourage them to avoid excessively stimulating the baby during an episode. It may also be possible to preempt crying episodes through increased carrying (Wolke 2001). Other interventions that may prove helpful are changes in the baby's diet as recommended by a pediatrician or family physician and the use of formula hydrolisates. Higher fiber-content formula has not been demonstrated to be effective.

EXCESSIVE AND PERSISTENT CRYING

The problem of excessive and persistent crying is important given its frequency, the state of suffering it reflects in the child, and its aversiveness to parents and others. An accurate diagnosis of the problem can help health care professionals design interventions to alleviate it. Crying is excessive when it lasts a relatively long time per episode or during a day, compared with the duration of crying in normal circumstances. That is, in a given day, the baby spends comparatively more time in a state of crying or in crying and fussing. Crying is persistent when it does not tend to diminish as months go by. As described earlier, in the section "Normal Crying," crying has a typical maturational curve, tending to be of less duration at the end of the first 6 months of life. Excessive and persistent crying is not a disorder in and of itself. It can be understood as a set of problematic behaviors in the infant or as a syndrome resulting from multiple causes. In this section, we discuss the most common excessive crying behavior and some mechanisms of intervention. This behavior is a final common pathway manifesting several difficulties and sometimes also serving as a marker of vulnerabilities in the infant that can be dealt with as soon as they are identified.

Excessive and persistent crying is both a mystery and a problem. When crying is so intense, lasts long, and is very difficult to extinguish, its adaptive value for the infant tends to disappear. When crying becomes the problem itself, there are negative consequences for the baby, the parents, and their relationship. This clinical presentation is what we face in infant mental health clinics and pediatric clinics. That is, parents are worried when their baby seems to cry excessively or is not easily soothed.

As noted earlier, colic is one explanation of excessive crying that has been advocated by the lay public and by health professionals as well. In some areas of the world, an infant who cries excessively is understood as the equivalent of a colicky baby. Excessive crying also has been called persistent mother-infant distress syndrome, which Barr (1998) defines as the minority of babies who, in the first 3 months of life, are diagnosed with colic and continue to manifest excessive irritability and crying for many months instead of following the usual course of improvement.

From the clinical point of view, there are infants who cry much more than 3 hours of accumulated time in a 24-hour period. In the infant mental health clinic, babies are brought in who cry most of the time or well above 3 hours per day. They most likely represent a small proportion of children, but they present a major challenge.

Epidemiology

Unfortunately, excessive crying is not rare. Some epidemiological surveys lead researchers to suggest it may affect up to 10% of infants in the first year of life (St. James-Roberts and Halil 1991). This prevalence has been found in infants in urban London and in an urban community in Denmark (Alvarez and St James-Roberts 1996). A recent study in the Netherlands of 1,826 infants in the first 6 months of life reported a prevalence of excessive crying of about 7.6%, while mothers described the baby as "crying a lot"(14%) and "difficult to comfort" (10.3%) (Van der Wal et al. 1998). The total prevalence for problematic crying (i.e., problematic for the parents) was 20.3% of mothers.

Excessive Crying as a Transactional Phenomenon

The discomfort parents experience in the presence of a crying infant has been shown by several elevated physiological measures in the mother that occur when she hears her baby cry (Corter and Fleming 1995). When crying is intense and long-lasting, it can even become unbearable for some parents. In the study in the Netherlands, Van der Wal et al. (1998) discovered a surprising number of mothers (2%–3%) who reported that they slapped or shook their baby in response to the crying. These responses occurred more frequently when the mother had a lower level of education. Excessive crying thus places infants at risk for maltreatment, neglect, or physical abuse (Crowe and Zeskind 1992; Mrazek 1993).

Even in the absence of abuse, the perception of a baby as inconsolable, unresponsive, and difficult may color the relationship and the caregiver's view of the baby for a long time after infancy (Papousek 1985). The lack of a positive response from the baby questions or challenges the maternal and paternal capacity to soothe and calm their baby and may lead to parental self-doubt or a perception that the parents are not doing a good-enough job.

Evaluation

Evaluation of the baby who cries excessively should include a hands-on assessment of the infant, in addition to a history of the crying problem and other behavioral manifestations. The direct examination of the child should assess specific sensitivities, motor patterns, language, mood, relatedness, and cognitive development. The relational context of the infant is crucial to understanding the problem. An occupational therapist experienced in sensory integration also can help get a picture of this processing of input and self-regulation abilities.

Causes and Phenomenology

In a review of 167 cases referred to our infant mental health clinic (Maldonado-Durán et al., in press), we found a high proportion of infants who met the arbitrary definition of excessive crying (defined as the presence of more than 3 of 10 possible symptoms related to fussing, crying, and irritability). Many parents bring in their babies when they are 18 months old. The baby's visit to the clinic at this age may have to do with the parents' realization that the colic has not gone away and with the fact that the baby has more mobility and intentionality and exhibits more intense expressions of anger that may prompt the parents to seek help. Among a previous group of 100 cases, more than half met that definition of excessive crying (Maldonado-Durán et al. 1998). The main causes of excessive crying found frequently in the clinical setting, described below, are medical illness, drug withdrawal, hunger, and gastroesophageal reflux. In the section "Regulatory Disturbances," we focus in some detail on such disturbances.

Medical Illness

At first, parents and the clinician should worry about whether the crying is related to an underlying medical condition. Infants are sometimes taken to the emergency room because of their intense crying, which could have a medical cause, such as an ear infection, a gastrointestinal condition, or a neurological disorder (e.g., hydrocephalus) (Poole and Magilner 2000) or migraines (Guidetti et al. 2000). A diagnostic workup can rule out immediate physical causes (Poole 1991), such as the sting of an insect. The team would examine the infant's skin and clothing, palpate large bones, and inspect the eyes (especially the corneas) and ears; perhaps the team would even conduct a rectal and neurological examination.

Drug Withdrawal

In the United States, up to 20% of all babies may be born having been exposed in utero to drugs or alcohol. These babies are at higher risk of negative effects from the mother's consumption of these substances during her pregnancy—effects ranging from transient behavioral alterations to physical malformations (Buchi 1998).

During the neonatal period (first month of extrauterine life), when the baby is constantly irritable, fussy, and crying, clinicians should consider the possibility of a drug withdrawal syndrome, even if the parents deny such use. The newborn may be addicted to a certain drug— such as alcohol, benzodiazepines, cocaine, or even inhalants (Jones and Balster 1998). The withdrawal syndrome consists of marked irritability, jerkiness, or convulsions. The drug-addicted baby in withdrawal may present as extremely sensitive to the slightest environmental stimulation, signaled by a hypertonic response to stimuli or crying when talked to, touched, or even approached closely (Bay 1990; Chasnoff et al. 1992).

The treatment depends on the severity of symptoms and the substance in question. It may include temporary protection from environmental stimuli and later gradual exposure. Sounds may have to be muffled. Visual stimulation may need to be reduced by dimming lighting to the minimum possible and covering the cot or incubator. Tactile stimulation and manipulation may also need to be reduced. Clustering care procedures, as described by Als (1998), may consist of performing various interventions (e.g., changing a diaper, changing position, administering medication, bathing) during short periods of time to respect the baby's behavioral states (e.g., sleep). The baby is positioned in a flexed posture, and swaddling may facilitate the child from having to cope with stimuli. Sedative medications may be useful in helping the newborn make the transition to a state of calm and being free of drugs.

Hunger

The neonate and young infant exhibit variations in how often they need to be fed. Breast-fed infants may need more frequent feedings than formula-fed babies because breast milk tends to be more diluted. Primates, therefore, have to breast-feed their babies more frequently than do other mammals, whose milk is more concentrated (Hinde 1989). Also, at times of distress or illness, the baby may need more frequent feedings.

Inexperienced parents or those whose personality makes them very organized may decide that the infant should be fed for fixed periods of time according to a timetable. To do this, the mother at times sets aside her intuitive responses, such as feeding a crying baby, to follow a rigid rule, such as feeding him or her only every 4 hours.

Parents with eating disorders may also worry excessively about the possibility that their baby could become fat. Some mothers with anorexia nervosa tend to see their babies as fatter than they really are. As a result of their fear that the child will become obese, they may restrict the quantity or frequency of feedings so that the baby experiences hunger and cries frequently and intensely (Maldonado-Durán and Sauceda-Garcia 1998b; Stein et al. 1994, 1996).

> Ms. J is a mother of twin babies who are 4 months old. Jokingly, she says she asked God for a baby and he gave her two, which is a lot for her. She complains that the babies cry all the time. On observation, it appeared obvious several times that the babies cried when they were hungry because they rooted for milk. But she would say it was not time for their feeding because they had just eaten (e.g., 3 hours ago). Several sessions later, she revealed her fear that they would become fat if she fed them "too much." She then said she has bulimia and had suffered a lot as a child because she was fat and was teased cruelly.

Gastroesophageal Reflux

The physical condition of gastroesophageal reflux may be encountered during the first 6 months of life, but it can also persist well into the second 6 months and beyond. It consists mainly of the return, or reflux, of gastric contents into the esophagus, leading to the frequent regurgitation of milk. As a result of this exposure of the esophagus to the acid contents of the stomach, the reflux can cause esophagitis. This condition occurs in about 3% of newborn babies (Sterling et al. 1991) or higher, up to 8% (Orenstein et al. 1999), and is more common in the premature infant (Joyce and Clark 1996). One manifestation is excessive irritability and crying (Strassburg et al. 1988, 1990). Other manifestations are refusal of feedings, frequent regurgitation or vomiting, Sandifer syndrome (persisting tilting of the head), near-death experiences from choking, and failure to gain weight (Maldonado-Durán and Sauceda-Garcia 1998a).

Gastroesophageal reflux should be considered in the differential diagnosis of excessive crying, particularly if the baby cries or regurgitates persistently during feedings, cries harder when lying down, or cries when pressure is exerted on the abdomen. The diagnosis is made through clinical phenomena and confirmed with continuous PH monitoring in the esophagus. There are various treatments, from "thicker" and more frequent feedings in smaller amounts to medications that promote gastric emptying and motility (e.g., erythromycin and cisapride) to surgery (funduplication) to prevent the return of gastric contents into the esophagus, to positioning the baby to diminsh the likelihood of reflux, for instance, on the belly (Orenstein et al. 1999).

Regulatory Disturbances

Several clinicians have pointed out the relationship between excessive crying and regulatory disturbances (DeGangi 1991; Greenspan 1992; Maldonado-Durán and Sauceda-Garcia 1996; Von Hofacker and Papousek 1998). The Zero to Three classification of infant disturbances contains a definition of regulatory disorders. Other authors, rather than referring to disorders, prefer the designation *regulatory disturbances* because it is unclear whether these problems are true disorders and because little is known about their etiology, clinical course, and delimitations with other infant disorders. We will refer to them as *disturbances* with the understanding that these syndromes are severe, interfere to a significant degree with the infant's adaptive abilities, and cause considerable suffering to both the child and the caregivers.

The infant with regulatory disturbances faces challenges very early on in life. Frequently, these difficulties include excessive crying, particularly when the regulatory problem is of one of oversensitivity. The infant with unusual patterns of sensitivity (of sensory integration) has difficulties organizing and maintaining a state of contentment for even a brief period of time. Very frequently, the child will also exhibit problems in other areas of functioning that require organization and self-regulation (e.g., sleeping, eating, attention span, level of motor activity, and emotional regulation).

The prevalence of regulatory disturbances in infancy is unknown; no epidemiological studies address this entity. In particular, no studies take into account the sensory and motor patterns that fall under the umbrella of sensory integration difficulties.

The clinical construction of regulatory disturbance or disorder is useful in several respects. It emphasizes or lends credibility to challenges that may be inherent in the infant from very early on. Identifying these challenges can be helpful for parents so that they can learn how to respond and adapt their caregiving to the uniqueness of their baby. The construction should not be considered as a way to label the child with a disorder, but rather as a ratification of parental perceptions that the baby faces difficult times that will require a number of accommodations and mutual adaptations. Caregivers may feel guilty or inadequate when their child is overly fussy, does not mold to their arms, is unable to feed properly, and cannot organize a state of contentment.

The Zero to Three classification suggests that there are four types of regulatory disturbance: 1) oversensitive, 2) undersensitive, 3) motorically disorganized, and 4) combined sensitivities. The last type meets the criteria for problems with self-regulation but does not fit into any of the first three categories. The regulatory disturbances most commonly associated with excessive crying are the oversensitive, motorically disorganized, and combined sensitivities types.

Oversensitive Type

In the oversensitive regulatory disturbance, infants have an unusually high sensitivity to the surrounding sensory world. They may be oversensitive to tactile, auditory, or visual stimulation.

A baby may respond to light touch (tactile stimulation) with an aversive response and not want to be held or touched. When the parent offers comfort (e.g., tries to hold the baby), the crying intensifies and seems to signal a preference for being left alone in the crib. The baby may show discomfort with certain textures of clothing, such as nylon or roughly textured material. Many infants also appear to be fastidious: they do not ever want their fingers to have any sticky substance on them, or they are reluctant to play with sand, plasticine, Play-Doh, or other substances that come into contact with their hands. The child with these sensitivities will frequently have excessive food selectivity or even food refusal due to the consistency and texture of certain foods. They may strongly dislike the sensation or cry when water touches their hair during a bath. Some authors refer to these patterns as *tactile defensiveness* (Sears 1994). Paradoxically, many of these infants also have a high pain threshold. Parents spontaneously report noticing that their child takes little note of knocks, falls, and so forth and appears extremely tough.

Very young infants who have difficulty becoming habituated to certain noises (auditory stimuli) may wake up easily on hearing them. When awake, the child may react to practically every noise, even hardly noticeable ones, in the environment and so become overstimulated. These stimuli may include voices, television, radio, appliances, and other common household noises (washing machine, blender, fans, and even computers and fluorescent lights). At times, the infant is able to tolerate a certain "dose" of noise, but the accumulated effect of several noises at a time may prove to be too much to maintain a state of calmness. Older children may cover their ears to muffle sound. This behavior may also be observed when a motorcycle goes by or an airplane flies overhead. Going to stores or being in social gatherings can usually result in temper tantrums and crying in the toddler who is too sensitive to sound.

Visual stimulation may also become an aversive stimulus. It may have to do with the intensity of light or the amount of visual objects in the surroundings. The infant may be very annoyed or cry when exposed to sunlight. This reaction may also occur indoors in brightly lighted areas or where there are complex visual patterns. In many cases, the infant becomes more irritable, upset, and demanding if there are intense colors, geometrical patterns, or many toys in the room. Such exposure can quickly lead to a loss of control, which suggests that the infant may be overstimulated. One infant for whom we consulted consistently became nauseated and gagged when exposed to bright sunlight. Another child had a tendency to become easily fussy and agitated. His room was packed with colorful toys, visual patterns, and so forth that his well-intentioned parents had purchased to provide early stimulation. These surroundings, plus other stimuli, maintained a state of constant agitation and activity in the child. When the parents implemented the treatment advice to take out many of the visual objects and allow the child to interact with only a few toys at a time, he managed much better.

Another manifestation of hypersensitivity is a short attention span, as if the baby responds to every input around and cannot focus and screen out other signals. Such hypersensitivity may surface only when the caregiver tries to interact with the baby through more than one sensory channel (e.g., talking, presenting the face, and rocking the baby all at once). It may also surface when vestibular system hypersensitivity may be present, that is, the baby becomes overstimulated when moved (e.g., carried or transported in a stroller or automobile) and easily develops nystagmus or nausea. Some infants have an aversion to the prone position and instead want to sit up from early on, hating to lie down on their back.

Motorically Disorganized Type

The unique functioning of the central nervous system does not limit itself to sensory areas alone. It also may involve motor patterns such as muscular tone, movement coordination, motor planning, and sheer amount of motor activity. Some infants even want to be in constant motion. The baby is unfocused and very active and often cries intensely or frequently because of frustration or because the parents limit his or her boundless need for activity, stimulation, and exploration. Bedtime, mealtime, and presence at places where the infant has to be calm are major challenges that may result in tears, temper tantrums, and parent-infant confrontations.

Hypertonicity is evident because the baby appears stiff when touched. The baby's movement patterns give an appearance of rigidity or whole-body movement rather than movement of a limb or a segment of a limb. Some infants seem to have a predominance for extensor patterns of movement; they arch their backs and are unable to mold to their parents' arms. In some cases of hypertonicity, the baby attempts to sit or walk at a very early age, giving the impression of precocity; the parents see a baby who is ready to take steps at 6 months of age or even earlier, or the toddler constantly walks on tiptoes.

With older infants, it is important to observe how they go about solving problems that involve movement (e.g., getting up on a chair, obtaining a toy). This function of motor planning shows how the child pictures in his or her mind certain motor patterns, sequences, and postures required to obtain a certain result. Sometimes a child older than 1 year seems to be completely at a loss about how to perform even the most trivial motor activity, such as getting a desired toy only a foot away. Apparently unable to picture what needs to be done to get the toy, the child becomes desperate and angry.

Motor coordination challenges often go unrecognized unless they are very severe. However, early recognition may enable parents to design interventions to help the child develop better coordination. The infant may misdirect movements, have a poor grasp of objects (e.g., a toy), or show immature motor patterns. A fine motor tremor in the fingers when attempting to hold something is often a manifestation, as are difficulties in "crossing the middle line" between the left and the right sides. So are other "soft" neurological signs such as tongue protrusion, constant mouthing of objects, and grimacing when attempting a motor activity. The child may fall often, stumble over things, and have poor equilibrium. Another manifestation is the delay in developing a clear preference for the left or right hand to carry out motor tasks. By age 4, the child may still be holding objects or drawing first with one hand, then the other.

Proprioceptive information is the awareness of one's body parts, particularly one's head and limbs; where they are located in space; and how they are positioned. Children who do not fully register this information are described as having hyposensitivity. They may appear more clumsy or, as sometimes described by parents, "like a bull in a china cabinet." The child may bump into things, cause frequent small accidents, step on toys, and fail to develop adequate strategies for avoiding such occurrences. Another behavior that occupational therapists view as hyposensitivity is the constant seeking of stimulation (Dunn and Brown 1997). The theoretical construct to explain this stimulus search is that the child is under-registering information and must seek more of it. It is thought that by eliciting stimulation, the child perceives it as more easily controllable. This process can be seen in the child who wants to touch everything and explore every object encountered. Such children may also frequently lie on the floor and roll over and over in a conspicuous pattern of seeking tactile body input. They may walk rubbing against the wall or they may "bounce off the wall" or "butt" people to seek intense pressure input.

Combined Sensitivities Type

Children often have combined sensitivities—that is, they are hypersensitive to some modalities and hyposensitive to others. Emotional states, level of excitement, motivation to perform an activity, and other states may also change these sensitivities. Parents often report that their child will react differently to someone from one day to the next.

INTERVENTION STRATEGIES

The choice of which interventions to use will clearly depend on the specific pattern of regulatory disturbance in the child and the caregiver's disposition to implement changes to alleviate the infant's discomfort and crying. The interventions have the goal of alleviating the excessive crying, not in and of itself but rather because it is a sign of discomfort in the baby.

The crying baby can be approached from several points of view. Some interventions can be attempted to alleviate the crying of infants in general. However, given the uniqueness of each child, it is a process of trial and error; what could be very effective with one baby could be counterproductive with another. Services like Cry-sis in London, a hotline for parents seeking advice from a volunteer when a baby is crying inconsolably, provide useful suggestions from experienced parents and emotional support for the caregiver of the crying infant. We have already described some interventions to alleviate crying associated with specific conditions. We focus here on the very sensitive infant because this is a frequent presentation of excessive crying in infants.

One of the most important issues in dealing with excessive crying may be a preemptive approach that circumvents episodes of intense and unmanageable crying. The caregiver can often learn to recognize signals in the baby that are a prelude to a stage of disorganization and chaos that produces an episode of long-lasting crying. When the precipitants or signals of overload are identified, the parent can intervene at that moment and support the baby so that the disorganization does not occur.

There are three main groups of interventions:

1. Techniques to prevent the baby from being overstimulated, overwhelmed, or uncomfortable (i.e., providing an adequate "sensory diet")
2. Maneuvers to help the infant cope with stimulation and become able to process it better
3. Interventions to improve the parent-child relationship (i.e., the fit between them), given the uniqueness of the baby

In clinical practice, these interventions are often implemented concurrently. There is little empirical information about the effectiveness of such clinical interventions. They are described as commonly used in dealing with very sensitive or motorically disorganized infants who have excessive and persistent crying.

Changing the Amount, Duration, and Quality of Stimulation

A general statement about altering one or more aspects of the stimuli that the infant receives is to closely observe the baby and his or her response to environmental stimuli or input (Dunn 1997). Only through careful observation and detailed questioning of the parents can we deduct what might be stimuli that precipitate overstimulation, overload, crying, fussing, irritability, or temper outbursts in the infant. For this purpose, the clinician observes the baby carefully in interaction with the surroundings and attempts to observe the response in the various sensory channels. By talking, presenting objects, and observing the infant's response to sounds and being held, the clinician can get clues to the baby's ability to self-organize and to what precipitates discontent or crying. It is very useful to observe the baby in natural surroundings (i.e., at home or day care) and conduct an ecological observation of the infant within a familiar environment. This approach can provide clues about what the child has to deal with in everyday life. It also aids in determining what can be modified or implemented in the real world of the child. The clinician can suggest ways to modify, in the home and at day care, some features that may be unsuitable to a particular child.

Parents or caregivers have much longer and detailed knowledge of the infant than has any clinician. Listening to their observations and asking detailed, specific questions about the baby's reactions to different stimuli and activities (e.g., bathing, changing diapers, feeding, going to bed, putting clothes on, going out) can provide clues to what is bothering the baby.

Another general principle is to monitor the baby to observe signals of overstimulation, overload, or aversive reaction to input. Identifying these signals can enable the observer to help the parent learn when the child needs a break from that sensory information so that he or she can terminate a certain activity or give the child an opportunity to rest before the child becomes upset and inconsolable. This close monitoring will preempt crises and help parents to read their child's signals of distress or discomfort, while there is still time to change settings or give the baby a rest. The parent becomes a "baby observer" with information about what to look for in his or her unique child.

The baby may prefer to have interactions in some sensory modalities more than others. Because he or she may tolerate auditory stimuli better than visual ones, the parent might approach the baby more easily by talking softly, singing, or using music or rhythmic, soft noise to engage the child in pleasurable interactions that will not be aversive.

Tactile Sensory Systems

Children who react against being touched or who fuss or cry when held may need frequent opportunities to rest from being held. Even a light touch is felt as aversive; some children prefer more deep touch—or even being squeezed rather than touched gently. Because a child can become more irritated when other people are around or get too close (invading the baby's personal space), monitoring for signs of overload and adding distance may be ways of preempting overstimulation.

The parent may observe the baby's response to different types of touch experiences, for example, with the material of clothes or bedding and the amount of physical touch the baby can tolerate. By not insisting on holding or carrying the baby continuously and, instead, holding the infant only until he or she has had enough stimulation, the parent may avoid an aversive reaction. Giving the baby the opportunity to lie in bed or close by, within visual or auditory distance but without being touched, may help the infant recuperate from previous stimulation.

Parents intuitively touch their baby lightly and lovingly. The infant, however, may feel that even this form of caressing is aversive, especially if the infant was born prematurely. So changing the manner of touch may help the baby process this stimulus better. Deep pressure and more intense touch may be tolerated much better than gentle touch. This preference appears to be why toddlers prefer rough-and-tumble play or why they seek intense contact with people.

Auditory Systems

The baby may be sensitive to certain tones, quality of noise, rhythmicity of stimuli (e.g., types of music, such as music with drums), or volume (decibels) and sheer amount of noise stimulation within a certain time. Although the baby may be able to cope with the voice of one person, the voices of two or more people may be too much and may precipitate crying. Television is a frequent presence in many households, sometimes from morning till night, as a part of the usual background. At times parents do not realize that the sound from the television being on constantly may overstimulate their baby. We visited the home of a toddler whose two young parents liked rock music (father) and television (mother), and both sources of noise were on simultaneously much of the time; yet neither parent correlated this constant noise with the toddler's tendency to become more "wild," unfocused, and irritable. When we pointed out this relationship, the parents turned off the stereo and television, leading not only to less noise but also to their increased availability for interaction with their child.

An intervention can include simply moderating the volume of the caregiver's voice or keeping it at a certain pitch. It may also include reducing the number of auditory stimuli occurring at one time (e.g., voice, television, radio, fan). For example, the parent can experiment in reducing the number of concurrent noises to which the infant is exposed, thus alleviating the child's tendency to become overwhelmed by them.

> William is a 9-month-old adopted baby. His parents, Mr. and Mrs. N, both in their mid-twenties, adopted William when he was 2 weeks old. He cries a lot, fusses frequently, and seems to be generally discontented. He does not like to be held, arches his back when held, and avoids eye contact. He often goes to a corner in the house or a room as if to protect himself. Worried about his crying and fussing, his adoptive mother sought consultation with another health professional. She was told that the baby had an attachment disorder and was given advice to hold the baby forcefully, which made him cry more. When she brought William to the clinic for a second opinion, however, there were obvious signs that he was attached to his mother because he cried whenever she left the office, looked for her and his father, and was quickly consoled when his parents returned. William would refer visually to them and go to them for emotional refueling. On examination, he would cover his eyes if others tried to make contact with him or if they got too close to his face. He would also avert his gaze, arch his back, and try to escape. If anyone insisted on contact with William, he would start crying. He was highly sensitive to noises and paid particular attention to the slightest noise in the office, the passing cars, the movement of a camera, and so forth. William's parents confirmed that he became very annoyed by intense noises and was easily scared by unusual ones.

The clinicians described William's pattern of hypersensitivity to the adoptive parents, noting that their baby was, indeed, quite attached to them. The clinicians noted that the mother spoke in a very high-pitched and intense voice that was somewhat bothersome even to them. On the third interview, Mrs. N noted that William had improved remarkably. He was much more content and did not cry as much. She felt that what had helped her the most was that she changed her voice when talking to William. She discovered that she was trying too hard to engage him: the more she talked to him and presented herself in front of him, the more he would try to avoid her and escape the interaction. As she started using a softer voice and talked less, he began to come more often to her, seemed better able to tolerate reciprocal interactions, and played with her for longer periods of time. She felt that their interactions were much more pleasurable for both of them, and she continued to search for ways to help William face and deal with the world of stimuli around him. Parents with a hypersensitive child like William can try to find a preferred sort of sound for their infant and then use it to gain his or her attention and promote reciprocal interactions.

Visual Sensory Channel

The baby may react intensely to stimuli that anyone else finds innocuous. It may be that sunlight or colorful, vivid visual patterns are too much for the baby.

> Ronny is a 10-month-old infant and an only child. His mother is from Burma and his father from China. They are in a good economic situation and have eagerly read about early stimulation of intellectual abilities and brain development (e.g., listening to Mozart's musical compositions). They sought consultation because their baby was extremely irritable, fussed practically all day, and did not eat well because he could not focus long enough. When a videotape made at home was observed by the evaluating clinicians, it became obvious that there was too much visual stimulation for this particular child. With the best of intentions, the parents had partially covered his bedroom walls with colorful images, cartoon characters, and geometrical patterns and had provided an enormous number of colorful toys. Clearly, Ronny could not focus on any one thing because he had an avalanche of input to his eyes. The parents were advised to reduce this stimulation because direct examination of Ronny revealed that he was very sensitive to visual stimuli. When the parents moved to offering just one or two toys at a time and made Ronny's environment less colorful, his irritability decreased and his ability to focus improved remarkably.

A similar problem may be encountered in some day care centers. To make the environment interesting, day care providers may display intense colors and lots of images. For some children, excessive visual stimuli may simply be too much.

Diminishing the patterns and intensity of colors and objects on the walls can be helpful. It may also prove helpful to reduce the intensity of light in the room. Fluorescent light, for example, can produce too much stimulation in some children. Some children are so sensitive to outside daylight conditions that they have to wear dark glasses and avoid direct exposure to the light.

In addition to having a fewer number of objects within sight, the infant may also benefit from having periods of rest from any form of visual input. Taking a break in a room with dimmed lighting and going to a corner of a room where not much is to be seen may be helpful. So is getting inside a "tent" or a "cranny." Many children seek this rest naturally, crawling under tables or other furniture to shelter themselves. These defensive maneuvers could be interpreted as bizarre behavior.

Parents worry a lot about eye contact. Although being able to look another person in the eye is a very desirable goal, doing so may not be easy for the infant. Some young children are aversive to direct eye-to-eye contact and try to avoid it. It is as though the face of another person is too much. A gradual move to eye-to-eye contact, rather than insisting on or forcing the contact, may result in the infant's gradual ability to tolerate it.

> After months of being fussy and irritable, Johnny was able to explain at age 2½ why he did not like looking at people. He found their facial features, wrinkles, eyebrows, warts, and nostrils somewhat scary. He looked intensely at these features in faces and preferred not to see them because the experience seemed so unpleasant.

Other sensory experiences may contribute to the feeling of overload and displeasure. There may be olfactory messages in the surroundings, of a particular person, or in a room in the house (e.g., a spot in the kitchen). The temperature in the room may also be a source of discomfort for the oversensitive child.

Helping the Infant Cope, Organize, and Regulate

Several techniques can actively provide support to the infant in facing the world of stimuli that must be dealt with in everyday life. The point of the intervention is not to reduce or eliminate the stimulus but, instead, to support the baby in coping with the stimulation, making it possible for him or her to manage the signals and maintain a state of well-being while doing so.

Swaddling and Containment

A variety of ways to touch, hold, and contain an infant can be attempted to reduce hyperreactions to stimuli in general. Swaddling is possible only with the very young infant. Techniques such as placing the arms in the midline, putting the hands near the face or mouth, or just touching the baby's body firmly can be an adequate alternative. Some clinicians believe that in the very young infant, swaddling may feel similar to the tight conditions in utero, particularly toward the end of the pregnancy.

The older infant may enjoy the sense of calmness and control provided by the caregiver while being held. Many infants who experience anxiety or are overwhelmed by the environment may cope better when they are held and contained. In practice, parents can play games with the child that involve rolling the child up in a blanket or placing the child in a hammock, two activities that provide the experience of containment. For the older child, parents can rely on the use of beanbag chairs.

Massage or Deep Pressure

There is some evidence that touching the infant, particularly the very young infant, may release substances (hormones or neurotransmitters) that promote the baby's weight gain and induce states of quiet alertness or calmness (Field 1995). Clinically, many children who are easily overstimulated, becoming hypertonic and restless, can be helped to cope with these states by being exposed to massage or deep pressure. Some techniques involve holding or containing the infant, carrying the infant in a sling, or even rolling up the child (especially if a toddler) in a heavy blanket or quilt. When the baby is making the transition to sleep, a heavy blanket can sometimes help achieve a state of calmness enough to induce sleep. Massage with the hands in the muscles of the upper and lower limbs and pressure on the palms may also be quite calming for the child.

Vibratory Stimulation

A variation of a touch intervention is vibratory stimulation. Occupational therapists believe that for most children and adults, vibratory stimulation is relaxing and soothing. It is why some parents find that placing a colicky baby in a child's seat on top of a working washing machine or dryer can help the baby calm down. Mild vibrating objects, such as "doodling pens," are readily available and can be applied gently to the infant's arms, legs, and back. The parents can then evaluate whether a strategy leads to a calming response.

Buccal Stimulation or Mouthing Activity

Infants like to explore objects with their mouth, which has a high concentration of tactile receptors at this stage of life. For many babies, this activity functions to promote self-organization, grounding, and pleasure. In the very young infant, it can take the form of nonnutritive sucking. In older infants, it may involve constantly mouthing their hands, toys, or clothing or chewing or biting on objects. The opportunity to mouth objects may allow the child to cope with other sensory challenges. In the older child or preschooler, parents may provide an object for the child to chew on to assist him or her in self-regulation; even gum may serve this purpose.

Vestibular Stimulation

Dieter and Emory (1997) postulate that vestibular stimulation—rocking or moving the infant in the air along horizontal or vertical axes—may induce a state of alertness and, at the same time, produce a calming and soothing response. Parents intuitively perform this soothing stimulation when they provide rhythmic motion to a crying baby to help him or her calm down. Such motion may release calming neurotransmitters that help the baby relax and focus better. When the infant appears to become overloaded with stimuli, this technique can help maintain a state of organization. In the toddler or 2-year-old, swings or other devices that rotate or gyrate around an axis can be used for the same purpose.

Auditory Stimuli

A variety of auditory stimuli, ranging from singing and talking to white or neutral noise, can be helpful. Some infants show a preference for auditory stimulation and are particularly responsive to someone who sings and talks softly to them. At times of distress, quiet singing, rhythmic vocal noise, or interesting noises may help the infant focus and "entrain" in that rhythm and regain a state of self-organization. Within a caregiving relationship, parents may use favorite songs or sequences, and the memory of previous pleasurable exchanges may help the infant calm.

White noise is a form of mild stimulation that can help the child who has difficulty turning down bodily stimulation. In addition to simple techniques for producing white noise (a fan set on low or a radio tuned to static), white noise machines are available today that feature rainfall, running water, wind in the trees, and so forth.

Physical Activity

A more agitated, restless, and unfocused child can be helped through physical activity to release accumulated energy or stimulation. The more energetic and active child may need an opportunity to release energy so that he or she can tackle a subsequent challenge. Parents can help by giving the infant relatively brief breaks to run, climb, jump, yell, and release energy; the breaks enable the child to tackle further demands for attention and self-control.

Biofeedback

In children 2 years old or older, biofeedback techniques may help them cope with their surroundings and achieve a state of calmness. These techniques include abdominal breathing, hand-warming exercises, and the tensing and releasing of muscles. They can be taught to a young child in simple form. If the child becomes interested, parents can present these activities as games to help the child calm down and can practice the activities with the child.

Mapping the Developmental Progression of Self-Organization, Regulation, and Coping

In addition to thinking about the infant's present status, sensitivities, discontent, and crying, as well as strategies to help the baby cope, it is important to consider a developmental plan with the general goal of helping the baby move forward with higher challenges. These challenges would be a greater flexibility in different environments, an increased ability to face new situations and demands, and an ability to maintain a state of self-regulation and balance. A developmental point of view provides a sort of "map" of what comes next in the child's adaptive and coping efforts (Zeitlin and Williamson 1994) and provides guidance on how to modify the next tasks for the baby.

Rather than thinking of treating the child or suggesting strategies of sensory integration for the baby, it is useful to think of the baby in relation to the caregivers. Maneuvers that could be implemented at home to enhance the child's ability to cope with the environment optimally are implemented as play interactions, as Greenspan (1992) suggests in his concept of "floor time." In the context of a partnership, mutually enjoyable interactions, and emotional comfort (Cummings and Davies 1996), it is likely that the baby's self-regulation will improve when compared with a state of tension, anxiety, pressure, or anger.

REFERENCES

Acebo C, Thomas EB: Role of infant crying in the early mother-infant dialogue. Physiology and Behavior 57(3):541–547, 1995

Als H: Developmental care in the newborn intensive care unit. Curr Opin Pediatr 10(2):138–142, 1998

Alvarez M, St. James-Roberts I: Infant fussing and crying in the first year in an urban community in Denmark. Acta Pediatrica 84(4):463–466, 1996

Baildam EM, Hillier VF, Ward BS, et al: Duration and pattern of crying in the first year of life. Dev Med Child Neurol 37:345–353, 1995

Bard KA: Parenting in primates, in Handbook of Parenting: Biology and Ecology of Parenting, Vol 2. Edited by Bornstein MH. Mahwah, NJ, Erlbaum, 1995, pp 27–58

Barr RG: The "colic" enigma: prolonged episodes of a normal predisposition to cry. Infant Mental Health Journal 11(4):340–348, 1990

Barr RG: Crying in the first year of life: good news in the midst of distress. Child Care Health Dev 24(5):425–439, 1998

Barr RG, Konner M, Bakeman R, et al: Crying in !Kung San infants: a test of the cultural specificity hypothesis. Dev Med Child Neurol 33:601–610, 1991

Barr RG, Rotman A, Yarenko J, et al: The crying of infant with colic: a controlled empirical description. Pediatrics 90:14–21, 1992

Barr RG, Chen S, Hopkins B, et al: Crying patterns in preterm infants. Dev Med Child Neurol 38(4):345–355, 1996

Bay J: Substance abuse and child abuse: impact of addiction on the child. Pediatr Clin North Am 37:881–904, 1990

Becker JC, Liebrsch R, Tautz C, et al: Shaken Baby Syndrome: report on four pairs of twins. Child Abuse Negl 22(9):931–937, 1998

Bensel J, Haug-Schnabel G: Primär exzessives Schreien in den ersten drei Lebensmonaten [Primary excessive crying in the first three months of life], in Handbuch der Kleinkindforschung [Handbook of Research in Early Childhood], 2 Auflage (2nd Edition). Edited by Keller H. Bern, Switzerland, Hans Huber, 1996, pp 45–61

Bensel J, Haug-Schnabel G: Nature meets nurture: excessive crying in a German sample. Paper presented at the Sixth International Workshop on Infant Cry Research. Lancaster, UK, July 1997

Brazelton TB: Implications of infant development among the Mayan Indians of Mexico. Hum Dev 15:90–111, 1972

Buchi KF: The drug-exposed infant in the well-baby nursery. Clin Perinatol 25:235–250, 1998

Chasnoff IJ, Griffith DR, Freier C, et al: Cocaine-polydrug use in pregnancy: two year follow-up. Pediatrics 89:284–289, 1992

Chess S, Thomas A: Temperamental differences: a critical concept in child care. Pediatr Nurs 11(3):167–171, 1985

Corter CM, Fleming AS: Psychobiology of maternal behavior in human beings, in Handbook of Parenting: Biology and Ecology of Parenting, Vol 2. Edited by Bornstein MH. Mahwah, NJ, Erlbaum, 1995, pp 87–116

Crowcroft NS, Strachan DP: The social origins of infantile colic: questionnaire study covering 76,747 infants. BMJ 314(7090):1325, 1997

Crowe HP, Zeskind PS: Psychophysiological and perceptual responses to infant cries varying in pitch: comparison of adults with low and high scores on the Child Abuse Potential Inventory. Child Abuse Negl 15:19–29, 1992

Cummings EM, Davies P: Emotional security as a regulatory process in normal development and the development of psychopathology. Dev Psychopathol 8:123–139, 1996

DeGangi GA: Assessment of sensory, emotional and attentional problems in regulatory disordered infants, Part I. Infants and Young Children 3:1–8, 1991

Dieter JN, Emory EK: Supplemental stimulation of premature infants: a treatment model. J Pediatr Psychol 22(3):281–295, 1997

Dunn W: The impact of sensory processing abilities on the daily lives of young children and their families. A conceptual model. Infants and Young Children 9(4):23–35, 1997

Dunn W, Brown W: Factor analysis of the Sensory Profile from a national sample of children without disabilities. Am J Occup Ther 51(7):490–495, 1997

Eibl-Eibesfeldt I: Human Ethology. New York, Aldine de Gruyter, 1987

Field T: Massage therapy for infants and children. J Dev Behav Pediatr 15(2):105–111, 1995

Greenspan SI: Infancy and Early Childhood: The Practice of Clinical Assessment and Intervention With Emotional and Developmental Challenges. Madison, CT, International Universities Press, 1992

Guidetti V, Galli F, Cerutti R, et al: "From 0 to 18": what happens to the child and his headache? Funct Neurol 15 (suppl 3):122–129, 2000

Gustafson G, Harris K: Women's responses to young infants' cries. Dev Psychol 26:144–152, 1990

Hinde R: Temperament as an intervening variable, in Temperament in Childhood. Edited by Kohnstamm GE, Bates JE, Rothbart MK. West Sussex, UK, Wiley, 1989, pp 27–33

Jones HE, Balster RL. Inhalant abuse in pregnancy. Obstet Gynecol Clin North Am 25:153–167, 1998

Joyce P, Clark C: The use of craniosacral therapy to treat gastroesophageal reflux in infants. Infants and Young Children 9(2):51–58, 1996

Lee K: The Crying Pattern of Korean Infants and Related Factors. Dev Med Child Neurol 36:601–607, 1994

Lehtonen L: Infantile colic. Turun Yliopiston Julkaisuja [Turku University Press] Annales Universitatis Turkuensis [Annals of Turku University, Turku, Finland] 151:1–51, 1994

Lucassen PL, Assendelft WJ, Gubbels JW, et al: Effectiveness of treatments for colic: systematic review. BMJ 316:1563–1569, 1998

Maldonado-Durán M, Sauceda-Garcia JM: Excessive crying in infants with regulatory disorders. Bull Menninger Clin 60(1):62–78, 1996

Maldonado-Durán JM, Sauceda-Garcia JM: Colico y Reflujo Gastroesofagico [Colic and gastroesophageal reflux], in La alimentación en la primera infancia y sus efectos en el desarrollo [Feeding in Infancy and Its Effects on Development]. Edited by Lartigue T, Maldonado-Durán JM, Ávila H. México City, Plaza y Valdez, 1998a, pp 189–206

Maldonado-Durán JM, Sauceda-Garcia JM: La madre con dificultades de alimentación y sus efectos en el bebé y el niño de edad pre-escolar [Mothers with eating disorder and effects in the infant and preschool age child], in La alimentación en la primera infancia y sus efectos en el desarrollo [Feeding in Infancy and Its Effects on Development]. Edited by Lartigue T, Maldonado-Durán JM, Ávila H. México City, Plaza y Valdez, 1998, pp 235–256

Maldonado-Durán JM, Holigrocki R, Moody C: Excessive crying, feeding and sleeping problems, and the caretaking environment. Paper presented at the Eleventh International Conference of the International Society for Infant Studies, Atlanta, GA, April 2–5, 1998

Maldonado-Durán JM, Helmig L, Moody C, et al: The Zero th Three diagnostic classification in an infant mental health clinic: its usefulness and challenges. Infant Mental Health Journal (in press)

Miller AR, Barr RG: Infantile colic: is it a gut issue? Pediatr Clin North Am 38(6): 1407–1423, 1991

Mrazek PJ: Maltreatment and infant development, in Handbook of Infant Mental Health. Edited by Zeanah CH Jr. New York, Guilford, 1993, pp 159–170

Murray A: Aversiveness is in the mind of the beholder: perception of infant crying by adults, in Infant Crying: Theoretical and Research Perspectives. Edited by Lester BM, Zachariah Boukydis CF. New York, Plenum, 1985, pp 217–240

Orenstein SR, Izadnia F, Khan S: Gastroesophageal reflux disease in children. Gastroenterology Clin North Am 28:947–970, 1999

Papousek M: Umgang mit dem Schreidenden Säugling [Dealing with the crying infant]. Sozialpädiatrie [Social Pediatrics] 7:294–300, 1985

Papousek H, Papousek M: Intuititive parenting, in Handbook of Parenting: Biology and Ecology of Parenting, Vol 2. Edited by Bornstein MH. Mahwah, NJ, Erlbaum, 1995, pp 117–136

Pickford EJ, Hanson RM, O'Halloran MT, et al: Infants and atropine: a dangerous mixture. Journal of Pediatrics and Child Health 27:55–56, 1991

Poole SR: The infant with acute, unexplained, excessive crying. Pediatrics 88(3): 450–455, 1991

Poole S, Magilner D: Crying complaints in the emergency department, in Crying as a Sign, a Symptom and a Signal. Edited by Barr RG, Hopkins B, Green JA. London, MacKeith Press, 2000, pp 95–105

Prior M: Childhood temperament. J Child Psychol Psychiatry 33(1):249–279, 1992

Sears CJ: Investigating and coping with tactile defensiveness in young children. Infants and Young Children 6(4):446–453, 1994

St. James-Roberts I, Halil T: Infant crying patterns in the first year: normal community and clinical findings. J Child Psychol Psychiatry 32:951–968, 1991

St. James-Roberts I, Bowyer J, Varghese S, et al: Infant crying patterns in Manali and London. Child Care Health Dev 20:323–337, 1994

St. James-Roberts I, Conroy S, Wilsher K: Clinical developmental and social aspects of infant crying and colic. Early Development and Parenting 4:177–189, 1995

Stein A, Woolley H, Cooper SD, et al: An observational study of mothers with eating disorders and their infants. J Child Psychol Psychiatry 35(4):733–748, 1994

Stein A, Murray L, Cooper P, et al: Infant growth in the context of maternal eating disorders and maternal depression: a comparative study. Psychol Med 26(3):569–574, 1996

Sterling CE, Jolley SG, Besser AS, et al: Nursing responsibility in the diagnosis and treatment of the child with gastroesphageal reflux. J Pediatr Nurs 6:435–441, 1991

Stifter CA, Braungart J: Infant colic: a transient condition with no apparent effects. Journal of Applied Developmental Psychology 13:447–462, 1992

Strassburg HM, Müller H, Greiner P: Chronische Unruhe un Gastro-ösophagealer Reflux beim Säugling [Chronic fussiness and gastroesophageal reflux in the infant]. Pädiatrische Praxis [Pediatric Praxis] 37:1–9, 1988

Strassburg HM, Haug-Schnabel G, Müller H: The crying infant: an interdisciplinary approach. Early Child Dev Care 65:153–166, 1990

Van der Wal MF, van den Boom DC, Pauw-Plomp H, et al: Mothers' reports of infant crying and soothing in a multicultural population. Arch Dis Child 79: 312–317, 1998

Von Hofacker N, Papousek M: Disorders of excessive crying, feeding and sleeping: the Munich interdisciplinary research and intervention program. Infant Mental Health Journal 19(2):180–201, 1998

Wolke D: Behavioral treatment of prolonged infant crying: evaluation, methods and a proposal, in New Evidence on Unexplained Early Infant Crying. Edited by Barr RG, St James-Roberts I, Keefe MR. St. Louis, MO, Johnson & Johnson Pediatric Institute, 2001, pp 187–208

Wurmser H, Laubereau B, Hermann M, et al: Excessive infant crying: often not confined to the first 3 months of age. Early Hum Dev 64(1):1–6, 2001

Zeitlin S, Williamson GG: Coping in Young Children. Baltimore, MD, Paul H Brookes, 1994, pp 86–87

11

Sleep Disorders in Infants and Young Children

Klaus Minde, M.D., F.R.C.P.C.

The phenomenon of sleep and its disturbances have been of interest to clinicians and laypeople since time immemorial. In the Middle Ages, sleep was thought to be a retreat of the spirit from the body, permitting other spirits or supernatural forces to enter (Riley 1985). Rational and scientific thinking changed this perception; during the past 100 years, two major explanations for the necessity and meaning of sleep have been advanced. The more popular one is the *restorative theory*. Dr. William Hammond (1873/ 1982), a psychiatrist in New York, first mentioned it, defining the purpose of sleep as follows: "The state of general repose which accompanies sleep is of special value to the organism in allowing the nutrition of the nervous tissue to go on at a greater rate than its destructive metamorphosis" (p. 9). He also stressed that for this reason, "in infants the necessity for sleep is much greater than in adults, and still more so in old persons" (p. 16). While we know today that the brain does not decrease its activity at night to the degree that Hammond suggested, contemporary understanding to some extent supports his restorative concept. For example, we know that brain protein synthesis occurs more during sleep or during the customary sleeping periods (Adams 1980) than at other times and that more amino acids are liberated in the late evening hours than any other time of day (Oswald 1980). In addition, there is evidence that an increase of slow waves during sleep brings about restoration of muscle (Griffin and Trinder 1978) and that rapid eye movement (REM) sleep restores our emotional well-being (Moruzzi 1965).

The other theory to explain sleep is called the *ethology* or *conservation theory*. In essence, it states that species survival depends on adaptation to the world at large as well as on defense against predators. Because our planet is dominated by a circadian rhythm of day and night and because most species can find food only during one part of the cycle, it makes ethological sense for the organism to be inactive when feeding is inefficient. Dement (1972) and Kellerman (1981) extended this notion, suggesting that the need for protection against predators may have contributed to the sleeping habits of humans, with one person watching to keep the others safe.

Group sleeping, however, also reinforces bonding and requires a sense of trust in others. Kellerman believes that fear of losing this protection is the basic cause underlying most psychologically determined sleep disorders. This association between the state of one's relationships and the quality of one's sleep is, of course, a very important aspect of the psychodynamic for understanding and treating sleep problems in both children and adults. Moreover, across cultures, bedtime settling, night waking, and issues such as who sleeps with whom and whether children are separated from adults at night are influenced by parents or other significant caregivers. The adults, in turn, are likely to follow cultural and societal practices as well as their own needs and feelings, ensuring that sleep-related phenomena have significant social impact (Adair and Bauchner 1993).

The dialogue between those who see sleep and its disorders as related primarily to the biological function of the central nervous system and those who emphasize psychological determinants is reflected in the multidisciplinary development of sleep medicine. Less than than 50 years has passed since Dement et al. (1957) first reported on the association between ocular and gross motor movements and certain sleep states in young college students. Since then, we have seen an increasing number of studies—assisted by enormous technological advances in the observation and measurements of sleep states—on sleep and its disorders in children. They have come from the fields of medicine, psychology, and the basic sciences, as well as from the psychoanalytic community. These studies ultimately led to the first comprehensive textbook on the principles and practice of sleep medicine for the child (Ferber and Kryger 1995).

In this chapter, I first provide an overall summary of the development of sleep in infants and young children. I follow this summary with a discussion of various types of sleep disorders, their epidemiology and classification, and clinical evaluation of sleep-disordered children and their families within their specific cultural context. Finally, I describe the treatment of common sleep problems.

BIOLOGY OF NORMAL SLEEP IN INFANTS AND TODDLERS

Sleep Physiology

Until 1953, sleep was thought of as a state characterized by lack of wakefulness and reduced arousal to stimuli. In that year, Aserinsky and Kleitman (1953) reported that sleep consists of two nonwakeful states best distinguished by the presence or absence of rapid eye movements (REMs). Since then, sleep in which eye movements occur is called *REM sleep* and sleep without eye movements is called *nonREM* or *NREM sleep*. NREM sleep is what we normally think of as sound sleep. It is divided into four substages that reflect the depth of sleep and the responsiveness of the organism to the environment. These stages can be identified on the basis of electroencephalogram (EEG) characteristics.

REM sleep is associated with rapid binocular eye movements, body twitches, and even short utterances. Most of our dreams also occur during REM sleep. In fact, it appears that REM sleep may be a compromise between the need for rest and physical restoration and the demand to be easily aroused and alert (Siegel 1990). For example, hibernating animals are typically in a REM-like state of sleep, and some species (e.g., the bear) can even give birth and suckle their young while spending much of their time sleeping (Thorn and Levitt 1981). Indeed, the heightened activation of central and autonomic nervous system processes during REM sleep seems especially important to newborns because of their as yet limited ability to process information during wakefulness. As Roffwarg et al. (1966) postulated more than 30 years ago, the high percentage of REM sleep in neonates (55% compared with 20% in young adults) may serve to stimulate immature neurons and synapses in the brain "internally" at an age when infants cannot yet make adequate use of outside stimulation.

Sleep Architecture

Sleep architecture refers to the structure and depth of sleep as it occurs during a specific sleep period. The architecture of infant sleep has been studied and recorded for some 20 years (Anders 1978), initially by making electrical recordings during a sleep period and more recently by recording the baby's movements from a watch-sized wrist sensor (Sadeh et al. 1991). The reader should understand some descriptors of sleep and its architecture:

- *Sleep onset* is the time when wakefulness changes to sleepiness.
- *Sleep period* defines the time from sleep onset to full and enduring arousal. It will, therefore, include brief wakings during the night. Naps are daytime sleep periods.
- *Sleep cycle* refers to the repeated episodes of NREM sleep followed by REM sleep. Sleep cycles last 50–60 minutes at birth and increase to 90–100 minutes in the adult (Anders 1979). Thus, a 12-month-old infant may go through eight sleep cycles in the course of a 10-hour sleep period and through one or two cycles during an average nap.
- *Bedtime* is the time at which purposeful wakeful activity ends, sleep conditions are established, and sleep is expected. Actual sleep onset may follow shortly thereafter or may be significantly delayed, the latter defining a key symptom of a sleep disorder.
- *Sleep hygiene* is a term used to define the habits that children acquire, often with the help of their caregivers, for falling and staying asleep. They may include bedtime stories, the teddy bear on the left and the doll on the right, and music with an activated mobile.

The typical architecture of an actual night's sleep by a 30-month-old toddler is shown in Figure 11–1. One can see from the figure that this youngster took only 9 minutes to fall asleep after being placed in the crib and then went through 10 cycles of quiet (NREM) and active (REM) episodes. There were also five periods of being awake, for a total of 60 minutes, and 5 minutes of out-of-crib time. The toddler's sleep period lasted from 19:17 to 7:04 (i.e., 11 hours and 47 minutes).

It should be emphasized that from the very beginning, the regulation of an infant's sleep cycles depends to an important degree on the parent-infant interaction. For example, newborn babies who sleep with their mothers in the hospital room spend more time in quiet (NREM) sleep and cry less often than infants who sleep in the newborn nursery (Keffe 1987).

DEVELOPMENTAL CHANGES IN SLEEP AND THE SLEEP CYCLE

The organization of sleep and waking states proceeds in an orderly fashion from birth on. At term, infants on average sleep 16.5 hours per 24 hours. Average sleep decreases to 14.25 hours at 6 months, 13.75 hours at 12 months, and 13 hours at 2 years (Ferber 1985). At the same time, nocturnal sleep increases from 8 hours at birth to 11 hours at 12 and 24 months. Thus, babies at birth are awake as much at night as they sleep during the day (Coons and Guilleminault 1982). They also go from wake-

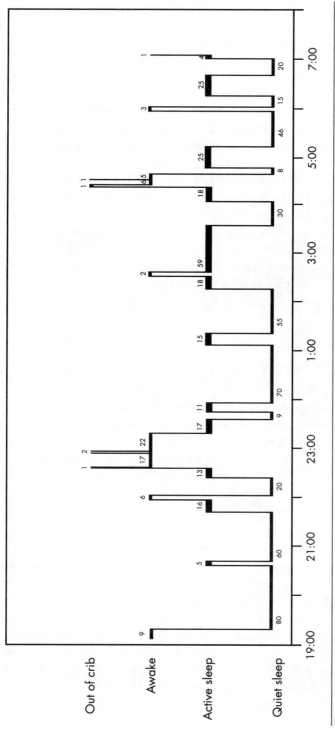

Figure 11–1. Sleep record.

fulness into active (REM) sleep for 15–20 minutes and then into quiet (NREM) sleep (Dreyfus-Brisac 1979).

As babies mature, their active sleep time becomes proportionally shorter, decreasing to 43% at 3 months and to 30% of total sleep time by 12 months (Anders et al. 1983). During the second half of the first year, infants also begin to move from periodic waking directly to quiet sleep, the pattern observed in adults. At that time, they also tend to move less rapidly from REM to NREM sleep (Anders et al. 1983). In addition, the organization of the sleep-wake cycle changes. From a seemingly even distribution of sleep and wakefulness during the day and night, infants begin to adapt to the light-dark cycle of our day and the recurring social cues that go with it. For example, by 6 months, the longest continuous sleep period during the night for an infant has lengthened to 6 hours, and there are comparatively longer waking periods during the day. At age 6–12 months, children usually require two naps per day. From then on until around age 3, they have only one nap. Figure 11–2 depicts the total daily sleep requirements in hours and the changes in the proportion of nocturnal versus daytime sleep taking place in the first 4 years of life.

IMPACT OF SOCIAL AND CULTURAL FACTORS ON SLEEP

Sleep is a physiological event as necessary to survival as eating and toileting. Yet all these functions are also intricately connected with the traditions and needs of other household members, leading to a wide range of sleep behaviors that can be considered normal for an individual youngster.

Feeding

Feeding and sleeping are closely associated in early life. Very young infants need to nurse or feed every 3–4 hours, and their short sleep periods, which are fairly independent of the light-dark cycle, are highly appropriate times for bringing food and rest together. There is, nevertheless, an ongoing debate about whether breast-fed babies require more frequent feedings than formula-fed ones. Nursing mothers tend to feed their infants more frequently (i.e., the mothers will not let their babies get very hungry). More frequent feedings can lead to more frequent night wakings, which may fulfill the criteria of a sleep problem (Elias et al. 1986; Zuckerman et al. 1987), although other authors have not found this association (Adair et al. 1991).

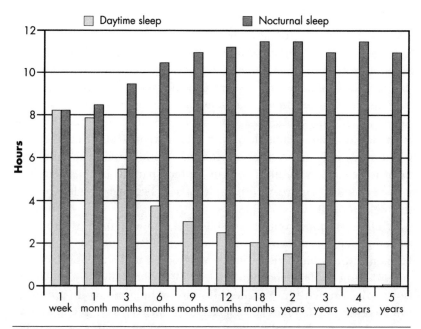

Figure 11–2. Average total sleep times during childhood.

During infancy, normal daytime sleep occurs in several discrete naps that decrease in frequency and length over time. At about age 4, daytime sleep decreases to just one brief daily nap, while nighttime sleep continues to increase.

Source. Adapted from Ferber R: *Solve Your Child's Sleep Problems.* New York, Penguin, 1985. Copyright 1985, Richard Ferber. Used with permission from the author and Simon & Schuster.

In North American culture, many children at 6 months of age are given some solid food at bedtime because the parents believe it will increase nighttime sleep. There is no evidence that this belief is true (Macknin et al. 1989), although most children at that age can go without a feeding for one 6- to 12-hour period per day, regardless of the consistency of their last feeding. In fact, night wakings beyond 6 months of age for a feeding are a learned response; that is, they may be normal for some babies but are not necessary for physical health or emotional well-being.

Co-Sleeping

Professionals in North America frequently suggest that young children should sleep alone, and that advice is followed, at least by middle-class parents. This is a relatively new development. One hundred years ago, most families in the United States and Canada slept together in one room (Thevinin 1976), and in a majority of cultures this practice persists (Burton and Whiting 1961).

One can justifiably assume that a practice like co-sleeping, which has a long history and is common in a significant number of cultures, may have been useful for infant well-being during the course of human evolution. Lozoff et al. (1984) examined this issue in great detail and found that regular co-sleeping (i.e., more than two to three times a week) is alive and well in the United States, at least among some ethnic groups. About 50% of African American infants, 21% of Hispanic infants, and almost 10% of white infants sleep with their parents (Lozoff et al. 1984). Children from families of lower economic standing co-sleep more frequently, regardless of ethnic origin. In fact, parents in those families tended to interact more with their children at bedtime as well as during the night (Lozoff et al. 1984).

While co-sleeping continues to be quite common, there is also good evidence that it is associated with increased sleep problems in healthy Hispanic, white, and African American children under age 4 (Madanski and Edelbrock 1990; Schachter et al. 1989). Specifically, African American co-sleeping children protested more at bedtime, and parents in white co-sleeping families considered their children's sleep behavior as especially conflictual and distressing (Lozoff et al. 1996). However, this situation was true only when children shared a bed with their parents; when children were just sleeping in the same bedroom as their parents, it was not related to sleep problems. There was also no relationship with social class (Lozoff et al. 1996).

It is not clear whether co-sleeping causes sleep problems or occurs in response to them, or whether other factors (e.g., general family stress) would explain both co-sleeping and troubles with sleeping. Mosko et al. (1997) provided intriguing data on this topic. Using sophisticated non-invasive technology, they observed 35 breast-feeding Latino mother-infant pairs when the babies were 11–15 weeks old. Twenty infants were routinely sharing a bed; the others slept alone. All mother-infant pairs were observed during a bed-sharing night and a solitary-sleeping night. The routinely bed-sharing infants showed more transient awakenings, even during deep sleep, than the solitary sleepers did. They were also breast-fed more frequently. McKenna et al. (1997) interpreted the frequent awakenings as potentially protective against sudden infant death syndrome (SIDS) because the babies were in constant body contact with their mothers and were less likely to develop apnea. This study suggests that co-sleeping during the initial weeks of life may provide some protection against SIDS, but such a pattern may lead to later sleep problems in some children.

Transitional Objects and Thumb Sucking

The term *transitional object* was first used by Winnicott (1953) to describe the inanimate objects (e.g., blanket, teddy bear, piece of cloth, or pacifier) toddlers use to comfort themselves in the absence of their mother or other primary caregivers. According to Winnicott, the transitional object serves as a substitute for the parent, and its removal can lead to distress. Because going to bed is a repeated separation from the primary caregivers, transitional objects often help children ages 9–36 months deal with the associated anxiety.

Here again, however, cultural differences occur. In Sweden, 45% of 4-year-olds use transitional objects, decreasing to 7% by age 14 (Klackenberg 1987). Wolf and Lozoff (1989) reported that transitional objects are used more commonly by children who fall asleep alone (57%) than those who fall asleep in the presence of a caregiver (30%). Italian rural children, who rarely sleep alone, also had little use for a transitional object (only 4.9% used one). The same was true for Korean children, of whom only 18% ever used one, compared with 64% of a matched U.S. sample (Gaddini 1970; Hong and Townes 1976). Thumb-sucking habits followed the same trend: 32% of children who fell asleep alone sucked their thumbs, whereas only 11% of the others did (Wolf and Lozoff 1989).

This variability obviously reflects different underlying principles of caregiving and suggests that many children experience some separation anxiety when they are expected to go off to sleep by themselves (Wolf and Lozoff 1989). In addition, some parents obviously use this daily event to teach their children strategies to cope with small adversities (i.e., these children soothe themselves with the help of a pacifier, blanket, or thumb), while other parents assume the responsibility of soothing their children to help them fall asleep.

Bedtime Routines

Children generally engage in social interactions along with bedtime preparations that facilitate the transition from wakefulness to sleep-onset. Many families develop bedtime routines or rituals with private and individualized context and meaning. For example, there may be a bath, special toys and washing rituals, followed by two stories; there may be a predetermined number of kisses or a special way of being tucked in. All these activities are helpful for young children; they value sameness and an unhurried pace of events that promises more of the same. The routines also aid them in conceptualizing that a night alone will be followed by a reunion with family the next morning and another day of fun and adventure.

SLEEP PROBLEMS IN CHILDREN: EPIDEMIOLOGY AND CLASSIFICATION

Sleep disorders are periodically classified by a special committee of the American Sleep Disorders Association and are published as the Diagnostic Classification of Sleep and Arousal Disorders (DCSAD). The latest revision, the International Classification of Sleep Disorders (ICSD), was published in 1990 (American Sleep Disorders Association 1990). The recommendations of this committee were incorporated into DSM-IV (American Psychiatric Association 1994) and retained in DSM-IV-TR (American Psychiatric Association 2000). They focus primarily on sleep disorders in adults, but modifications for pediatric populations have been published (Sheldon et al. 1992). Table 11–1 gives a summary of the classification.

As Table 11–1 shows, DSM-IV-TR differentiates between *dyssomnias*, or disruptions of the sleep process, and *parasomnias*. Parasomnias are sleep disorders in which behaviors that may be triggered by various parts of the brain disrupt ongoing sleep. A sudden apnea in an infant, or a mother's awakening her 9-month-old because she believes he needs a 3 A.M. feeding, will cause a dyssomnia; nightmares and periods of sleepwalking are parasomnias.

Parasomnias are uncommon in children younger than 36 months, but dyssomnias are common, although estimates of their prevalence vary somewhat between investigators because of different definitions of the term *sleep disorder*. Anders and Eiben (1997) stated that most infants do not meet the full DSM-IV criteria for an *extrinsic dyssomnia* or *primary insomnia*. He suggests that such children might be better classified as having "protodyssomnias," which are characterized by repetitive night wakings and inability to fall asleep.

Table 11–1.   Primary sleep disorders

ICD	DSM-IV-TR
Dyssomnias	
Intrinsic dyssomnia	Primary hypersomnia
Extrinsic dyssomnia	Primary insomnia
Parasomnias	
Arousal disorders	Nightmare disorder
	Sleep terror disorder
	Sleepwalking disorder
Medical and psychiatric sleep disorders	
Associated with medical disorders	Sleep disorder due to medical condition
Associated with neurological disorders	

Source.   American Psychiatric Association 2000; American Sleep Disorders Association 1990.

Moore and Ucko (1957) defined a good sleeper as an infant who sleeps from midnight to 5 A.M. for at least 4 weeks without being removed from the crib. These authors concluded that 70% of their normative sample of 160 children fulfilled this criterion by 3 months, and that almost 90% did so by 9 months. Jenkins et al. (1980), who followed 360 infants in a central borough of London at specific intervals for 2 years, found that about 20% of children woke regularly at night. In a follow-up report, these same authors provided interesting data on the persistence of sleep problems (Jenkins et al. 1984). They found that 50%–70% of poor sleepers at 6, 12, 18, 30, or 36 months continued to have problems at the subsequent appointment 6 or 12 months later. However, only 20% of children who showed sleep problems at 6 months still exhibited them at 3 years. Similarly, Beltramini and Hertzig (1983), who analyzed the sleep and bedtime behaviors of 133 children in the New York Longitudinal Study (initially directed by Thomas and Chess), reported that 30% of the children typically woke up one or more times per night during the first 4 years of life. More recent studies from Israel and New Zealand confirm these figures (Scher et al. 1987; Wooding et al. 1990).

These data are based on parental reports, and there has long been concern about the accuracy of such information. Specifically, two forms of error may distort the accuracy of reported sleep patterns in children. First, parents may base their judgment on the time an infant wakes up but fail to consider when the infant fell asleep. For example, an infant who sleeps from 7 P.M. to 2 A.M. may be labeled a "night waker," while the baby who sleeps from 10:30 P.M. to 5:30 A.M. is considered to "sleep through." Yet both infants have an uninterrupted sleep period of 7 hours. Second, many parents either do not notice or are not disturbed by their children's night waking and, therefore, do not report a problem (Scott and Richards 1990). Clearly, an accurate reporting system of sleep behavior and well-operationalized clinical criteria are needed to determine the presence and severity of a specific sleep problem.

Richman and her colleagues (Richman 1981, 1985; Richman et al. 1982, 1985) have done much to develop a recording system that defines the type and severity of sleep disorders in young children. They created a parental diary to monitor the following types of information for 1 week as follows:

• The time the child went to bed at night
• The time he or she went to sleep
• The times he or she woke up during the night
• The time the child went to sleep again
• How often the parents took the child into their bed
• The time the child woke up in the morning

At the end of the week, the scores were combined, giving the average number of wakings per night and their duration. Each item was then rated on a scale from 0 to 4, allowing for a composite sleep score from 0 to 24. Richman considered a score of 12 or above to reflect a serious sleep problem if the child displayed this behavior for more than 3 months.

This procedure was used to assess the sleep patterns of 771 children (ages 1 to 2) in a London suburb (Richman 1981). In this study, 20% of these children were found to wake up five or more times per week; 9.5% of the children woke up three or more times per night, were awake for more than 20 minutes per night, or moved into their parents' bed.

There is good evidence for the persistence of sleep problems in later childhood. For example, Zuckerman et al. (1987) followed 308 infants age 3 months with sleep problems and found that 41% still had difficulties at age 3, while only 26% of the sleep-disturbed 3-year-olds had not had trouble sleeping at 8 months. Kateria et al. (1987) found that 84% of 205 sleep-disturbed infants still had sleep problems at age 6.

In an investigation of a representative sample of 432 German children at ages 5, 20, and 56 months, Wolke et al. (1994) obtained similar results. Thus, 21.5% of all children had night-waking problems at 5 months, 21.8% at 20 months, and 13.3% at 56 months. One in four of the 5-year-olds regularly slept with parents. Children with night-waking problems had a 2.2- to 2.5-fold increased risk of remaining night wakers from one assessment period to the next, compared with nonwakers.

Scott and Richards (1990) published the latest estimate of sleep disorders in the United Kingdom, it involved 1,500 children ages 1–2. Of these children, 25% woke up at least five times per week, but only half their mothers considered their waking a serious problem. Not settling at night for more than 30 minutes was the second most common complaint in this sample, occurring in about 10% of children; in 70% it was associated with night wakings. Very early waking, which occurred more frequently in homes where two or more children shared a bedroom, was mentioned least often as a problem.

Work by our own group has added some new aspects to these findings (Minde et al. 1993). In a study of 58 children ages 12–36 months, 30 had a serious sleep disorder. We employed a time-lapse infrared video camera to record the children sleeping in their homes. This arrangement allowed us to compare various sleep parameters as they were reported by the parents and seen on videotape. Interestingly, the parents of the poor sleepers on average reported 2.8 wakings per night, while the video camera recorded 3.6 wakings. At the same time, mothers of good sleepers reported that they awakened only 0.5 times per night, while video records revealed a surprising average of 3.2 wakings. In other words, there was no difference in the incidence of interrupted sleep experience between the reported poor sleepers and good sleepers, thus confirming Anders's 1979 report. The only difference was that the good sleepers managed to go back to sleep without waking anyone, while the poor sleepers called out for assistance. Obviously such a calling-out routine in a young child can happen for many reasons, ranging from anxiety in the child to over-solicitous parenting practices. It is this great variety of outside contributing events and biological circumstances that makes the field of pediatric sleep medicine so complex and challenging.

ASSESSMENT OF SLEEP DISORDERS

The evaluation of a family with a sleep-disordered child is complex and must be carried out with tact and sensitivity. In many cases, disturbed nights have been a chronic condition for several months. Parents and children, therefore, present as exhausted, irritable, and helpless. Some parents express feelings of guilt and anxiety when they talk about wishing to have their evenings to themselves rather than to be constantly cuddling their infants or giving them drinks in the middle of the night. Parents may also be anxious or overprotective, trying to avoid upsetting their children in any way. Or they may interfere with their baby's settling patterns, checking on the baby excessively because of the need to reassure themselves.

Our experience suggests that the evaluation of a youngster's sleep problems should be done in the presence of both parents whenever possible. This approach establishes from the start that the child's difficulty is a family matter and needs to be assessed within that context. An initial assessment should include

- A detailed sleep history.
- A general developmental and medical history of the child.
- A complete social and psychiatric history of the child and family.
- A session during which the clinician can observe the parent-child relationship.
- In some cases, a formal developmental screening or physical examination.

Depending on the findings, a more detailed examination may be indicated, involving further psychological and specialized laboratory tests of the infant (e.g., EEG) or a psychiatric assessment of one or both parents.

Because the great majority of sleep problems are behavioral and reflect the parent-child relationship, a careful history of this aspect of the infant's life becomes particularly important. Although some pediatricians are interested in such an assessment, few pediatric residency training programs provide more than the most elementary training in this field (Mindell et al. 1994).

Sleep History

The following areas should be considered in assessing a sleep disorder. This approach is based on the sleep management manual developed by Douglas and Richman (1984).

Bedtime and Settling Procedures

This area includes bedtime routines. For example, when does the child get ready for bed? How and where does the child fall asleep (e.g., in the parent's arms or in the crib)? Does the child have ways to settle down (e.g., a pacifier or blanket)? What do the parents do when the child comes out of the bedroom later in the evening?

Night Awakenings

This area covers the number and length of awakenings per night. For example, how many times does the child wake? How long does the child remain awake? How does the family react to the wakings? How does the child settle again?

Daytime Naps

To learn the number of daytime naps, we may ask, How many naps does the child take during the day? How long are the naps? How does the child settle at that time? It is especially important to note possible differences between settling procedures and the child's sleep behavior during the night and during the afternoon nap.

Attempted Previous Solutions

We want to know how long the problem has gone on, especially because children show normal variations in sleep patterns. Difficulties of less than 3 months' duration occur in many normal children. We ask the parents, What do you think causes the sleep difficulty (e.g., an illness, anxiety triggered by a visit to grandmother)? How have you previously tried to change your youngster's sleep pattern (e.g., medication, let the child "cry it out")?

It is usually helpful to ask parents for a developmental description of these sleep patterns to understand how the disturbance developed over time. It is also important to record how this history is presented. Parents may disagree with each other on the troubling symptoms, or one parent may speak while the other is silent. Factual information is extremely important in assessing sleep disorders. Thus, statements such as "He has never slept more than 1 hour at a time" or "She wakes up 10 to 20 times every night" are not helpful and should be reformulated into the "usual" activities and patterns of the youngster. Ferber (1995) suggests asking about the onset, duration, character, frequency, and consistency of the sleep symptom and how long it has persisted in its current pattern. For example, when parents complain about night-time waking, it may be useful to know whether the child wakes gradually or suddenly, whether the child stays in the crib or bed crying softly or starts screaming, and whether the child comes into the parents' bedroom or into their bed.

Similar details must be sought when inquiring about the child's sleep environment. This inquiry covers data about the bedroom, including what its size is, whether it is dark at night or has a nightlight, whether it is noisy, whether it is close to the parents' bedroom, and whether the door is open or shut.

Bedtime rituals and routines must be assessed with equal thoroughness and their consistency ascertained. Some families have no routines and change the child's bedtime every day.

In helping parents focus their attention on the sleep behavior of their child, it is very useful to have them fill out a sleep diary for 1–2 weeks and bring it along for discussion. Such a document can also be helpful in assessing the benefit of specific interventions during subsequent treatment.

Developmental and Medical History of the Child

It is useful to know about the pregnancy and delivery of the child, as well as neonatal behavior (e.g., episodes of colic and feeding patterns and their regularity). One should also inquire about the infant's general ability to organize or modulate behavior. For example, some children quickly learn to soothe themselves when distressed by sucking their thumb or using other transitional objects; others have few or no means to do so. Many sleep-disordered children fall into the latter category, suggesting that treatment should include teaching the child how to calm himself or herself.

Hence, it is important to know how the youngster behaves during waking hours and whether problems are also exhibited then. For example, is the child miserable during the day or can the child amuse himself or herself and get along with others? Is the child enrolled in a play group or nursery?

Medical events may also affect sleep patterns. For example, epileptic attacks and severe mental retardation can interfere with normal sleep, as can allergies, intestinal disorders, and painful infections (e.g., middle-ear infection).

Social and Psychiatric History of the Child and Family

It is essential to obtain objective information about general aspects of the patient's family life. This information would include such data as the mother and father's personal backgrounds, an account of their families of origin, their work, the father's level of involvement in the care of the family, and whether the parents can confide in each other. We also want to know the parents' ideas about and methods of discipline, their ways of having fun, and their thoughts and ideas about the character and underlying personality of the baby.

It is also helpful to inquire about the parents' early relationships with their own parents; these experiences frequently serve as a model for the attitudes and feelings parents have toward their own children. For example, parents who describe their own families as "matter of fact" or "tolerating no unnecessary complaining" may get very angry about their toddler's wakefulness at night and consider unduly harsh consequences, such as locking the child in the bedroom and letting him or her cry it out.

Stresses experienced by the parents are also important. Are the stresses related to external events (e.g., work or finances), do they reflect difficulties between the couple, or are they triggered by memories of their own childhood? Have there been previous episodes of emotional difficulties in one or both parents? If so, did they require professional treatment and for how long? Did the mother suffer from postpartum blues or depression? If so, how did this affect her caregiving ability toward the patient? How much has the present sleep problem contributed to the family's stress? Do other relatives or siblings help care for the child? How successful are they?

Finally, it may be useful to inquire if other family members have had similar symptoms. Some familial tendencies have been established in sleepwalking, sleep terror, and head banging (Ferber 1988; Kales et al. 1980).

It is essential to obtain this information in a context of mutual respect and collaboration; the parents are our primary allies and co-therapists in dealing with the child's sleep difficulty. They should not be made to feel that they are seen as patients. This approach is not always easy and may require much patience and sensitivity.

Parent-Child Relationship

Once the formal sleep assessment interview with the parents is completed, it is important to evaluate the overall caregiver-infant relationship. The rationale here is that difficulties in settling or night-sleeping behavior usually also show themselves during daytime interactions between the child and his or her caregiver. Empirical investigations support this association (Minde et al. 1994; Richman et al. 1982). To learn about the parent-child relationship, it is best to observe the primary caregivers and the problem sleeper during a free play period and also while both partners are engaged in a structured task. For reliable results, this period does not need to exceed 10 minutes. The structured task may consist of having a snack together, looking at a book together, building something together, or demanding that an older toddler clean up after playtime. The request for the child to clean up often provides especially valuable data because the caregiver-infant dyad is under greater pressure.

When observing actual behavior, we often see difficulties in the actions of poor sleepers in a number of areas:

- *Joint attention or engagement.* The partners are not focused on the same activity or event.
- *Overall reciprocity.* There is little verbal dialogue or turn-taking activity when both partners are engaged in a mutually responsive way.
- *Overall organization or regulation of interactions.* The timing and pace of the interactions between the child and his or her parent may not be comprehensible to the observer because members of the dyad do not participate in and regulate each other's activity.
- *State similarity.* The parent's and the child's activity levels are poorly matched.
- *General mood during the interaction.* Expressions of anger or excessive control appear in either child or caregiver during play. For example, the parent may attempt to appease the child by not sticking to reasonable demands.

The presence of one or more of these interactive difficulties suggests that the parent finds it hard to set age-appropriate limits. This failure may have a specific motive (e.g., the mother may prefer the infant's company to her husband's or may use the infant's company as a replacement during her husband's absence) or may be related to past events or imme-

diate external stresses in the parent's life. Difficulties in two or more of
these interactive patterns suggest that the parent is not in tune with the
child and, therefore, may find it hard to set age-appropriate limits while
providing the child with a solid sense of security.

Formal Developmental Screening or Physical Examination

A formal developmental screening or physical examination should be
done only for children who have a history suggestive of specific difficulties. For example, children who snore excessively or have suspected apnea attacks should have their ears, nose, and throat examined. If there is
any suspicion of a seizure associated with excessive sleepiness, a neurological assessment should be conducted. Severe and questionable developmental abnormalities should also lead to a referral for further detailed
developmental testing.

SLEEP DISORDERS

The complaint of sleeplessness in young children usually comes from the
parents because children tend to be quite happy staying awake. In fact,
one of the four DSM-IV-TR criteria for primary insomnia requires that
the sleep disturbance cause clinically significant distress or impairment
in social, occupational, or other areas of functioning. These criteria obviously never apply to infants and young children, although their caregivers may experience clinically significant distress. On the other hand,
there are parents who report their children's sleep problems, such as
head banging or snoring; however, the problems may more accurately be
called sleep behaviors because they do not reflect pathological conditions (Stores 1992). Likewise, some children may exhibit normal sleep
patterns (e.g., they sleep from 7 P.M. to 3 A.M. without waking up), but
their behavior is nevertheless disturbing to their families. It is, therefore,
suggested that parental complaints about their children's sleep should
always be taken seriously, whether or not the sleep problem qualifies as
a disorder. The more common sleep problems that are sources of caregiver frustration are discussed in the section immediately below, using
the ICSD as a diagnostic guide.

Dyssomnias or Disruptions of the Sleep Process

Sleep can be disrupted by an intrinsic event, such as apnea, or by an extrinsic event, such as the child's inability to go to sleep in the evening or
go back to sleep after three or four normal waking periods. About 85% of

all sleep problems are extrinsic. Four different types of night-waking patterns qualify as extrinsic dyssomnia: a) sleep-onset association disorder, b) nocturnal eating (drinking) disorder, c) bedtime struggles or limit-setting disorder, and d) circadian rhythm or sleep-wake cycle sleep disorder.

The term *night waking* describes children who wake up during the night and call for their parents or go to look for them. It occurs more frequently with children with the following characteristics:

- Children who have a difficult temperament (Carey 1974; Minde et al. 1994; Richman 1981; Weissbluth 1981)
- Children whose mothers are depressed or are exposed to psychosocial stressors (Richman 1981; Zuckerman et al. 1987)
- Children who sleep in one bed with their caregivers (Lozoff et al. 1996)
- Children whose parents are present while they fall asleep (Adair et al. 1991; Johnson 1991)

Contrary to common belief, the gender of the baby and teething pains are not reliably associated with night waking. It is of interest that either these conditions are all directly under parental control (e.g., their presence at sleep onset or by co-sleeping) or the conditions cause or add to parental stress (difficult temperament). We believe today that the actual sleep problem in these cases is learned by the child because the parent initially responded maladaptively to the baby (e.g., checked on slight noises) and inadvertently taught the child to expect the parents' presence when falling asleep.

Sleep-Onset Association Disorder

The rather fancy term *sleep-onset association disorder* describes a condition in which children have learned to associate any sleep onset with specific bedtime rituals that must be executed by the caregivers. For example, a child may demand that the parent sing one song after another or that the mobile play music all night long. Whenever the child wakes up during the night, he or she will demand a repeat performance. When the parent obliges, the child quickly returns to sleep, thereby establishing the diagnosis of the "association" as the main problem.

This problem can be quite challenging. Even though many children demand only a minor intervention to return to sleep, such as being covered with a blanket, a parent who has to do this two or three times a night and is unable to get back to sleep quickly will find it very draining. Because young children rapidly learn new patterns, such a disorder can develop in otherwise well-functioning families. For example, after a toddler's brief illness that required special caregiving, the toddler wants the extra attention to continue for months thereafter. In other children, this behavior is caused by a fear of separation and reflects a much more serious problem in the parent-child relationship.

Nocturnal Eating (or Drinking) Disorder

Some children who are put to sleep with a bottle and given another bottle to help them back to sleep after their first night-waking period can wake up repeatedly because they are fed too much fluid. The reason for this association, which goes against the common advice that children should be soothed back to sleep with the help of a bottle, seems to be the discomfort created by a full stomach or an overly wet diaper. The condition, documented by various studies (Ferber and Boyle 1983; Richman 1981; van Tassel 1985), affects about 5% of children between 6 months and 3 years. It is not uncommon for young children to be given large quantities of fluids per night (8–42 ounces). As in a sleep-onset association disorder, the problem is a learned association between an extrinsic soothing mechanism (in this case, a feeding) and the ability to fall asleep. It should be stressed that asking for milk or juice during the night is not a reflection of a physiological need because by 6 months all full-term, healthy, normally growing children are able to obtain all their necessary food intake during the day.

Bedtime Struggles or Limit-Setting Sleep Disorder

Bedtime struggles are common in toddlers. According to the American Sleep Disorders Association (1990), 5%–10% of children are affected. Bedtime struggles often first occur when children are able to climb out of their crib or are moved from their crib to a bed (i.e., during their second or third year of life). It is as if the removal of the crib's barriers creates a feeling of freedom that must be tested at all costs. Because toddlers also go through a developmental phase highlighted by a strong urge toward autonomy, parents must be especially sensitive when they impose behavioral limits. Bedtime struggles arise most often when caregivers do not establish and maintain clear expectations regarding bedtime and sleep circumstances (e.g., making the child sleep in his or her own bed). Parental expectations are frequently challenged not only by the toddler's determination but also by the toddler's charm. Thus, toddlers in their third year often also learn how to influence adults through their increasingly competent "cute" language skills. Parents who find themselves enchanted by their youngsters' shenanigans may fail to realize that they are gradually losing control.

On the other hand, anxious parents may also find it hard to assess the validity of their child's complaints and ruses (e.g., extra water; one more story from dad; one night in two, I should sleep in mom's bed). They may initially go along with the child's demands, only to become angry later. This loss of parental control will, in turn, make the child more anxious and demanding (Daws 1989) and lead to more disturbed nights. Some parents do not recognize the need for consistent limit setting even when their own life lacks consistency because of unpredictable external stressors and demands. In extreme cases, parental depression, alcoholism, or drug abuse may deprive children of any meaningful daily routine. Sleep problems will be only one of many behavioral symptoms these children usually display in response to their chaotic lives.

Sometimes the child who cannot fall asleep at the prescribed time is physiologically not ready to sleep. For example, if 24-month-old Janie always has difficulty falling asleep when she is put to bed at 8 P.M., her subsequent struggles may be a schedule-related problem. If Janie's 5-year-old brother shares and uses her bedroom until his 9 P.M. bedtime and likes noisy games, one can well imagine that falling asleep at 8 P.M. may simply be impossible for Janie.

Circadian Rhythm or Sleep–Wake Cycle Sleep Disorder

The circadian system is the biologically programmed pacemaker that brings about predictable sleep-wake alternation. This system is functional at birth but not yet attuned to the day and night cycle of our planet until the child is 3 years old (Kleitman and Engelmann 1953; Parmelee 1974). Although dysfunctions can occur because of brain abnormalities (e.g., hypothalamic tumor) or blindness (i.e., day and night cues are not perceived), difficulties most often appear because the child's particular schedule conflicts with parental priorities. For example, Peter's mother may need to leave home by 6 A.M. to be at work by 7 A.M. and must, therefore, drop him off at day care at 6:45 A.M. But if Peter has only gone to bed at 9 P.M. the night before, he may not be ready to be awake at that time.

Other difficulties may be created by an excessively long nap time, which some caregivers appreciate because it allows them "to do something for myself." However, 2-year-old Cynthia, who sleeps from 2 P.M. to 5 P.M., will obviously not be ready for bed again at 7 P.M. for an 11-hour sleep period, although her caregiver labeled the long afternoon sleep a "late nap."

As can be seen, the diagnosis of this condition can best be made in light of the history of the child and the family, when the clinician is aware of the developmental sleep requirements of a young child. The clinician must also be able to recognize the presence of coexisting family problems that may cause parents to be insensitive to the child's efforts at getting needs met.

Parasomnias

Parasomnias are conditions in which sleep is disrupted by an event happening during sleep or exacerbated by sleep that results in peculiar nocturnal behaviors (Guilleminault 1987). They are subdivided into a) various arousal disorders and b) sleep-wake transitional disorders.

Arousal Disorders

Nightmares.   The most common arousal disorder, the nightmare, is a frightening dream followed by awakening and often by crying and agitation. Nightmares occur during active (REM) sleep and are most frequent between the ages of 3 and 5, when the incidence ranges from 20% to 25%. Terr (1987) believes that nightmares can also occur in preverbal children, especially if they have experienced severe traumatic events. She bases this assumption on the similarity of behaviors between these infants and older, verbal children. Since REM sleep at this age is more common during the later part of the night, nightmares occur more frequently then. They are equally common in boys and girls and are a normal feature of development if they occur occasionally. One reason for the occurrence of nightmares in toddlers is that most children in their third year of life become increasingly aware of the rules and regulations governing our society and try hard to observe them. At the same time, they are also cognitively capable of recognizing that they are often unable to do so. This makes them feel insecure or guilty to the extent that some may even believe that they disappoint their parents. Such anxieties can be reflected in young children's dreams, leading to nightmares.

Sleepwalking (somnambulism).   Sleepwalking occurs most frequently during the transition between two sleep cycles (e.g., from a deep NREM sleep to a more active REM sleep) early in the night. Children who sleepwalk usually do it in a calm manner, and infants may just crawl around in their cribs. Because there is often little noise associated with these episodes, they are not always even noticed by the parents. Although sleepwalking does occur in infants, it is more common—and also more risky—in older children. Infants or toddlers either stay in their crib or simply appear in their parents' bedroom, while older children may actually leave the house or hurt themselves by falling down stairs or over furniture. Infants and toddlers also rarely wake up fully during a sleepwalking episode, while older children usually awaken after their night travel.

Night terrors. Night terrors are episodes of crying and screaming accompanied by great agitation and, at times, attempts to get out of bed. They are far less common than sleepwalking in infants and toddlers. They are usually brief (1–5 minutes) and are not remembered, although some older children recall a sense of "something closing in," explaining the traditional lay term for this condition, *incubus,* that is, an evil spirit that lies on people in their sleep.

Sleep-Wake Transitional Disorders

Symptoms that occur primarily during the period when children first fall asleep in the evening or when they try to go back to sleep during the night are called sleep-wake transitional disorders. The most common conditions affecting infants and toddlers are the *rhythmic movement disorders* (RMDs). These are stereotyped movements that include head banging, body rocking, or head rolling, where the head moves from side to side. Toddlers on their hands and knees often perform body rocking. These movements last for 15–30 minutes and usually begin during the first 9 months of life. They rarely continue after age 2. In a population study in Scandinavia, Klackenberg (1971) indicated that by 9 months about 60% of children perform some type of RMD and 22% still do so at age 2. In most cases, these rhythmic movements are not associated with any neuropsychiatric condition and disappear all by themselves. However, they can at times be quite disturbing to others. Injuries are infrequent, although soft-tissue damage to the eyes and forehead has been reported in mentally retarded children (Thorpy 1990).

Sleep Disorders in Children With Medical Conditions

Several rare sleep disorders may affect children with medical conditions, especially infants and toddlers; therefore, such problems should always be considered in the differential diagnosis of any sleep problem in this age group. These include obstructive sleep apnea syndrome (OSAS), food allergy insomnia, respiratory conditions, and neurological and other disorders.

Obstructive Sleep Apnea Syndrome

Obstructive sleep apnea is caused by a collapse of the upper airway following a forceful inspiration against relaxed oropharyngeal muscles during sleep. The sudden hypoxemia disrupts both sleep pattern and brain metabolism. Such children have problems breathing while sleeping (96%), they snore excessively (93%), or they have apnea observed by their parents (80%). Other signs are an overly restless sleep (74%), frequent wakings (60%), and excessive somnolence and irritability (32%). The condition occurs most frequently in infants born prematurely, in infants with large tonsils, or in those with reduced muscle tone. The exact incidence of the disorder in young children is unknown because most studies on the condition include older children and no study has separately studied children under age 4. Clinically, however, many parents describe an early onset of some key symptoms of OSAS, such as snoring or breathing difficulties. For example, Frank et al. (1983) reported that 28% of parents retrospectively described OSAS symptoms in their affected children going back to the first few months of life. Other findings support this report. Guilleminault and Stoohs (1992) described 25 infants with an "apparent life-threatening event (ALTE)"; that is, they experienced one or more episodes that frightened an observer because the infant had a severe apnea and a change in color or muscle tone, and showed signs of choking and gagging. These infants still had home monitors at 9 months and showed smaller airway dimensions. They also had a positive family history of snoring and OSAS, a finding confirmed by others (Redline et al. 1992). If this condition is suspected in the young child, a referral should be made to the appropriate specialist.

Food Allergy Insomnia

Some sleep problems are caused by an allergic response to food allergens. This response begins in infancy, is more common in boys, and will often diminish between 2 and 4 years of age (Kahn et al. 1989). The improvement is due to the developing immune system that, in a more mature state, is often capable of managing a wider range of foreign proteins. A 6-week trial of a diet free of cow's milk may be able to normalize the infant's sleep pattern. If this does not help, an allergist may have to be consulted.

Respiratory Conditions

Chronic respiratory problems may lead to clinically significant difficulties in breathing and getting sufficient oxygen into the blood. Both factors can cause sleep problems. The most common respiratory problems are asthma, bronchopulmonary dysplasia (BPD), and cystic fibrosis. Asthma often appears by age 2 and is preceded by eczema.

There is also usually a positive family history. BPD is a form of lung disease that arises as a consequence of an acute lung injury in the newborn. It occurs more often in premature infants who have required mechanical ventilation after birth. Cystic fibrosis is a genetic condition that begins in infancy with progressive destruction of functional lung tissue. However, a clinically significant impairment of respiration is not usually seen dur-

ing the first 3 years of life. Each condition will be obvious to the discern-
ing physician and requires treatment by an appropriate specialist.

Neurological and Other Disorders

Sleep-related epilepsy, often of a temporal lobe origin, can occur in rare
cases. More frequent are cases of developmentally delayed children with
a sleep problem. Youngsters with this condition may show extreme forms
of head banging and body rocking because they lack an ability to organize their sleep patterns (Stores 1992). They also need less sleep than
normally developing youngsters (Piazza et al. 1996). Specifically, by age
3, they sleep 2 hours less per 24 hours than do children who are not developmentally delayed (i.e., 9.5 compared with 11.5 hours), and their
night sleep is decreased to only 8.5 hours. Here again, specialists should
be called in to help in the management of such children.

Although DSM-IV dropped sleep disturbances as a diagnostic criterion for attention-deficit/hyperactivity disorder (ADHD), some reports
associate it with night-sleep problems and accompanying increased daytime sleepiness (Palm et al. 1992). Because it is not easy to reliably diagnose ADHD in very young children, the data need further confirmation.

Finally, an affective illness in the mother may lead to significant sleep
problems in young children. Stoleru et al. (1997) studied 61 mothers
with unipolar or bipolar depression and assessed two of their children's
sleep patterns at four time periods (1–3 years, 5–8 years, 8–12 years, and
12–16 years). More than 55% of the youngest children were rated on the
Children's Behavior Checklist (Achenbach 1978) as having sleep problems. These difficulties persisted over 4 years while the mother's illness
remained active and usually involved both siblings eventually.

TREATMENT OF SLEEP DISORDERS

The management of sleep disorders caused by specific medical and neurological conditions depends on the individual case and often requires
consultation with an appropriate specialist. The dyssomnias—the problems most commonly encountered by clinicians who specialize in helping
families with young children— invariably require the active involvement
of the parents but respond well to behavioral treatment.

The rich literature on sleep disorders includes many articles and book
chapters that describe these conditions in considerable detail but give little or no space to their treatment. When remediation is mentioned—for
example, in the textbook edited by Ferber and Kryger (1995) or in the
excellent review article by Adair et al. (1993)—few treatment details are

provided, and recommendations are often limited to telling parents to handle their children differently or referring them to standard instruction forms or self-help books (e.g., Ferber 1985). This approach does not do justice to many families who consult professionals; sleep disorders are intricately associated with the parent-child relationship, and parents are often unable to follow instructions that seem outwardly reasonable and easy to execute.

A more comprehensive review of the treatment of sleep problems follows below. I first refer to specific modes of intervention that have been empirically tested. I then discuss what the active ingredients in each intervention might be. Finally, I provide a treatment scheme that addresses both the dynamic and the practical challenges that sleep disorders present.

Four distinct types of intervention have been evaluated in the literature: rapid extinction, graduated extinction, positive routines, and scheduled awakenings.

Types of Interventions

Rapid Extinction

In the rapid extinction form of treatment, parents are usually instructed to systematically ignore their child's cries for the duration of the night and to let them cry it out (France and Hudson 1990). In some studies, parents were allowed to make one cursory check on the child's safety, on hearing their child cry, but they were not to check again for the rest of the night (e.g., Rickert and Johnson 1988). In an older study (which fortunately involved only six children), the parents were even asked to administer one slap and, without talking, return the child to bed (Rapoff et al. 1982). In all these studies, the treated children did better than the untreated control subjects. However, a number of investigators combined the extinction procedure with specific bedtime routines (Rapoff et al. 1982; Seymour et al. 1989) or medication (France and Hudson 1990). Not surprisingly, a good number of parents (25% in the Rickert et al. study) refused to participate when they learned that their child might be assigned a rapid extinction type of treatment.

Graduated Extinction

The graduated extinction treatment was developed partly to allow parents some contact with their children whenever they cried during the night. Parents were usually permitted to briefly check on their children (e.g., for 15 seconds) (Adams and Rickert 1989), but they had to wait before they entered the room once the crying had begun (e.g., for 10 minutes) (Pritchard and Appleton 1988). Some authors have also suggested progressively increasing the parents' waiting time by 5 minutes after each consecutive checking (Durand and Mindell 1990), a strategy that Ferber (1985) also suggests in his book for parents. The idea here is to extinguish crying by teaching the child that more crying decreases parental contact. Again, all the cited studies have shown this type of intervention to be successful when study subjects were compared with children on a waiting list.

A study by Sadeh (1994) provides intriguing data. With T. F. Anders, Sadeh developed *actigraphy*—a sophisticated methodology for measuring sleep disturbances. The actigraph involves a watch-sized wrist sensor that records the infant's body movements and can reliably measure the waking state of a young child. Using this methodology, Sadeh randomly assigned 50 infants to graduated extinction or to a co-sleeping intervention. Parents in the graduated extinction program had to wait progressively longer before checking on their child. The co-sleeping intervention had one parent sleep in the child's bedroom for 1 week without any other involvement with the child during the night. Both forms of treatment resulted in significant improvement. However, one could argue that the co-sleeping arrangement was based on concretely reassuring the infant that mom or dad would not disappear during the night, while the extinction paradigm communicated that the child can sleep and survive without having a parent in the bedroom. The success of both treatment methods suggests that a more generic process may be responsible for the changes in these children's sleep patterns.

Positive Routines

The positive routines intervention requires parents to set up regular calm activities that the child can enjoy before bedtime. If the child throws a tantrum, the activities are discontinued and the child is put to bed (Adams and Rickert 1989). In some way, this intervention turns the bed into a place of punishment, which common sense would suggest has little therapeutic impact. Yet Adams and Rickert (1989) and Gailbraith et al. (1993) report positive routines to be effective in helping children sleep through the night.

Scheduled Awakenings

The scheduled awakenings intervention requires that parents initially record the spontaneous awakenings of their child until they can discern a pattern. Once the pattern has been detected, the parents are asked to awaken and console the child approximately 15 minutes before a typical spontaneous awakening is expected. The scheduled awakenings are then gradually decreased and totally stopped after 2–3 weeks with good results, especially in regular sleepwalkers (Rickert and Johnson 1988).

Although this form of intervention appears paradoxical, a variation of it has been used successfully by Piazza et al. (1996) in somewhat older mentally retarded children. Such children, as mentioned before, need less sleep than youngsters who are not mentally retarded, and they often show significant sleep disturbances. Piazza et al. found that such children do best if one establishes their regular sleep onset time and puts them to bed at this time. If the children are not asleep within 15 minutes, they are forced to get up again, play, and be active for another hour, after which they are put to bed again. If they still do not fall asleep within 15 minutes, another hour of activity is added until sleep onset is observed. This time then becomes the regular bedtime for the child during the subsequent 2 weeks; after 2 weeks, bedtime is gradually moved backward by 15 or even 30 minutes per day.

The idea here is to avoid the association of the bed with being awake. Piazza et al. found this treatment to be much more effective than traditional bedtime scheduling, in which mentally retarded children are kept in bed at night but not allowed daytime naps in the hope that they will be more tired the following evening. In fact, Piazza et al. found that retarded children were not more tired on the subsequent evening even if they had not slept for half the night for many days in a row. While Piazza and her colleagues used and tested specific intervention strategies in isolation, many clinicians have utilized a mixture of these behavioral strategies with good results (Minde et al. 1993; Richman et al. 1985).

Caregiver-Infant Difficulties and Sleep Disorders

What, then, is the central difficulty that must be addressed in treating children with persistent sleep problems, and why do different strategies work? I believe that for various reasons caregivers often do not know how to set clear limits, or do not feel comfortable setting limits, on their children's sleep behavior at night; they need help with limit setting. Once they understand that limits imply safety and predictability, and they decide to take charge of their child's behavior, a wide range of management techniques based on various learning paradigms will be successful as the children realize that mom and dad now mean business.

In my opinion, among the various reasons parents hesitate to set limits for their child are attachment problems, marital conflicts, and temperamental mismatches between parent and child.

Attachment Problems

In work with sleep-disturbed toddlers, we have found that all their mothers were insecurely attached to their own mothers (Benoit et al. 1992). Thus, their nonauthoritative behavior with their children was often an attempt to make up for the harshness and insensitivity of their own childhood. What they did not realize was the degree to which their failure to set limits reflected their own insensitivity to their children's needs (in this case, control over sleep behavior). This insensitivity was revealed in their expressed fear that they would traumatize their children if they did not immediately respond to even minor noises from their children's bedroom at night. However, at the same time, they often expressed disappointment and anger with their children, for example, by not taking them back to their own bed when they insisted on joining them in their bed at midnight. More deprived parents often would not even set up bedtime routines that involved themselves because the routines interfered with their wish to watch TV, and their 2-year-old just had "to learn to listen and do things on their own."

Marital Conflicts

In our experience, some 25% of parents with sleep-disturbed children present with marital conflicts. Mothers in these circumstances often join their child in their beds at night because they prefer to sleep with the child rather than the spouse. Others will allow their 4-year-old to breast-feed in public or will be so "in tune" with the child's emotional needs that they have few or no resources left for other members of their family. Such overindulged children become anxious and unsure of themselves and readily cooperate even with an unreasonable mother to keep her from being unhappy with them.

Temperamental Mismatch

Parents with an easy, forgiving temperament are at times unable to recognize that their child needs precise, well-established routines to function well. Their own tolerance for ambiguity and lack of structure does not prepare them to meet the manipulative challenges of a fast-learning toddler. The result may be a child who increasingly signals a need for containment through evening tantrums or nightly demands for a playmate.

Other dynamics and circumstances obviously lead to sleep disturbances as well. Children may respond to outside stressors such as parental illness or a new baby by not sleeping. In other families, a number of stressful phenomena combine, with the sleep problem only one of many complaints.

However, there is no doubt that a disturbed parent-child relationship forms a central aspect of most chronic sleep disorders. The treatment approach we suggest is, therefore, based on a behavioral model that acknowledges the dynamic implication of symptoms and behavioral challenges. Initially, this means that parents need to be assured that a child who is well loved and stimulated during the day will not be damaged or feel rejected if the parents set clear limits about sleep behavior at night (Minde et al. 1993). Early in our work, we had intended to use a more dynamic approach; we hoped that approach would allow parents to understand the underlying thoughts and feelings that interfered with their ability to establish clear and transparent limits to their children's behavior. However, we quickly learned that this was a very tall order and that children responded to their parents' new directions even when the parents themselves did not yet understand why they had such difficulties with their children.

Treatment Process

The general aim of our treatment approach is not to get the children to sleep more or wake up less often but to teach them to manage their sleep behavior independently without disturbing their parents' sleep. Certainly, many young children wake up several times during the night, but they can be encouraged to settle themselves down to sleep again without their parents.

An important aspect of our treatment philosophy is that we do not prescribe how children should behave at night (e.g., how many hours of sleep they should get or whether they should sleep in a crib or with their parents). The parents decide what aspect of the sleep disturbance will be tackled initially. For example, some parents do not mind having their children in bed with them at times; for other parents, a midnight breast-feeding is part of their own comfort routine. Yet they may want to learn how to settle the baby without a fuss in the evening and convey that they mean what they say. It is therefore important to discuss with the parents in detail their treatment hopes and expectations and proceed only when there is agreement about the changes the family seeks.

This approach usually precludes the treatment of marital or other psychological difficulties within the couple or family, at least initially, if the parents do not mention such issues. Although this approach appears to contradict the likely association between sleep difficulties and various forms of parental difficulties, we believe in respecting the parents' right to select a first target for change. Doing so often sets the stage for their trust and, in turn, allows them to hear and implement other therapeutic suggestions. Furthermore, young children often respond rapidly to even minor modifications in parental behavior. This response is especially true if the ensuing behavior is developmentally more appropriate or represents a decrease in the distortions previously associated with parental interpretations of the child's disturbed sleep behavior (Lieberman 1992). For example, a couple's acceptance of their child's frequent waking as a reflection of the child's somewhat precarious ability to organize the level of arousal rather than as a hurtful attack on the parents' need to sleep can result in an entirely new sequence of parent-child transactions.

For the actual treatment process, we proceed as follows.

After one or two evaluative interviews and a 1- to 2-week period in which parents complete a sleep diary to establish a baseline for their child's behavior, treatment sessions begin (Figure 11–3). These sessions include both parents but may be held either with or without the infant.

Initially, and with an attitude of consistent, responsive support, we review the sleep difficulties again. The review allows us to form an impression of the family's settling and bedtime routine and the interests and predictability of the child's day. During this part of the session, we often can form an impression of the quality of parental motivation to change and the character of any resistance. Often we can sense disagreements between the parents about overall child-rearing practices or issues about the mother's involvement with her child. However, we try to focus on the sleep behavior and areas of agreement and disagreement concerning it.

If the daytime activities of a child (and the family) do not occur in a predictable sequence, we offer information about how toddlers need a sense of control that can be provided through regular daytime activities, including set times for meals and naps. Once daytime routines have been established, the parents are encouraged to create new bedtime rituals. For example, if bedtime feeding was part of a ritual, we suggest that it be removed from bedtime to an earlier time and place (e.g., in the kitchen or dining room).

Only then is the sleeping problem itself tackled. Recommendations depend on whether a helpmate (e.g., the father) is available to the mother. When the father is available, he is encouraged to take over most of the bedtime routine, with perhaps a small part of the ritual assigned to the mother, or all of the night awakenings. This suggestion is based on our experience that fathers are often less hesitant about taking charge of their children's behavior. They also typically have less contact with the child during the day and so are less tainted by previous interactions with their child. The great majority of fathers collaborate most willingly and even enthusiastically, whereas the mothers often seem doubtful either of their husband's capacity to cope or of their own ability to tolerate the

Date: _____

	Monday	Tuesday	Wednesday	Thursday	Friday	Saturday	Sunday
Time went to bed in the evening							
Time went to sleep in the evening							
Time(s) woke during the night							
Time(s) went to sleep again							
How you handled the night wakings							
Time woke in the morning							
Time of naps							
Time you went to bed							

Figure 11–3.   Sleep diary.

new arrangement. In our experimental study, we managed to get more than 90% of the fathers actively involved in their children's bedtime management (Minde et al. 1993).

If the parents agree to the father's active involvement, we elicit his thoughts about how he might comfort the child. He is encouraged to use pets, words, sips of water, and the like to keep his child in bed. Parents typically start their new program on the weekend so that the stresses of work do not immediately await them the next day. They also are warned that they may expect 2 or 3 uncomfortable nights but will likely begin to see change within 3–4 days.

When the child cries consistently, we suggest that the parent in charge of the settling procedure use the gradual checking method of entering the child's room and providing soothing at regular intervals (e.g., every 5–10 minutes) until the child falls asleep. If the checking approach seems too difficult for a parent to accomplish alone, a shaping technique can be employed. For example, if the child is sleeping in the mother's bed, she might first move with the child into the child's own bed. Then she would sit up in bed, move to a chair beside the bed, and edge the chair farther away from the bed until the chair is finally outside the room. This gradual approach provides children with some externalized holding, which encourages them to find their own way of organizing their overall sleep behavior.

In our experience, an average of four sessions spaced over a 6- to 8-week period will significantly modify the sleep behavior of some 85% of troubled infants and toddlers. Asking parents to continue with their sleep diaries during that time can also help in the discussions because the diaries will highlight continuing difficulties or beginning improvements. Follow-up interviews up to 6 months after the end of treatment revealed virtually no relapses; indeed, there was continuing improvement in the child's overall behavior (Minde et al. 1994). Treatment failures occur more often in families in which either the parents are unable to establish routines or the sleep problem is only one aspect of other major family problems. In addition, the unwillingness of a father or helpmate (in case mother is alone) to participate in restructuring the nighttime routines often spells treatment failure. On the other hand, a successful resolution of sleep problems usually creates positive changes in other troublesome daytime behaviors displayed by these children (Minde et al. 1993). This overall improvement suggests that caregivers who learn how to deal with conflict around sleep will also inadvertently use their new skills during daytime interactions with their child.

SUMMARY

In this chapter, I provided an overview of the epidemiology, manifestations, and treatment of abnormal sleep behaviors in children up to 36 months of age, demonstrating that, like other behavioral disturbances in infancy, problems in sleeping often reflect a difficulty in the caregiver-infant relationship. Also highlighted was the contribution of biological vulnerabilities and specific developmental parameters to the form and type of symptoms. Finally, a treatment program for sleep-disturbed children was described based on an understanding of the dynamic and developmental needs of both infants and their caregivers. This program has been proven to deal successfully with the great majority of sleep problems after only a few therapeutic contacts.

REFERENCES

Achenbach TM: The child behavior profile, I: boys aged 6–11. J Consult Clin Psychol 46(3):478–488, 1978

Adair RH, Bauchner H: Sleep problems in childhood. Curr Probl Pediatr 4:147–170, 1993

Adair R, Bauchner H, Philipp B, et al: Night waking during infancy: role of parental presence at bedtime. Pediatrics 87:500–504, 1991

Adams K: Sleep as a restorative process and theory to explain why. Prog Brain Res 53:289–325, 1980

Adams LA, Rickert VI: Reducing bedtime tantrums: comparison between positive routines and graduated extinction. Pediatrics 84:756–759, 1989

American Psychiatric Association: Diagnostic and Statistical Manual of Mental Disorders, 4th Edition. Washington, DC, American Psychiatric Association, 1994

American Psychiatric Association: Diagnostic and Statistical Manual of Mental Disorders, 4th Edition, Text Revision. Washington, DC, American Psychiatric Association, 2000

American Sleep Disorders Association: International Classification of Sleep Disorders: Diagnostic and Coding Manual. Lawrence, KS, Allen Press, 1990

Anders TF: Home-recorded sleep in 2- and 9-month-old infants. J Am Acad Child Psychiatry 17:421–432, 1978

Anders TF: Night waking in infants during the first year of life. Pediatrics 63:860–864, 1979

Anders TF, Eiben LA: Pediatric sleep disorders: a review of the past 10 years. J Am Acad Child Adolesc Psychiatry 1:9–20, 1997

Anders TF, Keener M, Bowe TR, et al: A longitudinal study of nighttime sleep-wake patterns in infants from birth to one year, in Frontiers of Infant Psychiatry, Vol 1. Edited by Call JD, Galenson E, Tyson RL. New York, Basic Books, 1983, pp 150–166

Aserinsky E, Kleitman N: Regularly occurring periods of eye mobility, and concomitant phenomena, during sleep. Science 118:273–274, 1953

Beltramini AU, Hertzig ME: Sleep and bedtime behavior in preschool-aged children. Pediatrics 71:153–158, 1983

Benoit D, Zeanah CH, Boucher C, et al: Sleep disorders in early childhood: association with insecure maternal attachment. J Am Acad Child Adolesc Psychiatry 31:86–93, 1992

Burton RV, Whiting JWM: The absent father and cross-sex identity. Merrill-Palmer Quarterly 7:85, 1961

Carey WB: Night waking and temperament in infancy. J Pediatr 84:756–758, 1974

Coons S, Guilleminault C: Development of sleep-wake patterns and non-rapid eye movement sleep stages during the first six months of life in normal infants. Pediatrics 69:793–798, 1982

Daws D: Through the Night: Helping Parents and Sleepless Infants. London, Free Association Books, 1989

Dement WC: Some Must Watch While Some Must Sleep. San Francisco, CA, WH Freeman, 1972

Dement WC, Kleitman N: Cyclic variations in EEG during sleep and their relationships to eye movement, body mobility and dreaming. Electroencephalogr Clin Neurophysiol 9:673–690, 1957

Douglas J, Richman N: My Child Won't Sleep. Harmondsworth, Middlesex, UK, Penguin, 1984

Dreyfus-Brisac C: Ontogenesis of bioelectrical activity and sleep organization in neonates and infants, in Human Growth, Vol 3. Edited by Falkner F, Tanner J. New York, Plenum, 1979, pp 157–182

Durand VM, Mindell JA: Behavioral treatment of multiple childhood sleep disorders: effects on child and family. Behav Modif 14:37–49, 1990

Elias MF, Nicolson NA, Bora C, et al: Sleep/wake patterns of breast-fed infants in the first 2 years of life. Pediatrics 77:322–329, 1986

Ferber R: Solve Your Child's Sleep Problems. New York, Penguin, 1985

Ferber R: Familial headbanging. Sleep Research 17:176, 1988

Ferber R: Assessment of sleep disorders in the child, in Principles and Practice of Sleep Medicine in the Child. Edited by Ferber R, Kryger M. Philadelphia, PA,WB Saunders, 1995, pp 45–54

Ferber R, Boyle MP: Sleeplessness in infants and toddlers: sleep initiation difficulty masquerading as a sleep maintenance insomnia. Sleep Research 12: 240, 1983

Ferber R, Kryger M: Principles and Practice of Sleep Medicine in the Child. Philadelphia, PA,WB Saunders, 1995

France KG, Hudson SM: Behavior management of infant sleep disturbance. J Appl Behav Anal 23:91–98, 1990

Frank Y, Kravath RE, Pollak CP, et al: Obstructive sleep apnea and its therapy: clinical and polysomnographic manifestations. Pediatrics 71:737–742, 1983

Gaddini R: Transitional objects and the process of individuation: a study of three different social groups. J Am Acad Child Adolesc Psychiatry 9:347–365, 1970

Gailbraith LR, Pritchard L, Hewitt KE: Behavioural treatment for sleep disturbance. Health Visitor 66:169–171, 1993

Griffin SJ, Trinder J: Physical fitness, exercise and human sleep. Psychophysiol-
ogy 15(5):447–450, 1978

Guilleminault C (ed): Sleep and Its Disorders in Children. New York, Raven
Press, 1987

Guilleminault C, Stoohs R: From apnea of infancy to obstructive sleep apnea syndrome in the young child. Chest 102:1065–1071, 1992

Hammond WA: Sleep and Its Derangements (1873). Philadelphia, PA, JB Lippin-
cott, 1982

Hong KM, Townes BD: Infants' attachment to inanimate objects: a cross-cultural
study. J Am Acad Child Adolesc Psychiatry 15:49–61, 1976

Jenkins S, Bax M, Hart H: Behaviour problems in preschool children. J Child Psychol Psychiatry 21:5–17, 1980

Jenkins S, Bax M, Hart H: Continuities of common behaviour problems in preschool children. J Child Psychol Psychiatry 25:75–89, 1984

Johnson CM: Infant and toddler sleep: a telephone survey of parents in one community. J Dev Behav Pediatr 12:108–114, 1991

Kahn A, Mozin MJ, Rebuffat E, et al: Milk intolerance in children with persistent
sleeplessness: a prospective double-blind crossover evaluation. Pediatrics 84:
595–603, 1989

Kales A, Soldatos CR, Bixler EO, et al: Hereditary factors in sleepwalking and
night terrors. Br J Psychiatry 137:111–118, 1980

Kateria S, Swanson M, Trevarthin L: Persistence of sleep disturbances in preschool children. J Pediatr 110:642–646, 1987

Keffe M: Comparison of neonatal nighttime sleep-wake patterns in nursery versus
rooming-in environments. Nurs Res 36:140–144, 1987

Kellerman H: Sleep Disorders, Insomnia and Narcolepsy. New York, Brunner/
Mazel, 1981

Klackenberg G: Rhythmic movements in infancy and early childhood. Acta Pediatrica Scand Suppl 224:74–83, 1971

Klackenberg G: Incidence of parasomnias in children in a general population, in
Sleep and Its Disorders in Children. Edited by Guilleminault C. New York,
Raven, 1987, pp 99–114

Kleitman N, Engelmann TG: Sleep characteristics of infants. J Appl Physiol 6:
269–282, 1953

Lieberman AF: Infant-parent psychotherapy with toddlers. Dev Psychopathol 4:
559–574, 1992

Lozoff B, Wolf AW, Davis NS: Cosleeping in urban families with young children
in the United States. Pediatrics 74:171–182, 1984

Lozoff B, Askew GL, Wolf AW: Cosleeping and early childhood sleep problems:
effects of ethnicity and socioeconomic status. J Dev Behav Pediatr 17:9–15,
1996

Macknin ML, Medendorp SV, Maier MC: Infant sleep and bedtime cereal. American Journal of Diseases of Children 143:1066–1068, 1989

Madanski D, Edelbrock C: Cosleeping in a community sample of 2- and 3-year-old children. Pediatrics 86:197–203, 1990

McKenna JJ, Mosko DD, Richard CA: Bedsharing promotes breastfeeding. Pediatrics 100:214–219, 1997

Minde K, Popiel K, Leos N, et al: The evaluation and treatment of sleep disturbances in young children. J Child Psychol Psychiatry 34:521–533, 1993

Minde K, Faucon A, Falkner S: Sleep problems in toddlers: effects of treatment on their daytime behavior. J Am Acad Child Adolesc Psychiatry 33:1114–1121, 1994

Mindell JA, Moline ML, Zendell SM, et al: Pediatricians and sleep disorders: training and practice. Pediatrics 2:194–200, 1994

Moore T, Ucko LE: Night waking in early infancy, Part 1. Arch Dis Child 33:333–342, 1957

Moruzzi G: The functional significance of sleep with particular regard to the brain mechanisms underlying consciousness, in Brain and the Unity of Conscious Experience. Edited by Eccles J. New York, Cambridge University Press, 1965, pp 345–388

Mosko S, Richard C, McKenna J: Infant arousals during mother-infant bed sharing: implications for infant sleep and sudden infant death syndrome research. Pediatrics 5:841–849, 1997

Oswald I: Sleep as a restorative process: human clues. Progr Brain Res 53: 279–288, 1980

Palm L, Persson E, Bjerre I, et al: Sleep and wakefulness in preadolescent children with deficits in attention, motor control and perception. Acta Paediatr 81:618–624, 1992

Parmelee AH: Ontogeny of sleep patterns and associated periodicities in infants, in Pre- and Postnatal Development of the Human Brain (Modern Problems in Pediatrics, Vol 13). Edited by Falkner F, Kretchmer N. Basel, Switzerland, S Karger, 1974, pp 298–311

Piazza CC, Fisher WW, Kahng SW: Sleep patterns in children and young adults with mental retardation and severe behavior disorders. Dev Med Child Neurol 38:335–344, 1996

Pritchard A, Appleton P: Management of sleep problems in pre-school children. Early Childhood Development and Care 34:227–240, 1988

Rapoff MA, Christophersen ER, Rapoff DE: The management of common childhood bedtime problems by pediatric nurse practitioners. J Pediatr Psychol 7: 179–196, 1982

Redline S, Tosteson T, Tishler PV, et al: Studies in the genetics of obstructive sleep apnea: familial aggregation of symptoms associated with sleep-related breathing disturbances. Am Rev Respir Dis 145:440–444, 1992

Richman N: A community survey of the characteristics of one- to two-year-olds with sleep disruptions. J Am Acad Child Psychiatry 20:281–291, 1981

Richman N: A double-blind drug trial of treatment in young children with waking problems. J Child Psychol Psychiatry 26:591–598, 1985

Richman N, Stevenson J, Graham PJ: Pre-School to School: A Behavioral Study. New York, Academic Press, 1982

Richman N, Douglas J, Hunt H, et al: Behavioral methods in the treatment of sleep disorders: a pilot study. J Child Psychol Psychiatry 26:581–590, 1985

Rickert VI, Johnson CM: Reducing nocturnal awakening and crying episodes in infants and young children: a comparison between scheduled awakenings and systematic ignoring. Pediatrics 81:203–212, 1988

Riley TL: Historical overview and introduction, in Clinical Aspects of Sleep and Sleep Disturbance. Edited by Riley TL. Boston, MA, Butterworth, 1985, pp 1–7

Roffwarg H, Muzio J, Dement W: Ontogenetic development of the human sleep-dream cycle. Science 152:604–619, 1966

Sadeh A: Assessment of intervention for infant night waking: parental reports and activity-based home monitoring. J Consult Clin Psychol 62:63–68, 1994

Sadeh A, Lavie P, Scher A, et al: Actigraphic home monitoring of sleep-disturbed and control infants and young children: a new method for pediatric assessment of sleep-wake patterns. Pediatrics 87:494–499, 1991

Schachter FF, Fuchs ML, Bijur PE, et al: Sleeping and sleep problems in Hispanic-American urban young children. Pediatrics 84:522–533, 1989

Scher A, Tirosh E, Jaffe M, et al: Survey of sleep patterns of Israeli infants and young children. Sleep Res 16:209, 1987

Scott G, Richards MPM: Night waking in one-year-old infants in England. Child Care, Health and Development 16:283–302, 1990

Seymour FW, Brock P, During M, et al: Reducing sleep disruptions in young children: evaluation of therapist-guided and written information approaches: a brief report. J Child Psychol Psychiatry 30:913–918, 1989

Sheldon SH, et al. Differential Diagnosis, in Pediatric Sleep Medicine. Edited by Sheldon SH, Spire JP, Cory HB. Philadelphia, PA, WB Saunders, 1992, pp 185–214

Siegel JM: Mechanisms of sleep control. J Clin Neurophysiol 7:49–65, 1990

Stoleru S, Nottelmann ED, Belmont B, et al: Sleep problems in children of affectively ill mothers. J Child Psychol Psychiatry 7:831–841, 1997

Stores G: Sleep studies in children with a mental handicap. J Child Psychol Psychiatry 33:1303–1317, 1992

Terr L: Nightmares in children, in Sleep and Its Disorders in Children. Edited by Guilleminault C. New York, Raven, 1987, pp 231–242

Thevinin T: The Family Bed: An Age-Old Concept in Child Rearing. Minneapolis, MN, Tina Thevinin, 1976

Thorn BE, Levitt RA: Sleeping and waking, in Physiological Psychology. Edited by Levitt RA. New York, Holt, Rinehart & Winston, 1981, pp 261–296

Thorpy MJ: Rhythmic movement disorders, in Handbook of Sleep Disorders. Edited by Thorpy MJ. New York, Marcel Dekker, 1990, pp 609–629

van Tassel EB: The relative influence of child and environmental characteristics on sleep disturbances in the first and second years of life. J Dev Behav Pediatr 6:81–86, 1985

Weissbluth M: Sleep duration and infant temperament. J Pediatr 99:817–819, 1981

Winnicott DW: Transitional objects and transitional phenomena: a study of the first not-me possession. Int J Psychoanal 34:89–97, 1953

Wolf A, Lozoff B: Object attachment, thumb-sucking and the passage to sleep. J Am Acad Child Adolesc Psychiatry 28:287–292, 1989

Wolke D, Meyer R, Ohrt B, et al: Incidence and persistence of problems at sleep onset and sleep continuation in the preschool period: results of a prospective study of a representative sample in Bavaria. Prax Kinderpsychol Kinderpsychiatr [Practice of Child Psychology and Psychiatry] 43:331–339, 1994

Wooding AR, Boyd J, Geddis DC: Sleep patterns of New Zealand infants during the first 12 months of life. Journal of Pediatrics and Child Health 26:85–88, 1990

Zuckerman B, Stevenson J, Bailey V: Sleep problems in early childhood: continuities, predictive factors, and behavioral correlates. Pediatrics 80:664–671, 1987

12

Evaluation and Treatment of Eating and Feeding Disturbances of Infancy

J. Martín Maldonado-Durán, M.D.
J. Armando Barriguete, M.D.

Eating and feeding difficulties in infancy are common and, when severe, can be life-threatening. They usually lead to diminished weight gain or growth in stature. Eating in the first years of life is crucial. The brain develops at an extraordinary pace, as numerous recent studies have shown (Uauy et al. 1999; Vestergaard et al. 1999). It is essential to keep in mind that a child needs adequate nutrition to satisfy the demands of growth in general and the brain in particular. The scope of all eating and feeding disturbances is extensive. In this chapter, we discuss the most common problems and the methods for their clinical evaluation and treatment. An adequate evaluation of the presenting problem(s) leads to the design of appropriate treatment strategies. (We do not describe the normal development of feeding or the physiology of feeding because these aspects of eating in infancy can be found in a number of available resources [Bosma 1986; Tuchman 1994; Wolke 1994].)

The authors wish to thank Dr. Maria Ramsay of Montreal Children's Hospital for her guidance and consultation over the years.

Both DSM-IV-TR (American Psychiatric Association 2000) and ICD-10 (World Health Organization 1992) define feeding disorders in early childhood as only nutritional intake problems that lead to failure to thrive (FTT) or malnutrition. Our view is different. We contend that feeding disturbances or disorders are not synonymous with FTT or with stunted growth. Feeding disturbances can occur even in the absence of problems with nutritional intake. An infant may have difficulty sucking, chewing food, making the transition from liquids to semisolids, or behaving properly during mealtimes—the presence of any of these problems may not lead to a failure to thrive (Maldonado-Durán 2000). Often, this accommodation is due to compensatory strategies developed by parents to help their infant not become underweight. Nonetheless, the child faces difficulty, so the problem should be identified and addressed, preferably before it leads to severe underweight. Thus, feeding disturbances are manifestations of difficulty in the ability to request, receive, ingest, process, and maintain enough food in the body long enough for the body to grow.

FEEDING RELATIONSHIP AND FEEDING SITUATION

Eating and feeding are essentially social actions (Hoffmann 1998); that is, they are interactive (Barriguete et al. 1998a) as well as cultural (Barriguete et al. 1998b; Moro and Barriguete 1998). Both actions involve more than merely incorporating food, a nutritious action. Eating and feeding are each a facet of the total relationship between the caregiver and the baby. The baby also establishes a relationship with the food itself. As the baby takes the food, he or she also "takes in" the caregiver and the nature of the relationship. Thus, the nature of the interactions between babies and the persons who feed them has a powerful impact on the success or failure of the feeding, including the satisfaction and emotional rewards for both persons involved. Given the importance of feeding and nutrition, the quality of the interactions and involvement between the caregiver and the infant has a significant impact on the child's ability to be nourished.

Because feeding is a two-way phenomenon, both the baby and the caregiver contribute to the exchange with each other. If the baby, for instance, is unable to sustain sucking and turns his or her head away repeatedly, the mother may experience this as an act of rejection or as a sign that she is incompetent. Instead of an exchange of mutual satisfaction and joy, the feeding may turn into a conflicted, frustrating, unhappy, or painful moment for the participants. This consequence is common for the child with a physical condition—such as cerebral palsy—that affects the child's ability to eat: meals last much longer and are often fraught with conflict (Sullivan and Rosenbloom 1996).

The feeding situation is the actual encounter in which a person (the adult) offers food to the infant. It involves the setting where the feeding encounter takes place. Is it in front of the television or in a quiet environment? Is the positioning of the baby favorable to ingestion of food, or it is uncomfortable and painful? Is there a lot of tension or overstimulation in the environment, or is there an atmosphere of peace and comfort? These variables can have a powerful impact on the success of the feeding.

Failure to Thrive

There are several commonly accepted definitions of FTT. Compared with a normative group, a child who fails to thrive will weigh less than the third percentile, given the age of the infant and the growth norms for his or her social group (Tolia 1995). Another definition, frequently overlooked, is a significant drop in the baby's weight from its steady increase along a standard curve: FTT occurs when weight decreases by at least two standard deviations in the percentile curve from where it had been maintained (Ramsay 1995). This decline often goes unrecognized because children appear to have adequate weight when they are, for instance, in the tenth percentile. However, for an infant who had been developing in the ninetieth percentile up to age 4 months, a drop to the tenth percentile is a manifestation of FTT.

Failure to thrive occurs because of deficits in caloric intake relative to the infant's expenditure of calories, which causes the energy supply to be less than what is required to maintain an increase in weight. For infants, the daily demand is around 80–120 kcal/kg of ideal body weight, although this depends on the baby's metabolic rate and expenditure of calories (Barness and Curran 1996).

Growth Stunting

A problem more common than FTT is growth stunting (GS). This term refers to the failure of the infant to achieve a body length (stature) comparable to that of other children in his or her social group. Children are considered to have GS when their body length is below the third percentile of the norm. GS also is considered to be present when the attainment of height descends two or more standard deviations from where it had been progressing. This occurs when a child of normal weight for his or her age falls behind in height. (A child may have both FTT and GS.) GS is thought to be due to a lack of protein, which promotes growth in stature (Waterlow 1996). Although a child may be ingesting enough calories, it seems that the body economizes or saves energy sources (protein) and so sacrifices growth in height. GS is fairly common in developing countries, reaching perhaps 40%–60% of all children who live at the poverty level. It is often argued that the child is short because the parents are short. However, studies of the supplementation of calories for such children show that an improved diet leads to catch-up growth over the long term.

EPIDEMIOLOGICAL ISSUES

Feeding disturbances and disorders in young children are common, affecting 20%–30% of infants (Ramsay 1995). These disorders may surface at the beginning of extrauterine life or when the infant has to learn how to incorporate food into his or her mouth, and they may persist throughout childhood. There is evidence that such disorders do not usually improve spontaneously (Douglas and Bryon 1996). Yet primary health care workers often overlook such feeding problems (Skuse et al. 1994) unless they are very severe and cause serious problems with weight gain or result in the infant totally refusing to eat anything. Unfortunately, feeding difficulties tend to persist. When they do, they can lead to several negative outcomes: a persistent or worsening feeding problem, FTT, or GS (or all three conditions), as well as disturbances in other aspects of the parent-child relationship.

Two tendencies interfere with the adequate recognition of feeding problems in infants; they have to do with maternal attributions. One is that a child's small body size or weight is attributed to the mother herself being very small. Yet it has been shown in countries such as Egypt and Jamaica that young children who get enough protein in their preschool years will have a compensatory growth that helps them achieve a stature significantly taller than that of their parents. This finding leads to the conclusion that entire families or populations may be short mainly because of a transgenerational pattern of protein deprivation that interferes with sufficient growth. When this deficiency is remedied, height will increase in the next generation (Waterlow 1994).

Another problem is the inference that a baby's development of FTT is pathognomonic with maternal neglect or poor parenting techniques. Wolke (1996) calls this the "myth of maternal deprivation" (p. 4). In cases referred to the infant mental health clinic, there may be an over-representation of parents who have more difficulty taking care of their children, leading to the impression of maternal deprivation. However, community studies have failed to identify a close association between eating disturbances and poor parenting practices or maternal deprivation (Skuse et al. 1994).

In a survey by Leung and Robson (1994) in Alberta, Canada, around 15% of children who were 2–5 years of age had some sort of feeding disturbance according to their parents. Parental reports also noted diminished appetite or hunger in 24% of boys and 21% of girls. In a Nebraska study of preschool children (12,000 boys and girls), 17% of the children were reported by their parents to be excessively "picky" about food (Stanek et al. 1990).

Even so, FTT is not so rare: some recent surveys have shown that, even in industrialized countries, this disorder may affect 3%–4% of the open population of infants (Skuse et al. 1994; Wilensky et al. 1996; Wolke 1996). In reality, as shown by the British study (Skuse et al. 1994), the majority of such children are rarely referred to a pediatrician or physician for their problem.

Growth stunting is fairly common worldwide and even widespread in developing countries. Surveys in Middle Eastern countries (e.g., Pakistan and Egypt) and in Latin American countries suggest a prevalence of GS of 40%–60% among young children (Von Braun et al. 1993; Waterlow 1994). It has been suggested that children who have markedly stunted growth may also suffer in their cognitive development, have a less enthusiastic and exploratory attitude, and exhibit more irritability and apathy (Lawrence et al. 1991; Meeks-Gardner et al. 1999).

Obesity is also quite prevalent. It has been suggested that in the United States, this problem may affect 10% of all children (Flegal 1999; Troiano and Flegal 1998). It has been linked to dietary habits and diminished physical exercise in the lifestyle of families, as well as many hours of sitting and watching television per week (Lindquist et al. 1999). The prevalence of obesity seems to be on the increase in several industrialized countries (Flegal 1999).

COMMON FEEDING DISTURBANCES

Our approach to the description and characterization of feeding problems in infancy is phenomenological—that is, centered on what appears to be the main manifestations of disturbance rather than on a theoretical formulation of underlying psychological or emotional causes (Maldonado-Durán and Sauceda-Garcia 1998). Another classification (Chatoor 1997) emphasizes that issues of emotional development, such as problems in separation, individuation, and attachment, could be at the root of problems like feeding refusal (for the child who is affirming his or her autonomy in the area of eating). Chatoor considers psychodynamic issues to be at the root of the behavioral manifestation—feeding difficulties—in the infant and notes that they are in close correlation with psychodynamic difficulties in the caregiver, for instance, the need to soothe the child with food. Because there is limited empirical validation of this position, we take a different approach.

We believe that it may be easier for clinicians to look at and then describe what actually happens in the feeding situation, a readily observable phenomenon, and then develop clinical interventions based on those observations. These interventions may be psychodynamic in nature for those cases in which the issues proposed by Chatoor appear to be present and are a significant block to successful feeding. We propose assessing the situation along four main axes that roughly correspond to those proposed by the Zero to Three classification (Zero to Three 1994), although in this case the axes would all refer to feeding issues (see appendix to this chapter).

This classification can be kept in mind when assessing a child because each axis is rated separately (Maldonado-Durán et al. 1998). It is the equivalent of a more detailed qualification and formulation of the presenting problems:

- Axis I includes those feeding difficulties observed in the child that may or may not be the central problem or even the reason for referral.
- Axis II includes problems with the quality of the feeding relationship, which can only be evaluated by firsthand observation of the reciprocal interactions between the caregiver and the infant. A feeding relationship disturbance may be the primary problem but can lead to other difficulties. It may also be secondary to the child's difficulty, resulting perhaps from the caregiver's frustration with the challenges presented by the infant. Such is frequently the case with children who have medically based difficulties, such as cerebral palsy. Alternatively, there may not be a feeding disturbance at all. Instead, the child may have an eating difficulty that does not correspond in any way to the parent-child relationship around the issue of feeding and is not related to some major contribution from the primary caregiver.
- Axis III relates to the physical status of the child, which includes changes in height, weight, body mass index, and so forth, as a result of the feeding problem or concomitant with it. There may be no change in the body weight despite the existence of a feeding disorder. Alternatively, a feeding problem may be the result of an underlying physical

condition, such as an oral malformation or a body dysfunction (e.g., esophagitis or a heart condition leading to cyanosis during feedings).

* Axis IV includes stress factors related to family and cultural issues that affect eating. They may include the family's beliefs about feeding and eating and particular constellations having to do with a given family. Cultural factors may pertain to practices or myths within certain cultures. For example, "Girls should eat less to be thin" while "Boys should eat well to be strong" might be common to the overall culture of the United States. How and when children are breastfed and weaned also reflect cultural expectations. In Latino families, it is relatively common to prolong breastfeeding, compared with Euro-American families' patterns. For example, we have observed the Purépechas Indians from Mexico (an aboriginal group west of Mexico City) to permit their young children to continue breast-feeding until 3 years of age. Also, the children are fed in any place and on demand at any moment (Barriguete et al. 1998b). Bottle-feeding is allowed in many Latino families until age 2 or 3. Also, there are beliefs about "cold" and "hot" foods (referring not to their physical temperature or spiciness, but rather to a belief in the intrinsic property of a food) that should be proscribed at certain times. Some families are strict vegetarians for religious reasons and so feed the baby according to this code. There may be factors impinging on feeding, such as excessive stress and tension in the family, or a high noise level in the house (because of the stereo and television), that make it hard for the child to focus on feeding. Other feeding situations may also not be conducive to feeding.

Axis I: Problems Observed in the Infant

In all cases, the problem is considered a disturbance if the child does not exhibit the developmentally appropriate behavior for someone of the same age. Of course, several factors may be operating simultaneously. The clinician can note the most prominent symptom and add others as secondary issues. Overall, there are 10 categories of observable problems in the infant (see appendix to this chapter for more detail).

Appetite Disturbances

Appetite disturbances can be manifested as a lack of interest in either eating or the food itself as well as from the child becoming quickly satiated after eating just a little. The infant with an appetite disturbance may also hardly ever ask for food or may even seem to have no interest in feeding. Very young infants may sleep for prolonged periods without waking up to eat and without ever appearing to be hungry.

The appetite disturbances of excessive appetite or excessive appetite and thirst are seen more commonly in children in foster care situations (because of their history of emotional or food deprivation) or children under high stress (Gilmour and Skuse 1999). Such children appear not to feel the normal mechanisms of satiety, or if they do, it does not lead them to stop eating. Those who are older may constantly ask for food and then hide or hoard it.

Feeding Skills Disorders

Feeding skills disorders include difficulties with sucking (e.g., disorganized sucking, myoclonia, excessive fatigue, problems in lip control), with motor coordination, and with regulation of volume and speed of feeding. The very young infant may have difficulty staying awake and may fall asleep quickly after starting to suck.

Infants affected by sucking difficulties often seem unable to coordinate the muscles necessary for rhythmic and sustained sucking, which leads to frustration and slow intake of milk. Children affected by myoclonia develop rhythmic contractions of the perioral muscles that interfere with sucking or with sustained suction. Infants who become excessively fatigued appear to tire easily and often have to rest repeatedly while feeding; they take a long time to ingest even an ounce of milk or may even avoid continued sucking. Similarly, infants with problems in lip control (e.g., poor sealing of lips or difficulty positioning lips) struggle to ingest food and often cannot prevent either liquids or solids from coming out of the mouth once they have been consumed. Food is lost, leading to diminished total food intake despite the infant's expenditure of energy. Also, the negative pressure necessary to suck liquid from the breast or a bottle is diminished because of the lack of adequate "sealing" around the nipple. Another phenomenon is difficulty in positioning the lips to "clean the spoon," which is seen when the infant tries to ingest puréed foods or semisolids (Ramsay et al. 1993).

Motor coordination problems involving the toddler's hands and fingers can lead to a feeding skills disorder when the toddler is unable to get food from the plate to the mouth. This situation may occur because of difficulty in gathering the food with the hand, fingers, or utensils that are hard to manage (spoon, fork). The child may also have difficulty moving the food from the hand, fingers, or spoon into the mouth due to diminished proprioceptive input, that is, the child does not register the location of his or her mouth.

A third area of feeding skills disorders involves difficulty in regulating volume and speed of feeding. The child struggles with ingesting boluses that are too large for his or her mouth and cannot possibly be processed, so they must be spit out to avoid choking. Children affected by this difficulty may not know when to stop introducing food into the mouth; they keep ingesting more and more so quickly that it cannot be adequately mixed with saliva and chewed, so they must expel it. At times, the problem is the opposite: the child may take a long time between one mouthful and the next or may introduce excessively small boluses that prolong the feeding process.

Food Processing Difficulties

The main difficulty that infants have in processing food in the mouth involves chewing difficulties. Those with hypotonic muscles may find purées, semisolids, or solid foods difficult to chew. As a result, they may become exceedingly tired. At times, the chewing mechanism is not well adapted for processing some consistencies. Initially vertical, chewing becomes rotatory in the second year of life and thus gives the infant a more efficient way to manage meat, which is one of the most difficult foods to process. This, together with sensitivities in the oral mucosa, is often manifested by difficulty in progressing in the ability to manage increasing consistency in the food. For instance, an infant 1½ years of age may eat only liquids and spit out any lumpy or solid foods.

Swallowing Difficulties

Swallowing difficulties typically involve problems in coordination between breathing and swallowing. They particularly affect children who have some form of neurological compromise. These children may lack input on when to swallow, thus mistakenly attempting to do it while breathing, which leads to a choking episode.

In some cases, the infant or toddler may exhibit purposeful reluctance or resistance to swallowing. The child's practice of saving food between the teeth and cheeks has been referred to by some parents as "chipmunk" behavior. The child may hold the food there for several hours or even overnight without actually swallowing it, but perhaps chewing it more in a form of self-soothing behavior.

Another swallowing problem involves excessive nauseous reflex. The child is extremely sensitive to textures and stimulation in the oropharynx. Foods of thickening consistency may produce enough stimulation to generate frequent gagging or vomiting of the food about to be swallowed.

Food Refusal

The problem of food refusal has been called *infantile anorexia*. This term should be reserved for the infant who struggles for autonomy and control of the feeding situation (Chatoor 1997; Hoffmann 1998; Mazet and Stoleru 1996). Toward the end of the first 6 months of life, the infant typically attempts to gain more control of the feeding, which at times leads to conflict with the caregiver. As a result, the child may use any of several maneuvers designed to prevent the intake of food (Hoffmann 1992):

• Protruding the tongue purposefully to avoid food
• Keeping the mouth open so the food will fall out
• Spitting out the food
• Turning the head away persistently to avoid being fed
• Closing the lips deliberately to avoid being fed
• Arching the back or tilting the head backward, bending the body forward, sliding down in the chair, escaping from the chair, etc.

Posttraumatic Feeding Disorder

Posttraumatic feeding disorder is a condition that Chatoor (Chatoor et al. 1988) says requires the etiological antecedent of trauma during feeding. It could be in response to such situations as having previous choking episodes, being painfully fed with a nasogastric tube, and being force-fed. When a baby constantly resorts to maneuvers similar to the ones described in feeding refusal, it can be surmised that a painful association has been made between the traumatic experiences and feeding.

Mealtime Behavior Problems

In mealtime behavior problems, there is no primary motor coordination problem in the infant nor a clear refusal of food. Instead, the behavior is problematic because of the length of the meal (too long or too short) or because of two main problem areas that affect the parent or infant: a) concentration and physical activity and b) anger and frustration.

Problems with concentration and physical activity can often occur during meals. Infants may become disorganized during feedings, which can lead to overstimulation. As a result, the sucking effort can lead to excessive motor activity, constant shifting of position, and crying. Often the infant is literally unable to focus on the feeding, which becomes very frustrating for the child and the caregiver (Maldonado-Durán et al. 2002). Older toddlers with concentration difficulties are more likely to try several things at once (e.g., playing, jumping, walking, eating). They cannot focus on the activity at hand, which leads to prolonged meals or meals that are often interrupted. Caregivers who attempt to prevent all this activity in the child are likely to cause frustration and conflict.

To convey anger and frustration at the caregiver, these young children may use food as a weapon. They may pour liquid on the carpet just to challenge the person feeding them. Other maneuvers include throwing food or a cup or plate at the caregiver or a wall. The children may also spit at or spray liquid on the person who is feeding them.

Food Selectivity

Excessive food selectivity that affects toddlers leads them to decide they will eat only one or two kinds of food, possibly because they have an innate high sensitivity to textures, odors, or flavors. Being sensitive to textures means that the child rejects foods with a certain feel, such as solids or semisolids, because they produce an unpleasant sensation in the mouth. As a result, the 2-year-old does not progress in a normal way to handle thicker or more solid consistencies, preferring only liquids or "mushy" foods. This also may be the result of the child's prolonged lack of experience in processing foods, as with one who has been tube-fed for months or even years.

The child with a high sensitivity to odors or flavors has intense *neophobia,* or difficulty in accepting new odors and flavors. This sensitivity may trigger aversive behavior, such as gagging or even vomiting, when the food is introduced into the mouth. This reaction often occurs in the child with other signs of "sensory defensiveness."

Pica

Pica is the actual ingestion by the child, purposefully and repeatedly, of foods that are not considered edible by his or her cultural group. Such behavior should not be confused with the usual exploratory behavior of infants but, rather, as a disorder when it indicates a pattern of duration longer than 2 months in an infant older than 1½ years of age. The child actively seeks the material to be ingested, with the most common patterns being geophagia (dirt) or coprophagia (feces), as well as eating peeled paint from walls and cigarette butts. Pica may be associated with iron deficiency, as is often the case in geophagia, or with being deprived of stimulation, interaction, and supervision by adults (Lacey 1993). It is more common in children who live in institutions (e.g., orphanages).

Rumination

There are two patterns of rumination (merycism): the classical type and voluntary vomiting. The classical type involves ingesting food and then maneuvering it to make it go from the stomach back to the mouth again, where the child plays with the material in the oral cavity before re-ingesting it. This process may be repeated several times for self-stimulation and self-soothing as well as for a pleasurable activity (Brunod 1989). Rumination is also particularly common in institutionalized children deprived of human interaction and stimulation.

Toddlers who develop voluntary repeated vomiting methods can easily bring food up from the stomach and vomit it. This maneuver is clearly voluntary because the child can often be seen attempting to regurgitate by contracting the stomach and breathing deeply or by using a hand or other tool to stimulate the oropharynx and provoke the nauseous reflex. A successful episode of vomiting produces observable satisfaction.

Axis II: Feeding Relationship Disturbance

The true feeding relationship disturbance is one that is clearly maladaptive, of long duration, and rigidly maintained. It should be diagnosed only when the clinician has witnessed actual feeding interactions and distinguishes any of several main patterns of interaction, from underinvolvement to excessive anxiety to control or domination and inadequate feeding. Such observations supplement the statements about feeding from parents or caregivers.

Underinvolvement is a common pattern in feeding, partly because of the prevailing tendency for the parent and the child to have a distant feeding relationship. Parents or caregivers may feed inadequately, fail to maintain a predictable routine, or lack sensitivity to the infant's hunger cues.

Lack of feeding involves not offering enough or adequate food. The parent may dislike food or forget to feed the child. Feeding may be inconsistent and unpredictable, and there may be no overall routine for when, where, and what to feed the baby. The infant's cues and requests for food may even be ignored.

Excessive anxiety may be exhibited by the caregiver about feeding, caloric intake, dehydration, intoxication, illness, and so forth, resulting in either overfeeding or underfeeding. The emphasis here is on feeding the child well as the main or only way to convey love and affection. The caregiver who is excessively focused on feeding will experience considerable anxiety if the child is not hungry or refuses a meal. Such parents pay close attention to caloric intake and strive constantly for well-balanced meals.

A parent may overfeed his or her infant because of a fear of loss that is linked to a history of previous losses, such as postnatal loss or a death during the parent's childhood. In contrast, a parent may underfeed the child because of a parent's fear or misperception that the child might be or become fat. The parent's own painful memories of being overweight as a child may cast a shadow over the infant.

In a controlling relationship, the parent's agenda, desires, beliefs, and preferences almost exclusively take center stage and dominate what is offered to the child, regardless of the child's individuality, unique preferences, or vulnerabilities. The caregiver intends to control how much the child should eat, all the types of food ingested, and the timing (whether the child is hungry or not, satiated or not) and duration of the feeding. When control is an issue, there may even be a pattern of physically forcing foods into the child. The feeding situation becomes a battlefield, in large part due to a locking of wills, with a clear contribution by the parent.

Inadequate feeding techniques may be due to a lack of experience or a lack of information about food preparation, feeding, and nutritional needs. The caregiver unwittingly offers inappropriate foods or foods with insufficient calories or proteins. At times, parents do not provide enough calories or proteins because they give the child an excessive amount of juices that have a high volume but little nutritional value. Parents may not know how to prepare formula, or they may not have had any exposure to infant feeding. The parent who lacks a repertoire of maneuvers to manage the feeding challenges of the baby may give up too easily, thinking, for instance, that an infant who is taking a rest from feeding must be satisfied. This pattern commonly occurs in very young parents with little experience in caring for infants, in parents with limited problem-solving abilities, or in parents with multiple disruptions early in life such as those caused by growing up in foster homes.

Axis III: Medical Conditions as a Cause or Consequence of Feeding Difficulties

On Axis III, which delineates the medical conditions prior to or subsequent to feeding difficulties, the clinician notes any medical conditions or effects of substances that are pertinent to understanding the feeding difficulty and the status of the child and the parent-child relationship. A medical condition will sometimes be the root of the feeding problem or a consequence of it. Thus, it will be related to the resulting FTT, GS, or obesity that results from feeding problems.

Physical causes of feeding problems include cerebral palsy and related conditions or other neurological or neuromuscular conditions (e.g., altered appetite, motor coordination, feeding skills, and self-regulation in general); perceptual abnormalities, including visual and auditory impairments; and disorders of relating and communicating. The feeding problems may also be caused by general medical disorders leading to poor feeding endurance or interfering with the ability to eat; dysmorphic disorders; effects of chemical compounds or medications; and gastro-esophageal reflux.

General medical disorders may have physical causes. Chief among these are hypoxia during feedings (due to a cardiac condition), cerebral palsy, or even myasthenia gravis (leading to low muscular strength). Dysmorphic disorders, such as cleft lip or palate (macroglossia) or both, are conditions that involve a physical malformation in the oral cavity or in another associated structure. These disorders are almost always associated with a failure to thrive (e.g., Turner syndrome) or obesity (e.g., Prader-Willi syndrome).

Chemical compounds and medications (e.g., carbamazepine or valproic acid) can produce long-term effects on infants via in utero exposure. Other medications in current use (e.g., diazepam and other sedative or anticonvulsant medications, which can lead to muscular hypotonia) can also affect infants.

As a cause or consequence of a feeding problem, gastroesophageal reflux causes pain during eating. It is also associated with repeated regurgitation or vomiting.

Though the three main physical consequences of feeding problems are FTT, GS, and obesity, these conditions may also be the result of other physical conditions that are a cause or consequence of a feeding problem. Thus clinicians should look beyond the immediate physical cause for a possible underlying feeding problem or beyond the immediate feeding problem to a possible physical cause.

Axis IV: Stress Factors Related to Family and Cultural Issues

Although an extensive review of stress factors related to family and cultural issues is beyond the scope of the chapter, some of the main issues involved have been outlined earlier in this chapter, and further references can be consulted for this specific area (Moro and Barriguete 1998; Moro and Nathan 1999).

EVALUATION

An evaluation of the child, the feeding problem, the feeding relationship, and the caregiving environment is best done with a multidisciplinary treatment team that brings a variety of complementary expertise into play. If using a multidisciplinary team is not feasible, the primary clinician should at least be able to consult with specialists who can add their perspectives on the existing situation.

Multidisciplinary Team

In addition to a mental health clinician, a multidisciplinary team might include experts from the disciplines of nutrition, occupational therapy or speech therapy (or both), and pediatric neurology or pediatrics. Other specialists who might be included are physical therapists, a pediatric gastroenterologist, and a geneticist. The contributions of the team members would include the following:

- A nutrition specialist can best evaluate the current status of the patient, his or her caloric intake, the adequacy of protein being ingested, and the minimum nutritional requirements for resuming weight gain or growth.
- An occupational therapist or speech therapist can best evaluate factors such as sensory integration difficulties and the quality of movements involved in food intake, chewing, and swallowing. This therapist may be able to provide suggestions on positioning or on techniques to help the neuromuscular functioning of the systems involved in eating. Recommendations might note the need for special studies, such as the use of radiological or other imaging techniques, to examine the child's swallowing mechanism.
- Depending on the specific situation, a pediatric neurologist or a pediatrician may be required for consultation on health issues. Such a pediatric specialist can best deal with identification of and recommendations for managing malnutrition, FTT, GS, and so forth.
- The mental health professional can conduct a hands-on evaluation of the child, the parent-child relationship as a whole, and the feeding relationship in particular. This evaluation would also make note of the parents as individuals.

Evaluation Requirements

The patient evaluation requirements include a narrative of the feeding problem, a food diary, a growth curve, direct observation, a clinician's observation of the feeding relationship, and assessment of imaginary and fantasmatic interactions.

Narrative of the Feeding Problem

A key part of the patient evaluation process is the narrative account of the feeding problem. This historical account reports when the problem started or was noticed, how long it has lasted, how severe it is, and what its multiple effects are. The narrative should also include information about the "total child," i.e., any additional problems in the infant in other areas of functioning—for example, sleeping, irritability, mood, motor functioning, unique sensitivities, ability to relate, and ability to communicate.

The quantity, quality, consistency, and variety of what the child actually eats should be assessed and compared with his or her overall developmental level. It could be that a child is taking in enough calories and proteins at age 1½ by exclusively drinking fluids, yet the child is unable to eat semisolid or solid foods. This pattern of eating would be a problem in the child's maturing ability to process foods. Thus, the mere counting of calories and proteins would be misleading, as would focusing on the child's weight and height as the sole issue.

Food Diary

A food diary can be helpful in assessing how much a child is eating. This daily record of what and how much is eaten also should note when and where food is eaten, how long it takes for the meal, and what the other preferences of the infant are.

Growth Curve

An evaluation of the growth curve for weight and height can help indicate when the child's problem started. Changes from the norm in the growth curve should reveal when the weight gain started to decline or become stationary or when the growth in stature started to falter.

Direct Observation

Any observation of the child should involve watching the child's performance during sucking, drinking milk from a cup, taking in puréed food or solids, chewing, and swallowing. The observation of eating-related behavior gives the clinician firsthand information about the infant's eating patterns and problems. Such an observation of the "total child" goes beyond simply watching a few feeding situations. At times, the clinician trying to feed the child provides the firsthand experience of what difficulties the infant has in managing to eat.

Observation of the Feeding Relationship

For a more realistic evaluation of the problem, the observation of the feeding relationship should be as naturalistic as possible. If feasible, conducting a home observation or acquiring a home videotape of the typical events during a meal could be of much value to a patient's evaluation.

In compiling this information, the clinician can begin to see the multidetermined nature of the problem and the complexity of the interacting factors. It is important to assess not only those areas where there are challenges but also all the areas where there are strengths. Noting the strengths of the child and the family allows these elements to be better utilized in the child's treatment. Psychodynamic issues may be at play in the infant and the parent and in their relationship. The issues need to be understood because they can have a powerful impact on the clinician's perception of the problem, as well as on the family's motivation for change and the child's actual feeding experiences.

Assessment of Imaginary and Fantasmatic Interactions

The clinician tries to explore or assess the preconscious and unconscious perceptions and fantasies of the baby in the caregiver's mind. *Imaginary interactions* are preconscious thoughts and fantasies. *Fantasmatic thoughts* are rooted in unconscious meanings of the child in the mind of the parent or caregiver. Some clues are provided by the emotional tone; verbalizations; attunement issues, such as the choice of the baby's name; and the possible distortions of the baby due to the mental contents in the parent. Imaginary and fantasmatic interactions are often rooted in trigenerational-historical patterns in families (Lebovici 1998).

COMMON PROBLEMS AND APPROPRIATE INTERVENTIONS

The treatment strategy will depend on the family's priorities and the therapist's recommendations, though the physical health and nutritional status of the child are the primary considerations. The child's health and nutrition (e.g., severe malnutrition or dehydration) both have an impact on determining whether to treat the patient in an ambulatory clinic or in a hospital. The strengths of the family are especially crucial: parents should be motivated and interested in improving the situation, open to change, and willing to try new maneuvers. It is necessary to establish a good therapeutic alliance so that parents can feel understood and heard, while the therapists guide them to be more receptive to suggestions. Interventions can be directed primarily toward the child or the caregivers, but they can also be focused on the exchanges taking place during the feeding situation. At times, it may be necessary for the child to begin changing his or her behavior first, which helps the parent feel more optimistic and better able to implement some changes.

In this section, we highlight some common feeding problems and then discuss appropriate interventions. Even when the various interventions are described separately for different problems, they may be implemented simultaneously or consecutively, or even in a different order, depending on the nature of the situation.

Poor Appetite

A poor appetite may be noted from the beginning of extrauterine life and become more evident later. Some infants do not appear to perceive hunger as much and so do not ask for food. In these situations, one may need to wake the baby periodically and offer food. Some clinicians (M. Ramsay, personal communication, September 1999) use cyproheptadine (Periactin) to stimulate the infant's appetite, when doing so seems appropriate. Although there are no efficacy studies on the use of cyproheptadine in infants, this medication is known to stimulate hunger in adults through its serotonergic mechanism.

Sucking Difficulties

One of the various factors that may cause sucking difficulties is generally low muscle tone in the baby, which can lead to easy fatigue and a low intake of milk per feeding. The infant also may too quickly and regularly fall asleep while sucking. If the infant has a low ability to seal his or her lips around the nipple while breastfeeding, the mother should position the baby to hold the nipple with the lips around the areola (rather than just the nipple) to help "seal" the oral cavity and create more effective negative pressure. The baby may at first need assistance to initiate or continue the sucking activity: gently stimulating the lips and chin, moving the nipple in contact with the mouth, and giving an opportunity for a rest may all promote continued sucking. If the infant is being bottle-fed, using a bigger nipple or one with a larger opening will allow better passage of milk and facilitate the process. If the baby dozes off, he or she may need to be gently awakened to continue feeding.

Behavioral Disorganization During Sucking or Feeding

The problem of behavioral disorganization often is due to the baby's excessive sensitivity to sensory stimulation in the surroundings, as well as the rather high demands for self-control, organization, and concentration required by sucking or feeding. The infant may become overstimulated during the act of sucking or swallowing. At times, young infants may find unacceptable the mere recumbent position suggested for breast-feeding or simply being held. In these situations, reducing the amount of environmental stimulation may be helpful: turning the television down (or off), reducing other noises in the room (voices of people, other background noise), and helping the parent to not otherwise stimulate the baby so much (e.g., by not rocking, showing one's face, or talking to and stroking the baby all at the same time). In addition to reducing auditory input, it may be wise to reduce visual overload (e.g., reducing the amount of light in the room or the number of visible objects at the time of feeding). These "breaks" from stimulation with quiet time may assist the newly distressed infant in recuperating and being able to deal with more stimuli.

In addition to the general idea of reducing sensory input, a complementary strategy is to actively help the baby cope better with stimulation. Other techniques are deep pressure massage, oscillatory or vestibular (rocking, swinging) stimulation, or vibratory stimuli. Containing the baby with the arms (exerting some pressure) during feedings may help the baby to spend energy mostly on sucking rather than on moving and exploring the surroundings and, thereby, trying unsuccessfully to self-organize. The appropriateness of these measures is suggested by the child's positive response. Each child has a unique profile of sensitivities, so a technique that is successful with one child may prove ineffective or counterproductive with another.

Conflicts of Autonomy and Control During Feeding

Some infants have a more marked tendency to manifest a need for autonomy, that is, to explore, control, and exert their will. Normally, this desire becomes a theme in the infant's life around 9 or 10 months of age. But wanting to be autonomous can produce conflict when the infant tries to do things his or her own way rather than according to the caregiver's expectations or wishes. As Hoffmann (1998) pointed out, babies at this age want to explore the food, experiment and play with the food and the caregiver during the feeding situation, and hold the spoon or feed himself or herself. This desire for control requires the parent to "let the child be" and engage in a give-and-take where the creativity and exploratory wishes of the child can be respected. Some children who may not have had this opportunity may need to experience this mastery over their food; otherwise they might tend to be more oppositional in this area and other areas of life. For example, the baby may not accept being spoon-fed by the parent but instead wants to feed himself or herself, even if barely able to control the spoon. He or she may want to hold the plate or see the food or the spoon fall to the floor repeatedly. Some degree of control on the part of the child may help produce a compromise with the caregiver or parent, resulting in a combination of feeding oneself and being fed.

Excessive Food Selectivity and Poor Acceptance of New Textures and Flavors

The child with excessive selectivity will eat only one or two foods (e.g., chicken nuggets or macaroni and cheese) because of sensitivity (to textures, touch, flavors, odors, or all of these). This sensitivity causes the young child to feel "safe" only with a very restricted range of foods. Occupational therapy techniques along the lines of sensory integration may diminish the child's overall sensory defensiveness (using techniques of desensitization, a gradual increased tolerance of stimuli). Also, impregnating plastic or wooden toys that the toddler plays with (e.g., plastic cars or balls) or even daubing his fingers and hands with substances having new odors and flavors may help expose the child more subtly to new sensations in these channels. These foods may be gradually introduced into the child's diet as he or she becomes less sensitive or less aversive.

Ramsay (1998) described a technique of introducing very small amounts of the new food into the child's mouth then trying to create a positive interpersonal climate on its acceptance. Aversive behaviors on the part of the baby are not reinforced and may be ignored, while accepting behaviors are positively reinforced with praise or a cheerful attitude on the part of the caregiver or therapist. This intervention is an adaptation of a technique described as "mood modification behavioral therapy" (Stenberg and Hagekull 1997, p. 209), in which the focus is to change the association between feeding and conflict, or anger and defiance, and instead introduce a more positive and encouraging response to the trial of new foods and flavors.

Lack of Progression to the Processing of Higher-Consistency Foods

Even after 1 year of age, children with a food processing difficulty do not accept foods of a higher consistency than liquids or mushy, puréed foods. In most Western cultures, puréed foods are introduced into the baby's diet of milk and other liquids around 6 months of age. At 8–10 months, the baby will move on to semisolid foods and then, later on, to solids in small pieces, which can be managed with a vertical chewing motion. During the second year of life, rotary chewing develops to process higher consistency foods, such as meat. Difficulties with overall muscle tone, weakness in the muscles involved in chewing, or sensitivities in the mucosa may lead to the nonacceptance of foods with a higher consistency. The parent or caregiver who is aware that the infant struggles with these consistencies may continue to offer only the low-consistency foods as an adaptation. Progression may require the very gradual increase of foods with a slightly higher texture or consistency, as well as practice in the management of them. Such a gradual exposure and progression should lead to the eventual acceptance of solid foods. Exercises like mouthing a plastic object or a toy may help the child improve muscle coordination and strength. Depending on the individual child, other activities may be prescribed by a speech or occupational therapist. If a clinician evaluates a 2-year-old child who continues to take only liquids or purées, it may be useful to gradually start a program of offering slightly higher-consistency foods as the child masters each step.

Posttraumatic Feeding Disorder

The main problem with a posttraumatic feeding disorder is its connection with the memory of previously difficult or traumatic events related to feeding. There may be an association between feeding and pain, vomiting, near-choking, or tube feeding. In coping with a posttraumatic feeding disorder, a technique of gradual approximation and desensitization can be tried. At first, the child may be able to tolerate being near the food or near the spoon without attempting to introduce it in the mouth, instead exploring, experimenting, or playing with these items. Further on, the child may be able to have it touch his or her lips or mouth, receiving positive reinforcement for each new achievement. As the infant's anxiety gradually diminishes, he or she will be able to tolerate the introduction of food in the mouth, perhaps still without chewing or swallowing. The gradual approximation and positive reinforcement associated with less fear may eventually alleviate the problem.

With an infant who is older than 1 year (depending on the child), cognitive-behavioral play therapy techniques may be used to help alleviate anxiety. A puppet or stuffed animal can be placed near the baby and "fed" in play. The puppet may exhibit some of the behavior displayed by the infant and also "voice" some feelings of fear, concern, or caution in a very simple theatrical—largely visual and auditory—representation of the conflict at hand. The therapist or parent may then propose an alternative behavior and reassure the puppet that it is safe to try the new food and convince the puppet to eat now (or after another refusal is acted out). Humor can be used to minimize the fearful sensations experienced by the puppet. The child is invited to take part and to display different roles, be it the person who feeds or the one who is fed (the stuffed animal or puppet). The activity helps the child gradually express his or her fears and master anxiety.

Problem Behavior During Meals

A frequent scenario with toddlers is their apparent lack of interest in eating, accompanied by difficulty in getting them to actually sit down and eat. The typical problem behavior may proceed in the following manner: The child sits down for a minute or two, gets off the chair (or asks to get down), goes off to play elsewhere, and then comes back shortly for another spoonful of food. If actually sitting, the child may just play with the food, throw it on the floor or at the parent, or experiment with pouring liquid on the food or on the floor. The child may be excessively active and have difficulty inhibiting motor behavior long enough to sit down and actually eat. The child with these challenges often also has problems with some of the fine motor skills required for self-feeding, which can be frustrating.

At times, the amount of stimulation and interaction that is acceptable for many children may be excessive for a particular child. Having the child sit on the parent's lap (if culturally acceptable) or near the parent and reducing the environmental stimulation (e.g., turning off the television or radio and dimming the intensity of light) may help the child to sit for a longer period of time. Engaging the toddler in a conversation or a social exchange and also eating alongside the child may help the child to eat, perhaps imitating the adult. A relaxing activity prior to the meal (e.g., deep pressure or body massage) may help the child to be able to remain calm and sit longer. We are much more likely to motivate the child to go along with our wishes to eat together, and we will create a mostly cheerful exchange by engaging the toddler in pleasant reciprocal exchanges rather than insisting on compliance or getting angry.

A less common but equally important scenario is the toddler who manifests angry behavior toward the parents during mealtime. This behavior may consist of throwing food at the parent or the wall; deliberately pouring liquids on the floor or carpet; and even throwing the plate, drinking glass, or utensils. Such intentional actions should be distinguished from the occasional temper outbursts that any child may have during meals, even those resulting in the child throwing a plate when frustrated about something specific. When children deliberately throw the food after having been told not to, they may be purposefully provoking the parent to *do something*. This behavior should be seen in the context of the overall parent-infant relationship. Why is the child so angry, and why is that anger being expressed this way? What are other parent-child transactions like? Why this particular battlefield? A transactional-dynamic understanding of the situation will help create a therapeutic recommendation. In the long run, this approach may be better than just focusing on eliminating the child's angry or undesirable behavior.

By ascertaining the reason for the conflict and the child's expressions of anger, the therapist will be better able to suggest an intervention. The child may be angry at the parent due to a recent separation because of the parent's work schedule (e.g., seeing the parent little and being in day care for long hours), the birth of a sibling, or a recent move. The child's anger may be related to the quality of the parent-child relationship; for example, it may reflect a struggle between a very sensitive child and a rather forceful and matter-of-fact parent. In this particular case, an intervention suggesting a more diplomatic (soft) or empathic approach on the part of the parent may help create a better climate in the relationship overall, thereby reducing the child's angry expressions during mealtimes.

Difficulties in the Feeding Relationship

We have described the general notion of evaluating the total child and not just the feeding difficulties he or she might present. But it is also important to evaluate the caregiver-infant relationship as a whole and the feeding relationship in particular.

Each relationship between the infant and those who take care of him or her is unique and has specific features. The nature of one relationship, such as with the mother, does not necessarily determine the quality of another relationship, for instance, with the father. Also, as suggested by the Zero to Three classification of parent-child relationships (Zero to Three 1994), each relationship has several areas of interaction and only some of them may be affected. When there is a relationship disorder, most areas are negatively affected in the interaction between the infant and the caregiver (e.g., psychological involvement, actual interactions, emotional warmth, rhythmicity of interactions). The smaller the number of areas that are negatively affected in the parent-infant transactions, the better the quality of the relationship is.

INTERVENTIONS

We have already described some of the main manifestations of a troubled feeding relationship. Here we offer some suggestions for intervention when there is difficulty in these reciprocal interactions.

When a significant problem is due to an inadequate feeding technique, the clinician faces a dilemma. There may be information that the parents may not have and would like to have. However, it is necessary to be careful not to convey the message that the expert knows everything and the parents are doing everything wrong. This may alienate the parents permanently; they might feel criticized, judged, or even attacked. Information and suggestions regarding feeding can only be provided if there is a positive exchange between the clinician and the parents. After an investment has been made in developing this relationship, information regarding the baby's nutritional needs, such as how to prepare a bottle and how to hold the baby in different ways, may be welcome information that the parents could "take in" and implement. A common situation is diluting formula too much due to fear of overloading the baby. Parents may also give the child insufficient food because they are trying to follow a rigid schedule. The clinician's giving permission to modify feeding to the changing needs, demands, and states of the baby at different times or in different days may free adequate intuitive parenting interventions.

The problem may actually be in the caregiver's not knowing when to have mealtimes or how to prepare foods that are different from formula or milk. Many young parents do not have any experience with cooking or with actually having mealtimes when the family eats together. In many busy families, everyone eats separately and perhaps even in front of a television, leaving little opportunity for a social exchange during the meal or for the sharing of time and food. Children may be fed alone, without social interaction from a parent or caregiver, with the plate simply being put down in front of them. In many families, the concept of a family meal is unknown. Suggesting that the infant may eat better within a social exchange with the parents or family members may help some feeding problems. Toddlers are quite prone to imitate those around them: they may be motivated to taste new foods like the ones their parents eat, to "feed their parents" (putting food in the parent's mouth) and to be "fed by their parents" in an enjoyable exchange. Indeed, playful interactions may be an excellent vehicle to decrease the tension around meals or mealtimes and to help the parents enjoy the child in this area of their interactions.

A frequent concern in the feeding relationship has to do with issues of control. Mealtimes can easily become a battle of wills between parent and child, sometimes because the caregiver wishes to exercise excessive control during meals. Parents inherit a number of cultural prescriptions or family traditions or myths on what, when, where, and how to feed young children. When these prescriptions do not fit the unique characteristics of a child, they can intensify conflicts. Some common prescriptions are

- Children should eat everything on their plate (i.e., "clean the plate") and not waste food.
- Children should taste at least one mouthful or bite of every item on their plate.
- Children should not play during mealtimes.
- Children should not talk during meals.
- Dessert is allowed only after everything else on the plate is finished.

These very well-intentioned rules may or may not be adequate for an individual child. Particularly in the toddler years, a parent may misread the child's food selectivity as an attempt to control and manipulate the situation. A child could be punished for not tasting everything or for gagging or vomiting when forced to taste a certain food. Although parents wish to convey a message to the child by not giving in, being consistent, and not allowing the child to get up until the plate is empty, doing so can prolong the meal to an hour or longer. Frequently, well-intentioned and "experienced" relatives or friends advise parents that the child is spoiled and needs to be punished and that the parents need to be consistent with the punishment. Thus it may be a relief for parents to learn that it is an illusion to think that they really can make children eat. This behavior cannot be forced, even when parents try. Children have an enormous repertoire of behaviors they can use to not accept food or to expel it afterward, even when it is introduced forcefully. Indeed, parents really have control only over certain aspects of the feeding situation: what is offered, where, and when. Thus, parents could be helped to realize that feeding is a mutually cooperative activity that requires voluntary participation from both parties. The therapist may assist parents in feeling "relaxed" about those cultural prescriptions and in adapting expectations to the unique features of their child, adapting to who the child really is.

Another common situation is that parents and many health care professionals think that children know intuitively what is best for them. Many believe that if children were left to their own devices, they would—on their own—select a well-balanced diet and whatever else is "good for them" in the long run. But available evidence suggests that this is not so (Birch 1990, 1991, 1998). When left to their own choices, children tend to select sweet and highly fatty foods above all else. It therefore appears that the best route is to establish a compromise between what the child's preferences are and what he or she needs to ingest in order to grow rather than letting the agenda of the child or the parent be the sole dictating force. Also, by using dessert as the reward for eating, caregivers convey the implicit message that the only good thing is the dessert and that other foods are just necessary evils (Birch 1987). It may be better to offer dessert as a part of the meal rather than as a reward.

Parents who experienced deprivation early in life or who were maltreated themselves may find it difficult to set limits, even believing that they are hurting their children by denying some requests. Also, when a parent has lost a previous child or has had other losses early in life, there may be an unconscious association between feeding and protecting the baby because feeding is equated with making sure the child will be healthy and have a better chance for survival. The same line of reasoning can develop with a young child who suffers from a chronic illness (e.g., cystic fibrosis, arthritis) because the parents may have difficulty frustrating a child who is already suffering.

In Western cultures, there is an increasing preoccupation with being overweight, and parents are afraid of obesity in their child. Caregivers may struggle with their own sense of not having enough self-control, being fat, or feeling inadequate because they do not fit a cultural standard of thinness, youth, and health. This may lead parents to protect their children from similar dangers by ensuring that they will be thin. They may feel unconsciously proud if their child is underweight or "hardly eats anything" as they think they are helping the child not to suffer the stigma that they have encountered. They may unwittingly discourage the child from eating at mealtimes or not have mealtimes at all for the same reason, and they may also praise the child for being thin and beautiful.

The parent with an eating disorder may experience conflicts around feeding and with the child's body image. At times, mothers who suffer from anorexia nervosa may even perceive their baby as being overweight when, in reality, the baby is underweight (Stein et al. 1996). A female patient with anorexia nervosa came to our outpatient service because she was afraid that her baby might also suffer from an eating disorder. When we explored the mother's representation of her baby during the therapeutic consultation, she was very explicit: "When I saw my baby for the very first time, I saw his face with my father's nose, my husband's ears, and with my cheeks." In general, she did not like that resemblance, particularly to herself. This description alerted us to the fact that the patient did not really "see" her baby but instead had a perception of the child that was overshadowed by her fears and previous experiences.

SUMMARY

Food intake and feeding constitute an enormously charged area in which many "ghosts" (Fraiberg et al. 1975) can make their presence felt, because the process of feeding is much more than introducing calories or nutrients into the baby's body. Feeding and eating can bring many challenges to the baby and to the parent. Recognizing the problem for what it is may be the first step in remedying the situation. Mental health professionals are in a unique position to recognize and identify the problems and to validate parental concerns or their preoccupation with how their baby eats (or doesn't eat).

A clinician can support parents in validating their concerns and assist them in trying different strategies of intervention. As an outsider, the clinician is in an advantageous position to observe and evaluate the contributions of the baby and the parents, as well as the fit between them, to the presenting problems. Through the vehicle of a positive therapeutic alliance, the clinician can have a great impact on a patient's treatment, such as preventing failure to thrive or growth stunting, supporting the parent's creativity and intuitive strategies to feed the baby, and proposing modifications and adjustments depending on the baby's response.

REFERENCES

American Psychiatric Association: Diagnostic and Statistical Manual of Mental Disorders, 4th Edition, Text Revision. Washington, DC, American Psychiatric Association, 2000

Barness LA, Curran JS: Nutrition, in Nelson Textbook of Pediatrics, 15th Edition. Edited by Nelson WE, Behrman RE, Kliegman RM, et al. Philadelphia, PA, WB Saunders, 1996, pp 141–184

Barriguete JA, Lebovici S, Salinas JL, et al: La consulta terapéutica en algunas alteraciones de alimentación del lactante [Therapeutic consultation for some infant feeding disturbances], in La alimentación y sus efectos en el desarrollo [Feeding and Its Effects on Development]. Edited by Lartigue T, Maldonado-Durán M, Avila H. México City, Editorial Plaza y Valdez and Asociación Psicoanalitica Mexicana, 1998a, pp 391–406

Barriguete JA, Moro MR, Aguilar C: Étude préliminaire des soins précoces mere bebé (crianza) chez les P'urhe: aers une ethnopsychanalyse périnatale [A preliminary study of early mother-baby interactions among the Purépechas: towards a perinatal psychoanalysis], in Psychiatrie Perinatale [Perinatal Psychiatry]. Edited by Mazet P, Lebovici S. Paris, Presses Universitaires de France, 1998b, pp 471–488

Birch LL: The acquisition of food acceptance patterns in children, in Eating Habits, Food Physiology, and Learned Behavior. Edited by Brookes R, Popplewell D, Burton M. Chichester, UK, Wiley, 1987, pp 107–130

Birch LL: Development of food acceptance patterns. Dev Psychol 26:515–519, 1990

Birch LL: Children's preferences for high-fat foods. Nutr Rev 50(9):249–255, 1991

Birch LL: Development of food acceptance patterns in the first years of life. Proc Nutr Soc 57(4):617–624, 1998

Bosma JF: Development of feeding. Clin Nutr 5:210–218, 1986

Brunod R: Jeux interdits du nourrison: a propos de six cas the merycisme graves [Forbidden games in the infant: six cases of severe rumination]. Psychiatrie de l'Enfant [Child Psychiatry] 32(2):451–494, 1989

Chatoor I: Feeding and eating disorders of infancy and early childhood, in Textbook of Child and Adolescent Psychiatry, 2nd Edition. Edited by Wiener JM. Washington, DC, American Psychiatric Press, 1997, pp 527–542

Chatoor I, Conley C, Dickson L: Food refusal after an incident of choking: a posttraumatic eating disorder. J Am Acad Child Adolesc Psychiatry 27(1):105–110, 1988

Douglas J, Bryon M: Interview data on severe behavioural eating difficulties in young children. Arch Dis Child 75:304–308, 1996

Flegal KM: The obesity epidemic in children and adults: current evidence and research issues. Med Sci Sports Exerc 31:S509–S514, 1999

Fraiberg S, Adelson E, Shapiro V: Ghosts in the nursery: a psychoanalytic approach to the problems of impaired infant-mother relationships. Journal of the American Academy of Child Psychiatry 14(3):387–421, 1975

Gilmour J, Skuse D: A case-comparison study of the characteristics of children with a short stature syndrome induced by stress (hyperphagic short stature) and a consecutive series of unaffected "stressed" children. J Child Psychol Psychiatry 40(6):969–978, 1999

Hoffmann JM: A proposed scheme for coding infant initiatives during feeding. Infant Mental Health Journal 13(3):199–205, 1992

Hoffmann JM: De quien es la Cuchara? La relacion de alimentacion padres-bebe [Whose spoon is it? The parent-infant feeding relationship], in La alimentacion y sus efectos en el desarrollo [Feeding and Its Effects on Development]. Edited by Lartigue T, Maldonado-Durán M, Avila H. México City, Editorial Plaza y Valdez and Asociación Psicoanalitica Mexicana, 1998, pp 101–120

Lacey EP: Phenomenology of pica. Child Adolesc Psychiatr Clin N Am 2:75–91, 1993

Lawrence M, Lawrence F, Durnin JV, et al: A comparison of physical activity in Gambian and UK children aged 6–18 months. Eur J Clin Nutr 45(5):243–252, 1991

Lebovici S: L'arbre de la vie [The tree of life], in Psychopathologie du nourrisson [Infant Psychopathology]. Paris, Eres, 1998

Leung AKC, Robson WLM: The toddler who does not eat. Am Fam Physician 49(8):1789–1792, 1994

Lindquist CH, Reynolds KD, Goran MI: Sociocultural determinants of physical activity among children. Prev Med 29(4):305–312, 1999

Maldonado-Durán JM: A new perspective on failure to thrive. Zero to Three [Bulletin of Zero to Three] 21(1):15, 2000

Maldonado-Durán JM, Sauceda-Garcia JM: Los problemas de la alimentación en la primera infancia [Feeding problems in infancy], in La alimentacion y sus efectos en el desarrollo [Feeding and Its Effects on Development]. Edited by Lartigue T, Maldonado-Durán M, Avila H. México City, Editorial Plaza y Valdez and Asociación Psicoanalitica Mexicana, 1998, pp 133–162

Maldonado-Durán JM, Holigrocki R, Moody C: A proposed classification for feeding disorders. Infant Behavior and Development 21 (special ICIS issue): 120, 1998

Maldonado-Durán JM, Helmig L, Karacostas V, et al: Implicazioni diagnostiche e terapeutiche nella valutazione clinica dei disturbi alimentari e della regloazione nella prima infancia [Diagnostic and therapeutic implications in the evaluation of feeding and regulatory disturbances during infancy]. Psichiatria dell'infanzia e dell'adolescenza [Psychiatry of Childhood and Adolescence] 69:61–77, 2002

Mazet P, Stoleru S: Psychopathologie du nourrisson et du jeune enfant [Psychopathology of the Infant and Young Child]. Paris, Masson, 1996, pp 120–124

Meeks-Gardner JM, Grantham-McGregor SM, Himes J, et al: Behaviour and development of stunted and nonstunted Jamaican children. J Child Psychol Psychiatry 40(5):819–827, 1999

Moro MR, Barriguete JA: Aspectos transculturales de la alimentación del lactante [Transcultural issues in infant feeding], in La alimentacion y sus efectos en el desarrollo [Feeding and Its Effects on Development]. Edited by Lartigue T, Maldonado-Durán M, Avila H. México City, Editorial Plaza y Valdez and Asociación Psicoanalitica Mexicana, 1998, pp 337–362

Moro MR, Nathan T: Ethnopsychiatrie de l'enfant [Child ethnopsychiatry], in Nouveau traité de la psychiatrie de l'enfant et de l'adolescent [New Textbook of Child and Adolescent Psychiatry], Vol 3. Edited by Lebovici S, Diatkine R, Soule M. Paris, Presses Universitaires de France, 1999, pp 423–443

Ramsay M: Feeding disorder and failure to thrive. Child Adolesc Psychiatr Clin N Am 4(3):605–616, 1995

Ramsay M: La fisiologia de la alimentacion en el lactante: Su significado en la identificacion, proceso diagnostico y tratamiento [The physiology of feeding in the infant: its meaning in identification, diagnostic process, and treatment], in La alimentacion y sus efectos en el desarrollo [Feeding and Its Effects on Development]. Edited by Lartigue T, Maldonado-Durán M, Avila H. México City, Editorial Plaza y Valdez and Asociación Psicoanalitica Mexicana, 1998, pp 83–100

Ramsay M, Gisel EG, Boutry M: Non-organic failure to thrive: growth failure secondary to feeding-skills disorder. Dev Med Child Neurol 35(4):285–297, 1993

Skuse D, Wolke D, Reilly S: Socio-economic disadvantage and ethnic influences upon infant growth in inner London, in Clinical Issues in Growth Disorders: Evaluation, Diagnosis, and Therapy. Edited by Prader A, Rappaport R. Tel Aviv, Freund Publishing House, 1994, pp 56–70

Stanek K, Abbott D, Cramer S: Diet quality and the eating environment of preschool children. J Am Diet Assoc 90(11):1582–1584, 1990

Stein A, Murray L, Cooper P, et al: Infant growth in the context of maternal eating disorders and maternal depression: a comparative study. Psychol Med 26(3):569–574, 1996

Stenberg G, Hagekull B: Social referencing and mood modification in 1-year-olds. Infant Behavior and Development 20(2):209–217, 1997

Sullivan PB, Rosenbloom L: An overview of the feeding difficulties experienced by disabled children, in Feeding the Disabled Child. Edited by Sullivan PB, Rosenbloom L. Suffolk, UK, MacKeith Press, 1996, pp 23–32

Tolia V: Very early onset nonorganic failure to thrive in infants. J Pediatr Gastroenterol Nutr 20(1):73–80, 1995

Troiano RP, Flegal KM: Overweight children and adolescents: description, epidemiology and demographics. Pediatrics 101(3):497–504, 1998

Tuchman DN: Physiology of the swallowing apparatus, in Disorders of Feeding and Swallowing in Infants and Children. Edited by Tuchman DN, Walter RS. San Diego, CA, Singular Publishing Group, 1994, pp 1–25

Uauy R, Mena P, Valenzuela A: Essential fatty acids as determinants of lipid requirements in infants, children and adults. Eur J Clin Nutr 53(Suppl 1):S66–S77, 1999

Vestergaard M, Obel C, Henriksen TB, et al: Duration of breastfeeding and developmental milestones during the latter half of infancy. Acta Paediatr 88(12):1327–1332, 1999

Von Braun J, McComb J, Fred-Mensah BK, et al: Urban Food Insecurity and Malnutrition in Developing Countries: Trends, Policies and Research Implications. Washington, DC, International Food Policy Research Institute, 1993

Waterlow JC: Causes and mechanisms of linear growth retardation (stunting). Eur J Clin Nutr 48(Suppl 1):S1–S4, 1994

Waterlow JC: Linear growth in children, in Nutrition in Pregnancy and Growth. Edited by Porrini M, Walter P. Basel, Switzerland, S Karger, 1996, pp 45–54

Wilensky DS, Ginsberg G, Altman M, et al: A community-based study of failure to thrive in Israel. Arch Dis Child 75:145–148, 1996

Wolke D: Sleeping and feeding across the lifespan, in Development Through Life: A Handbook for Clinicians. Edited by Rutter M, Hay DF. Oxford, UK, Blackwell Scientific, 1994, pp 517–557

Wolke D: The myth of maternal deprivation. The Signal [Newsletter of the World Association for Infant Mental Health] 4(3):4, 1996

World Health Organization: The ICD-10 Classification of Mental and Behavioural Disorders: Clinical Descriptions and Diagnostic Guidelines. Geneva, World Health Organization, 1992

Zero to Three: Infants, Toddlers and Families: Diagnostic Classification of Mental Health and Developmental Disorders of Infancy and Early Childhood (DC:0–3). Arlington, VA, Zero to Three, 1994

APPENDIX

Proposed classification of the phenomenology of eating difficulties in infants and young children:

Axis I: Problems observed in the infant
1. Appetite disturbances
   A. Lack of appetite
      1) Few requests for food
      2) Little interest in feeding
      3) Prolonged periods of sleep
      4) Little apparent hunger
   B. Excessive appetite or excessive appetite and thirst
      1) Lack of normal mechanisms of satiety
      2) Failure to stop eating when satiated
2. Feeding skills disorders
   A. Sucking difficulties
      1) Disorganized sucking
      2) Myoclonia during sucking
      3) Excessive fatigue with sucking; excessive sleepiness while sucking
      4) Problems in lip control (e.g., poor sealing of lips, difficulty positioning lips to "clean the spoon")
   B. Motor coordination problems
   C. Difficulty regulating the volume and speed of feeding
3. Difficulties in processing the food in mouth
   A. Chewing difficulties
   B. Inability to manage higher-consistency textures, delay in development of food processing mechanism
4. Difficulties in swallowing
   A. Purposeful reluctance or resistance to swallowing
   B. Excessive nauseous reflex
5. Food refusal ("infantile anorexia")
   A. Using purposeful tongue protrusion to avoid introduction of food
   B. Keeping the mouth open so the food would come out
   C. Spitting out the food once it has been introduced
      1) Persistence in turning head away to avoid food in the mouth
      2) Purposeful closing of the lips to avoid food being introduced

3) Arching the back or tilting the head backward, bending the body forward, sliding down in the chair, getting away from the chair, etc.
6. Posttraumatic feeding disorder
7. Mealtime behavior problems
   A. Problems with concentration and physical activity during meals: inability to focus on eating, inability to sit still, or disorganization while trying to eat
   B. Use of food to convey anger and frustration
8. Excessive food selectivity
   A. High sensitivity to textures
   B. High sensitivity to odors or flavors
9. Pica
10. Rumination (merycism)
    A. Classical type
    B. Voluntary repeated vomiting

Axis II: Feeding relationship disturbance
1. Underinvolvement
   A. Failing to feed the child
   B. Offering insufficient or inadequate food
   C. Forgetting to feed the child
   D. Using an unpredictable pattern of feeding
   E. Ignoring the infant's requests and cues for food
2. Excessive anxiety over feeding
   A. Focusing on feeding, caloric intake, dehydration, intoxication, illness, etc.
   B. Using feeding as the main or only channel to convey love and affection
      1) Overfeeding due to fear of loss
      2) Overfeeding to overcome a history of previous losses (e.g., postnatal loss, deaths in the parent's childhood)
      3) Underfeeding due to fear the child is fat or may become fat
      4) Feeling anxious if the child is not hungry, refuses a meal, or pays excessive attention to calories
3. Controlling relationship
   A. Disregarding the child's individuality, unique preferences, or vulnerabilities because of an overriding parental agenda, desires, beliefs, or preferences
   B. Controlling how much the child should eat, all types of foods ingested, and timing of food (regardless of child's hunger)

   C. Physically forcing foods into the child
   D. Turning the feeding situation into a battlefield, due to a lock-
       ing of wills with a clear contribution by the parent
4. Inadequate feeding technique
   A. Lacking experience or information about food preparation,
       feeding, and nutritional needs
   B. Unwittingly offering inappropriate foods or foods with insuf-
       ficient calories or proteins
   C. Misunderstanding an infant's taking a rest from feeding as
       satisfaction

**Axis III: Medical conditions as a cause or consequence of feeding diffi-
culties**
1. Causes of feeding problem
   A. Cerebral palsy and other related conditions
   B. Other neurological or neuromuscular conditions (altering
       appetite, motor coordination, feeding skills, and self-regula-
       tion in general)
   C. Perceptual abnormalities (visual or auditory impairment)
   D. Disorders of relating and communicating
   E. General medical disorders leading to poor feeding endur-
       ance or inability to eat (e.g., hypoxia during feedings, due to
       a cardiac condition, or myasthenia gravis [low muscular ac-
       tivity])
   F. Dysmorphic disorders
       1) Turner syndrome (associated with FTT)
       2) Prader-Willi syndrome (associated with obesity)
       3) Cleft lip or cleft palate, or both
       4) Macroglossia
       5) Effects of chemical compounds or medications (long-
           term effects of in utero exposure to carbamazepine or
           valproic acid)
       6) Effects of presently used medications (e.g., diazepam
           and other sedative or anticonvulsant medications that
           can lead to muscular hypotonia)
       7) Gastroesophageal reflux
2. Consequences of feeding problem
   A. Failure to thrive
   B. Growth stunting
   C. Obesity

Note: Axis IV describes psychosocial situations outside those in the feeding relationship that, nevertheless, may contribute to the present eating problem (e.g., religious ideas, family myths, environmental factors obstructing feeding). Clinicians may want to add a description of the problem to their records, or even to create an Axis V, to indicate the level of development the child has reached in his or her eating abilities (e.g., vertical chewing, rotatory chewing, interest and ability to eat a variety of foods).

IV

Illustrative
Case Examples

13

A 3-Year-Old "Monster"

Richard J. Pines, D.O.

Consultants
Efrain Bleiberg, M.D.
Peter Fonagy, Ph.D., F.B.A.
Serge Lebovici, M.D.
Susan McDonough, M.S.W., Ph.D.
Lucile Ware, M.D. (Moderator)

In this chapter, I present a case involving a difficult child in the context of a multiproblem family. The discussion focuses on diagnostic issues and treatment approaches to this situation. The case involved four sessions, three in a clinical setting and one in the parents' home. With parental consent, all four sessions were videotaped.

Four sections make up the chapter:

1. A detailed narration of the case
2. The observations of the clinicians (Dr. Pines and Dr. Maldonado) who worked with the child and his family
3. Excerpts from the videotapes presented to a panel of consultants (Efrain Bleiberg, M.D., Peter Fonagy, Ph.D., F.B.A., Serge Lebovici, M.D., Susan McDonough, M.S.W., Ph.D., and Lucile Ware, M.D.)
4. Observations and suggestions of the consultants

Overall, this case presentation emphasizes the differences in the consultants' points of view, understanding, and recommendations to highlight the various ways of approaching a difficult case of a child in a multiproblem family.

> My son is a "monster"... Some days I just don't want to live with him...
> Nobody can help me with my child... My boy is totally out of control...
> Why is my child this way?
>
> Mother of 3-year-old boy

Parenting a child with special needs and behavioral problems is often extremely difficult. The acting-out child usually struggles both at home and in other settings. Working parents or parents who are just looking for some daily relief may find it difficult to locate an appropriate day care facility. Because of the severity of their aggression, mood liability, social skill delays, and other difficulties, these children are often misunderstood, shunned, and treated inappropriately. They are more likely to be referred for mental health consultation and treatment because they are disruptive and difficult compared with more passive and compliant children.

Mental health professionals may feel baffled by the challenges of a child described as a "monster." They may also feel overwhelmed by a parental expectation that the child should behave well. The case of a little boy, whom I will call Jacob, is representative of the difficulties encountered by the child, parents, day care staff, and mental health professionals. There are questions about the diagnosis and understanding of the child's difficulties, and discussants are asked to give advice on the most appropriate interventions. The case of Jacob also epitomizes a frequent situation encountered in the infant mental health clinic: The patient is an "impossible" young child who is part of a family that faces other problems, and there is a sense of immediacy in the request for intervention.

At the time this case was discussed, the evaluation and treatment process had unfolded for approximately 1 month. Jacob and his family had been involved in four sessions—three in the clinic and one in the parents' home. With parental consent, all sessions were videotaped. The case and videotape excerpts were presented to a panel of expert consultants, who were asked to offer their understanding of the case, not necessarily in terms of a standard nomenclature (e.g., DSM-IV-TR or Zero to Three), but from a psychodynamic or systemic perspective. They were also asked how they would suggest approaching the challenges of this particular child and family. As will be seen in the case study that follows, the family requested highly practical and realistic recommendations that could be readily implemented in order to alleviate their urgent sense of need for immediate changes in Jacob's behavior.

Jacob K, a 3-year-old biracial boy, was referred to our infant mental health clinic for evaluation by the nursing staff of the city's health department. His mother, Ms. K, is involved with this department through the Women, Infants, and Children (WIC) program, where she receives milk supplement and health care services for her youngest child, a 1-year-old girl. After Ms. K discussed with the nurses the enormous difficulties she was having with Jacob, they advised her to contact our clinic. During telephone contact to set up the first appointment, Ms. K said she was desperate for help because her son was a "monster," totally out of control, defiant, and extremely aggressive. She felt exhausted after fighting with him all day. She and her husband (Jacob's adoptive father) had tried "just about everything" to control Jacob with several discipline methods, but "nothing has worked." The first appointment was set up within 1 week of the initial phone call, followed by three subsequent appointments approximately 1 week apart. The first three sessions were held in the clinic office, and the fourth was conducted in the patient's home. The author and Dr. Martín Maldonado-Durán were both involved in every session.

Mr. and Ms. K came to the first session with Jacob, their two older boys (ages 4 and 6), a younger boy (age 2), and their baby girl. Ms. K took the lead, saying she was very upset and would welcome any feedback on what she could do for her son, who was "tearing her family apart." She made it clear she wanted immediate advice and did not want to wait for a long and complicated evaluation before receiving some suggestions.

Ms. K said Jacob was highly aggressive and frequently lashed out at those around him, including her, his adoptive father, his brothers, and his peers at the day care center. During these episodes of anger, Jacob shouted, bit people, kicked, and threw things. His outbursts, which lasted as long as an hour, occurred several times a day. During one such outburst, Jacob stabbed and killed a family pet bird with a letter opener.

These rages occasionally appeared unprovoked, but most of the time they were set off when Jacob did not get his way or when he was otherwise frustrated. Both parents felt Jacob acted this way because he wanted to be the center of attention. They wondered whether he was trying to manipulate them to get one-on-one interaction. Ms. K said she had tried time-outs, but Jacob would fight them and get up from the chair. Spanking did not work either because he became more angry and hateful afterward. She had sent him to his room for periods of several minutes, but he threw things around the room, destroyed toys, and kept coming out of the room anyway.

When angry and out of control, Jacob was difficult to soothe. Both parents felt he had very little patience and a bad attitude. They remarked that he seemed to be afraid of nothing. He did not appear to fear threats of punishments or even physically dangerous situations.

Ms. K said her son had a "very high pain threshold" and rarely cried, even when physically hurt or injured. He might get into dangerous situations and have "no regard for his personal safety." For instance, he might jump from furniture, climb on the stove, or leave the house and try to cross the street by himself. The parents saw Jacob as full of energy and in a state of constant activity for most of the day; he "never slows down."

Mr. and Ms. K were also concerned that Jacob spoke few discernible words and only a few two-word sentences (e.g., "All gone" or "I done"). He spoke to them mostly in a sort of jargon that was difficult to understand. They perceived him as quite clumsy; he would bump into walls, step on toys, and make loud noises constantly when playing with toys.

Regarding Jacob's early development, Ms. K described the conception, pregnancy, and birth as extremely difficult and stressful. Jacob was conceived after a brief affair with a man 13 years older than Ms. K. She described this man as a "father figure." She initially thought the man was Caucasian but later discovered he was from a multiracial background (Mexican, Native American, and Caucasian). She admitted being upset about this fact because of her experience with her biological father, who is also of both Mexican and Native American descent. Ms. K felt her pregnancy with Jacob was the most difficult of those she had undergone with her five children. She had felt a lot of guilt and shame during the pregnancy. When Jacob was born, she looked at him, cried, and thought, "I don't want him . . . he doesn't look right . . . his feet are too big." (Toward the end of the first session with the family, Ms. K proudly held up her baby girl and said, "Isn't she beautiful! I finally had a girl. Now I can stop having kids." She then stated that after her daughter's birth, she'd had a tubal ligation.)

Ms. K hypothesized that Jacob's problems were related to his biological father's ethnic background and to the fact that he had "Indian within him." She felt "it has to be from his father's side of the family . . . people in my family are not that way." She immediately added that she was only hypothesizing and "grasping at straws" because she desperately wanted some explanation for why Jacob acted this way.

Ms. K said her pregnancy with Jacob was a precipitant of her second divorce. When Jacob was born, DNA testing was performed to confirm his biological father's paternity. Mr. and Ms. K stated that Mr. K was "the only father Jacob has ever known." Jacob never had contact with his biological father and was adopted by Mr. K several months after his birth.

When discussing developmental milestones, Ms. K noted Jacob was not yet toilet trained. Jacob often imitated her when she was doing housework, and he also imitated his father shaving. Jacob was exhibiting sleep terrors (*pavor nocturnus*) approximately three or four times a week. The parents stated that Jacob did not have any medical problems, nor did he take any medications. When we discussed Jacob's strengths, the parents said, "He can be cuddly and sweet, even lovable, when he wants to be . . . he is good with his baby sister . . . and is curious about things."

The Family

Ms. K is 28 years old and now a stay-at-home mother. In the past, she worked outside the home as a waitress in a local bar. Jacob's adoptive father is 29 years old and Caucasian. He works for an insurance company in the mortgage foreclosure department. He said he likes to extend his work hours to nights and weekends because he does not want to be home to deal with the family struggles. Ms. K feels some of their current marital problems are related to Mr. K working long hours and coming home late. Mr. and Ms. K felt they married too soon, after a short relationship—"a little more than a one-night stand." When their relationship began, Ms. K was still married to her second husband.

The four other children in the home are three boys (ages 6, 4, and 2) and a girl (age 1½ months). Four of the five children have different fathers; the two youngest are from the current marriage.

Parents' History

Ms. K had a very difficult childhood and early life. Her parents divorced when she was 10 years old. She described her father as a "jerk" who never gave her the attention or love she wanted. After he divorced her mother, he left home and did not have any contact with the children during the next 3 years. Ms. K said she had not spoken with her father for the past 6 years. Ms. K's mother eventually remarried, and that marriage lasted approximately 13 years. Ms. K said she became close to her stepfather, but he also "walked out," and the family abruptly lost contact with him. She stated her stepfather "turned out to be a loser." At some point, Ms. K reflected on her childhood and said all she really had wanted as a child was to be "daddy's little girl" but never had the experience. It was very important for her to keep her husband now so her daughter would grow up with a father.

Ms. K further reflected on her numerous dysfunctional relationships with men. She had lived with five different men, marrying three of them. She had major problems in all these relationships. She also mentioned she lacked trust in "counselors," and that only after much thought and ambivalence had she sought help for Jacob. On the other hand, she said she was currently seeing a therapist (a woman) who was also doing some marital work with her and Mr. K. When speaking of their marriage, Ms. K stated she often felt that Mr. K was her "sixth child" because she was always having to care for him; she felt he was an extremely dependent man.

Mr. K's mother had passed away, leaving him a significant sum of money that enabled him to buy a large home for his current family. He proudly said he'd paid cash for the home. Like Ms. K, he was divorced and had other children, but he had not maintained contact with them. He said that for many years his relationship with Ms. K had been purely platonic. They became sexually involved while Ms. K was pregnant with Jacob.

Mr. K admitted he worked long hours and weekends partly to avoid confrontations with Jacob and Ms. K. Both parents agreed that Jacob seemed "worse" when Mr. K was around. Mr. K attempted to discipline Jacob by yelling at him and spanking him. Both parents felt Jacob listened more to Mr. K because of his deeper, louder voice.

Observations of the Clinicians

Jacob was a tall, slender, handsome boy who appeared well developed and well nourished. At times he seemed bewildered and confused by his surroundings. He used very little spoken language in his communication and, instead, pointed to things he wanted or sometimes just got them himself. Jacob used some difficult-to-understand jargon, often rambling on for extended periods of time. Frequently, neither the clinicians nor his parents could understand what he was saying, although he did use some intelligible words, such as "bye-bye," "hi," "dog," "okay," and "yes." The clinicians noticed that at times he tried to imitate his parents' speech, attempting to reproduce the sounds they were making. He had a communicational intent.

During the first session with the family, Jacob and his brothers had several disagreements. During some of them, Jacob quickly resorted to pulling hair and pushing, laughing loudly afterward. To engage in symbolic play, he needed an enormous amount of support and a very quiet setting with few distractions. Most of the play interaction was initiated by the clinicians rather than by Jacob.

VIDEOTAPE EXCERPTS PRESENTED TO PANEL

Session 1

Setting: Clinic office
Present: Mother, Father, Jacob, and three of his siblings

The children are actively playing with toys in the office while the psychiatrists talk to the parents. There is a lot of noise in the background, and on a few occasions Jacob can be heard shouting at his siblings. The mother makes several comments about Jacob:

> Yesterday he hit me so hard in the head that I could not believe it . . . He doesn't care who you are . . . He will go after you if he's mad.
>
> He's been dismissed from several day care centers . . . Last week he got into a fight with another boy and drew blood.
>
> I don't think he likes me . . . I think he's out to get me . . . I think he wants to see how far he can go before I make him leave . . . He's driving me crazy.

Ms. K also commented on her feelings about her current husband:

> I get angry with him . . . He works all day until 6:00 P.M. and comes home without a lot of understanding for me . . . He doesn't know how I feel being left home all day long constantly fighting with a 3-year-old.

Session 2 (5 days later)

Setting: Clinic office
Present: Mother and Jacob

Ms. K states:

> I've never had a real father . . . My biological father was a horrible man
> . . . I am embarrassed saying this . . . I have never told this to anybody,
> but you are a doctor so it is OK . . . I'd give anything to have a real father
> . . . I would like to be daddy's little girl . . . Even my stepfather was a loser
> . . . That's why it's so important for me to stick with this [marriage] . . .
> I am doing this for my daughter.

While Ms. K is reflecting on this, Jacob is quieter and more focused on exploring toys.

Session 3 (10 days later)

Setting: Clinic office
Present: Mother, Jacob, infant sister, and the two clinicians

Video scene: Jacob is busy playing with the dollhouse on the floor, interacting with the two clinicians. Ms. K. and the baby sister are sitting on a sofa watching these interactions. Mother states:

> He doesn't like being touched . . . Sometimes he does like it when his
> older brother body slams him.

Later Jacob moves to the sofa and is praised for being nice to his sister. He then inadvertently pulls on her hair and is scolded by his mother. After the scolding, Jacob moves away from his mother, who comments on his sensitivity to being reprimanded. Finally, Jacob settles on the floor with his head resting on the lap of one of the clinicians. His legs are extended toward the other clinician. We start discussing a possible intervention strategy (i.e., using deep pressure massage to soothe Jacob). One of us demonstrates this technique by applying deep pressure (squeezing) to Jacob's legs. Jacob seems to enjoy this, taking off his socks spontaneously. This action prompts us to continue the intervention. Jacob's anxiety level decreases noticeably, he appears more relaxed, and he lies very still and seems less angry overall.

Ms. K comments:

> Jacob, you are so lucky . . . You have two doctors massaging you and giving you all that attention.

Later on, she says she is going to try this technique at home.

Session 4 (4 days later)

Setting: Jacob's home
Present: Mother and Jacob

One of the clinicians is interacting with Jacob as the other one observes. They are in Jacob's room, where they play with several toys (e.g., small dolls, stuffed animals). We attempt to evaluate whether Jacob can pretend play because this symbolic ability is crucial to determining his diagnosis and prognosis. One of us pretends to be drinking from a cup, eating a piece of bread, and feeding a baby doll. At first, Jacob appears confused and is very quiet, observing the psychiatrist. Eventually, he begins to imitate the clinician's behavior, still seemingly unsure of what he is doing. After several minutes, Jacob becomes more involved in the play and actually chuckles and laughs, but he does not display any "spontaneous" pretending. Most of his pretending is a direct imitation of the sequences and actions shown to him by the clinician. Nevertheless, he has genuine pleasure in the play he is sharing with the adult who is engaging him. It is notable that Jacob's speech is very difficult to understand. He says very little. On the other hand, he seems to enjoy the interaction and, with prompting, is able to pretend and play. He is fully engaged in this reciprocal exchange and is truly playing.

CONSULTANTS' OBSERVATIONS AND SUGGESTIONS

Dr. Efrain Bleiberg: It is clear the therapists are helping this mother to play and to engage in symbolic exchanges with her child. It can be seen in the interaction with the clinicians. First, the child allows himself to be touched and then later engages in play.

The mother has some difficulty experiencing this child as a person with his own inner life and inner states. This difficulty makes it impossible for her to see the child as a person in vivo. That is, she is unable to read the child's intentionality, a process Dr. Fonagy has described as being important to development. This difficulty may interfere with the child's ability to acquire a self-reflective function. One striking aspect about this mother is that she is trapped in an impossible dilemma. She wants to be cared for by a father who has never been available to her. Another is how much this boy looks like his mother in terms of facial features, facial expressions, and gestures.

Certain cues can give the impression that some people have a tendency to avoid mentalizing. In this case, the mother seems to engage with her child in mostly negative interactions with little opportunity for reflection on his feelings and internal states. She expresses almost no joy in her son's productions, which may be due to her idealizing the hateful relationship with her biological father. She thought Jacob's father would fulfill the role of a protective, benign father vis-à-vis a little girl who is vulnerable and needs admiration and love, but he does not. So Jacob is perceived as a "monster." Later the mother comments on how lucky the child is to get so much (fatherly) attention from the two doctors.

From the last sequence (session 4), we see that this child can acquire some symbolic abilities, which would allow him to develop more appropriate human responses. These types of children are at risk—tremendous risk. This child is giving some ominous signs that he cannot mentalize and cannot reflect (e.g., he does not feel pain). Not only does he use aggression to deal with experiences, but he also shifts consistently away from feelings. Any type of vulnerability is perceived as dangerous. He escapes into a narcissistic, predatory, antisocial type of destructiveness, which is what the clinicians are trying to prevent.

Acknowledging her own pain is what will allow this woman to embark on the seemingly impossible task of coping with her child. It is what needs to happen in order for her to see the child as a human being rather than as a monster. She needs to see her own pain, deprivation, sadness, and losses epitomized in her questions: "Who provides me with a massage?" and "Who will give me deep relaxation?"

A fundamental piece of the intervention is to begin to talk with the family. In addition, as Dr. Pines and Dr. Maldonado have already begun to do, there is a need not only to model for the mother ways to make the relationship with Jacob more rewarding but also to show her how to play with Jacob and help him relax, calm down, and organize his experience. This approach would allow an appropriate outlet for his difficult feelings instead of forcing him to discharge them through motor aggression. He needs to begin to symbolize. To facilitate this process, there should be some discussion of Jacob's needs. It would be difficult to talk to the mother directly about her projections. I feel it is great that the therapists can play with the child and help to relax him. But what would give his mother a break and allow her to relax? Going through the back door, without talking to her as a patient directly, may be the answer. To connect to Jacob, she first needs to deal with her own needs, issues of abandonment, rage, and disappointment.

Dr. Susan McDonough: I would suggest a relational-focused approach to deal with some of the presenting issues. It may well be that parallel processes need to occur simultaneously, a process between the mother and the therapists and a process between the mother and the child. Dr. Bleiberg spoke about the mother's neediness and her deprivation, and how important it is for her to be fueled and then to fuel her children. I agree with this need.

I was also struck by the child's behavioral problems, particularly by his developmental delays. I suspect these delays go beyond what might be encountered in an emotionally impoverished environment. He is speaking in one-word utterances at age 3. He has disorganized patterns of behavior. I would suggest referring the child for evaluation to the school district staff; the evaluation usually comprises, at the least, an occupational therapy assessment, language evaluation, and cognitive testing. He seems to have extreme sensitivities, especially tactile ones. It would make it very difficult for his mother, father, and anyone else who is not tuned in to this child's differences to know how to relate to him in a way that is not overstimulating or counterproductive. I would like to raise the possibility that, biologically, he is a vulnerable child. The language delay, in particular, seems remarkable, and it would make communication between a very busy and overwhelmed mother and her child quite difficult.

It is hard to find gratifying experiences with him. I think that, while it is certainly important to be attentive to the dynamics of the parent-child relationship, the two psychiatrists actually tried to put some parameters around the stimulation this child was receiving, such as one-to-one interaction and an adequate level of stimulation. He calmed down, focused, and was more available to the clinician's overtures to engage him in play. In the meantime, Jacob's mother is very interested in how to provide her infant daughter with the environment she herself always wanted, but she has four other children to attend to. When the mother was able to be less distracted, we could see her watching Jacob interact with the doctors. She took some delight in this scenario, although she might also have been quite envious of it.

I was also struck by the physical similarities between Jacob and his mother. She identifies with Jacob as the reincarnation of this terrible man (her father)—but she protests perhaps too much. Overall, this case is fascinating.

Dr. Bleiberg: Regarding the issue of vulnerabilities in the child, it does not really matter how scientifically true this situation is or is not. The acknowledgment or confirmation that her son has inherent vulnerabilities might be helpful to Ms. K; it might help her feel a little more comfortable with the formidable challenge of rearing Jacob.

Dr. McDonough: Perhaps by helping her feel less guilty, the therapists' work with Ms. K might be more successful for helping the child achieve what he is capable of. She might develop some insight into her own contributions to Jacob's difficulties without becoming paralyzed by a sense of guilt. She would then understand that he may have some biological vulnerabilities that would make this child difficult for any parent. Such understanding might free her to try to engage with her son in a way that is unsuccessful.

Dr. Bleiberg: I have found it helpful to become ignorant of the extraordinary complexities about how children develop problems because we really do not know much about that. It might be helpful to say to the mother, "I do not know how you do it . . . you really have a tough challenge." In fact, one of the dangers is that the mother is looking at these two doctors, who are so competent and loving, and she might feel, "Please do it to me (massage me) . . . I could not possibly be that competent." I am more inclined to take the opposite position. I would be more likely to say, "My God, how did you survive? We have all these diplomas on the wall and all this training, . . . but we only work with the child for 1 hour, and then we are gone (like the husband) . . . With all of the resources we have, we would struggle much with a child like Jacob. How do you do it?"

Dr. Serge Lebovici: This family is very difficult; all the things one sees are a bit overwhelming. It is hard to sort out where to start. One aspect that should not be overlooked is that the mother has a baby in her arms. The mother may find it quite difficult to give this baby appropriate attention. I would focus on ways she could give this baby the necessary attention she deserves. I would help her to work more effectively with the baby. Her needs should not be put in the back seat, despite the many demands on the mother and the needs Jacob has.

I was also very impressed by how helpful the massage was to Jacob. After the massage, he was able to hold his sister more appropriately and engage in pretend play more effectively. The massage seemed to help reduce his chaotic experience. He was able to play symbolically, perhaps for the first time. This result illustrates the importance of working with the individual child, as well as with the parents. In Jacob's case, the massage may be an experience of being contained, highlighting for the little boy his body-ego and reassuring him that there are boundaries and that others are there to support him. I think the technique is one the mother might use in the future; it also illustrates the importance of paying attention to the uniqueness of each child.

Dr. Peter Fonagy: I am not in much disagreement with the previous observations and comments. But I would like to make a few provocative comments, the first concerning the aggression Dr. Bleiberg touched on. The main symptom that is disturbing about this young child is that he keeps attacking other children, as we saw in the first session with his siblings and as we learned from his history. We know that of all the symptoms a child could manifest at this age, the only one with bad prognostic indicators is this kind of aggression. One therapeutic approach is to agree with the mother's theory that the aggression is biological (i.e., largely genetic) and the child has some developmental delays because of "bad genes or a bad father." Although we would all agree the situation is overwhelmingly complex, aggression is something we can understand as a desperate defensive maneuver by the child to protect a very fragile sense of self or self-representation. When the child's sense of self is intruded on—for instance, through touch (something that most of us welcome rather than fight)—Jacob has to protect both himself and his self-representation. This line of reasoning suggests the problems of this child and his family should be considered a byproduct of a whole range of complex processes, some of them biological.

The next point is that the importance of "the body" in such children is immense. You have to understand why the deep pressure massage that works for this child may not work for another 3-year-old. Dr. Lebovici suggested massage was an organizing experience. When you do not have adequate mental representation, the body becomes the host for most of the self-experience that would normally be reflected on mentally. For Jacob, the massage is qualitatively different: it is actually an organization of his internal world. If you observe the massage as a microanalytic sequence, you notice odd little behaviors in the videotape. When the left leg is being massaged, the right leg "wants" a part of it and moves over. It is almost as if a real jealousy state exists between the two legs. In actuality, it is the same body, but for this child it may not be.

Dr. Bleiberg: I think Dr. Fonagy has given a very elegant formulation of this child's experience and how he copes. The point I would like to emphasize refers less to how the child experiences life, because I see the therapeutic task as trying to help this mother and family behave differently with the child. I agree with the formulation of how Jacob experiences his own body, his sense of urgency, and his difficulty with choosing and directing his own being. His own behavior is limited, and he needs to defend it with aggression. He has a tendency to experience bodily what other children would experience symbolically.

There is, however, the risk of emphasizing too much or too exclusively biological factors or complex mechanisms, such as a gene, to explain the child's problems. If emphasizing biology is done, Jacob's mother might believe even more firmly her son was born a psychopath, and she is justified in putting on him all of her rage and disappointment and her sense of his being out of control. How do we provide her a different formulation from the standpoint of interventions? What can we offer this mother and father and their family? The father is volunteering for every shift possible; his home life has become his work, and his work has become his home. The context in which this woman receives or fails to receive emotional support may or may not allow her to mentalize the child. How do we make sense of this situation and understand what needs to be done about it to provide them practical assistance? We need to help them develop ideas about what to do in a way that allows them to hear our interpretations without becoming more defensive. We need to help this mother begin to see her child with less entrenched negative views. We need to engage the family therapeutically while also defining the problem, all without exacerbating their difficulties or blaming the parents. An unspoken issue here is that the mother is at home with the child all the time. She "needs" the biologically based problem in the child. It alleviates her feeling of being incompetent, that she has tried but failed.

Dr. Lebovici: I agree with this assessment. This child acts with his body because he cannot act with his mind. There is a mandate for this child, a mandate to bring his family to treatment. The boy's responses, especially to the massage from the clinicians, show the effectiveness of having an active male involved with him in various interactions (i.e., the massage and the pretend play). Neither of these males has been a part of this child's life before. These interactions also illustrate the usefulness of conducting treatment with two individual clinicians. This treatment is often practiced in Europe because two therapists can share in the observation and interpretation and help each other with their reactions to individual children and families. Aside from the obvious economic factors that come into play in such a situation, we find this model of using two co-therapists helps each clinician sharpen his or her observations, see what the other does not capture, and support the other in this difficult therapeutic work.

Dr. Lucile Ware: One should be careful not to make the parents feel even guiltier; guilt is an occupational hazard of just being a parent. It would be important to also focus on the parents' competence, noting what they are doing well and helping them feel understood in their plight, not just with Jacob but also overall with how they are conducting their family life. Only then can they be ready to hear some practical suggestions.

Dr. McDonough: I would like to see this situation as an opportunity to assist the parents rather than just to add to their burden. I would like to select some segments of the videotape and present them to relieve the mother and, to a certain extent, the father from feeling so burdened. Jacob is a very challenging child; even with all of the psychiatrists' training and experience, it took time for them to find a way to achieve a positive encounter with him. One wonders whether Jacob is a child who from birth might have been more challenging rather than just a product of poor parenting. The mother appears to have parented her other children very successfully. I also appreciate Dr. Lebovici's concern about the infant daughter. It is hard for this mother to hold her two children in her mind at one time.

In terms of practical advice, the notion that the child seems to present some challenges that differ from those of the other children may be helpful. Thus, the mother and her husband could learn to behave differently with this boy. I would go with this notion of suggesting special activities to do with him, such as having special times together or rubbing him with lotion at naptime. When the mother thinks of these things spontaneously, I would compliment her on her marvelous insights and how she can capture what her little boy needs. I would encourage her to try this approach. It may also be helpful to the parents for the therapists to explain that this child can be exhausting for a family because of the energy it takes to raise him (perhaps more than is required for other children with two parents).

Dr. Lebovici: The two psychiatrists took obvious pleasure in the boy—one in conducting the massage, the other in playing with him. This therapeutic maneuver appears to be well accepted by the mother, who can see these males as interested in her son, interacting playfully with him, and commenting on his strengths, which she had not seen before. This interaction brings to mind her description of the absent father and the bad father who abandoned Jacob's mother. In a way, it is a corrective experience for the mother to see two males take pleasure in interacting with her son.

Dr. McDonough: One could use the videotape examples we saw today to show this mother how these interactions were pleasurable for the boy. One could select several segments and then discuss each one with her. This mother seems empty of feelings of competence. One would really have to work hard systematically to build up her feelings of self-worth. There is so much work to do that I am not certain why she should not be the patient.

Dr. Bleiberg: She did not come as the patient.

Dr. McDonough: Perhaps a relational focus could guide the treatment.

Dr. Bleiberg: This boy needs parents with a greater sense of competence. How does one get them to that point?

Dr. McDonough: Working with the mother could be a part of the treatment plan. I am concerned about the amount of energy it takes to work with the child and the parents. Is there any way we could be helpful to the therapists in helping the mother?

Dr. Bleiberg: This mother did start her own therapy process some months ago. She has lots of personal issues to work on in addition to her parenting concerns. From a clinical and practical standpoint, the question is how best to communicate with Ms. K so she can acknowledge her own need for help. This acknowledgment could occur more easily if the therapists did not focus on her psychopathology but, instead, talked about what she might be able to do with her son with some assistance. One of the wonderful aspects of life is that it offers opportunities for real reparation. As mental health professionals, we get into this field because of the desire to help people heal. By not explicitly focusing on this mother's own deprivation but by indirectly helping her understand the internal workings of her son, we may get closer to helping her address her own needs and her own experience. Perhaps there are some issues with which one could help her to get assistance for herself. What about including the adoptive father and getting him to play and deal with the boy?

Dr. Fonagy: The key intervention here is to teach the mother and father how to play with their child. As one saw clearly, by joining the child's pretend world, the psychiatrists fostered the child's integration of a psychic equivalent to understanding mental states by integrating the concrete world and the fantasy world. The fantasy world can be terribly frightening, but these two worlds can be brought together within the context of play when the child plays with a grownup. To me, what was heartening about this case was the extent to which the child could join in. When he did so, he seemed much more human. It would be helpful to help the mother get over her inhibitions about entering the pretend world of her child. Such an achievement would be practical and perhaps even enormously efficacious. It would be wonderful if all seven family members could pretend-play together.

SUMMARY

Jacob presented a number of difficult behaviors that were very disconcerting to his parents and were dealt with mostly by his mother. The intense relationship between mother and child was full of negative and unpleasant interactions. Through the interventions described in this chapter, Mr. and Ms. K were able to understand the meaning of Jacob's behavior in a different way. Their original theory was that he exhibited purposeful and angry behaviors to annoy his parents and siblings. Understanding his vulnerabilities and difficulties with sensory integration helped them move away from that idea. They started to implement techniques of soothing and monitoring Jacob's level of stimulation and overload. The parents not only gave him less negative feedback; they also attempted to praise him when he did not react aggressively. Jacob became more motivated to get along with them and please them. Mr. K made a conscious effort to come home earlier to participate in family interactions and be more involved in parenting. Later, Jacob was enrolled in a special preschool program where he could receive occupational and language therapy and also be part of a small group of children in the classroom. Mr. and Ms. K continued their couples therapy and eventually reported that, although Jacob was still a challenge, his angry behavior had diminished considerably and they were enjoying him more.

Ms. K appeared to believe someone had listened to her; this belief allowed her to move away from direct confrontations with Jacob and assume a more parental and containing role with her son. She also was able to begin speaking more openly about her own unmet childhood needs and realize some of them would never be met. Instead, she could try to provide for her children what she felt she had not received herself. As her husband felt less criticized, he became more supportive and involved and was better able to nurture her emotionally. The therapists left the door open for further consultation if the family required it in the future.

14

Physical Abuse and Neglect in the First 6 Months of Life

A Parent-Infant Psychotherapeutic Approach

Charles Millhuff, D.O.

Consultants
Kathryn E. Barnard, R.N., Ph.D.
Alice Eberhart-Wright, M.A.
Elizabeth Fivaz-Depeursinge, Ph.D., P.D., M.E.R.
Hisako Watanabe, M.D., Ph.D.
Lucile Ware, M.D. (Moderator)

In this chapter, I present and discuss a case that focuses on the diagnostic issues, treatment approaches, and additional efforts that may be required to provide effective treatment and care of a maltreated child. The chapter is organized into six main sections:

1. Presentation of the case
2. Discussion of the assessment and treatment planning issues

3. Descriptions of the first office visit by the child and her stepgrandmother, clinicians' visits to the grandparents' home and the day care
facility where the child spent most weekdays, and visits with the biological mother both in the clinic and in her home
4. Presentation of the formulation and outcome of treatment
5. Observations and suggestions of the consultants
6. Conclusion and case follow-up

The consultants—Kathryn Barnard, R.N., Ph.D., Alice Eberhart-
Wright, M.A., Elizabeth Fivaz-Depeursinge, Ph.D, P.D., M.E.R., and
Hisako Watanabe, M.D., Ph.D.—were presented simultaneously with details of the patient's history and treatment, including videotaped clips
from several clinical interviews. Their comments here are from a panel
discussion focusing on issues of diagnosis and intervention. The child
was seen at the infant mental health clinic at Menninger, where the consultants saw the clinical material and discussed with each other.

Katie was only 4 months old when she was diagnosed with a closed fracture of her left femur. The suspected cause was physical abuse by either
her mother or her mother's boyfriend. Katie was then assessed in the
emergency room, where she had been taken by her mother, and was immediately placed in the temporary care of the state's child protective
services. The mother said she did not know how the injury had happened.

Katie had been living at home with her 2-year-old half-brother,
Tommy; her mother, Carla; the mother's boyfriend, Jimmy; her maternal grandmother; and other extended family members on the maternal
side. The hospital's emergency room staff reported the child's situation
to child protective services because they thought the fracture was due to
physical abuse. Child protective services immediately placed Katie and
Tommy in a different home, that of their natural maternal grandfather
and his wife, Ms. P, who technically was Katie's stepgrandmother.

After a few days of this arrangement, which was a formal foster placement of Katie and Tommy, Ms. P became increasingly concerned about
a number of Katie's unusual behaviors. Katie screamed whenever her
diaper was being changed or whenever Ms. P left the room, even if only
for a moment. The stepgrandmother described Katie as acting intensely
"scared." Katie also acted extremely withdrawn and cautious whenever
new people were introduced into her environment.

In addition, at the first sight of a feeding bottle, Katie would start to
shake and cry, and when given the bottle, she would drink the contents
voraciously. She would suck so hard she would cry in frustration because
she became too agitated to suck well enough to drink the milk. Her
stepgrandmother and others also noticed Katie's clearly limited range
of affect; as Ms. P put it, "This baby doesn't smile."

Prior to Katie's fracture, the stepgrandmother was already concerned about neglect. While caring for Katie on evenings and week-

ends, she observed severe diaper rash, reddened cracked skin in the folds of her neck, and poor hygiene overall. She and others suspected Katie's mother commonly propped a bottle in Katie's mouth and then left Katie and her half-brother, Tommy, unattended for lengthy periods of time.

Katie was 5 months old when she arrived in our office for a mental health evaluation. The child protective services staff were concerned about the effects of the trauma on the baby and wanted to know what the grandparents could do to help Katie cope. The stepgrandmother welcomed this recommendation for a mental health evaluation. Ms. P said she had "forgotten many things" about taking care of young children, and she was concerned because of Katie's continued screaming, insecurity, and intense fears.

Katie was brought to her initial appointment by Ms. P and Katie's social worker from the referring social service agency. Because an evaluation and treatment would address several complex issues, we began by examining various domains of Katie's development, such as cognition, language, and emotional, social, and biological areas (e.g., sleep-wake cycles, eating patterns, motor coordination). We were particularly interested in how neglect and trauma had affected Katie's development. Further interventions involved visits to the various environments in Katie's world, including her stepgrandmother's home, the day care facility, a social service agency, and the home of her biological mother, who wanted to reintegrate Katie and Tommy into the family and in her care.

It was important to gain an understanding of not only the risk factors in Katie's life but any protective factors as well. Treatment primarily involved educating the grandparents, the mother, and the day care provider about Katie's special needs, focusing on Katie's current relationships so they could better meet those needs. We modeled various interventions and attempted to support and validate the experience of her caregivers. The effect of therapeutic work with Katie and her caregivers was demonstrated by her improved emotional regulation and ability to relate to others and to enjoy these relationships. Finally, this process helped clarify the readiness of the patient's mother for future primary caregiving responsibilities for her children.

ASSESSMENT AND TREATMENT PLANNING

Initial Office Visit

When Katie first arrived at our office with her stepgrandmother and the child protective services social worker, it was obvious her usual affect was of frozen watchfulness. It had been a week since her leg cast had been removed, but she still seemed to passively accept just lying in her baby carrier or to sit quietly on someone's lap.

Katie's motor coordination was ratchety and unsteady. She had a high muscular tone, and when picked up, she would stiffen, her whole body moving in the air as if made of one piece. She appeared mechanical and unable to relax. She tended not to bend her legs or arms, and she carried herself rigidly, with few natural movements of exploration or play. When presented with a toy, she did not reach for it; in fact, she seemed to have limited interest in even observing its movement across her visual field. Social reciprocity was noticeably absent, and she was generally silent or nonresponsive throughout much of our interview. Her muscular tone was high. She tended not to bend her legs or arms, exhibiting few natural movements of exploration or play. Only after we worked with her and her family for some time was she able to start moving and to express herself more freely.

We noticed when Katie was fed with the bottle, she would take up to eight sucks in a burst of feeding and then hold the bottle midline above her body. When feeding, Katie had a myoclonic movement in her jaw. She tended to gulp milk extremely fast, and she became almost disorganized trying to drink it. All her body limbs moved, she seemed unfocused and desperate, her breathing was very rapid, and she tried to drink the milk as quickly as possible.

Katie seemed to be the most connected to her stepgrandmother, who handled her carefully. From the beginning, Ms. P made statements about something being "wrong with this baby." She mentioned Katie often became frightened and upset, causing her whole body to shake. At such times, Ms. P usually felt exasperated because of her inability to console Katie enough to ease her discomfort. Ms. P's voicing of these concerns led to a discussion about what might actually have happened to Katie before she was removed from her mother's care.

Ms. P was very troubled and sad about the neglect and physical pain she suspected Katie had endured. She was extremely angry at the biological mother and whomever else may have been involved in Katie's sustaining a fracture.

From observing the present interaction between Katie and her stepgrandmother, we began to realize Ms. P was indeed struggling. She said it was difficult to remember the parenting techniques she had used with her two boys, both now grown. Ms. P also seemed quite emotionally distant from the baby. She would place Katie on the floor with her bottle propped up, and she tried hard to sculpt the position of Katie's hands so she could learn how to drink from the bottle by herself as quickly as possible. Ms. P appeared very capable of feeding, changing, and bathing Katie. However, there was little joy in the process, and she appeared to keep an emotional distance from the baby.

Ms. P seemed apprehensive about the special circumstances of Katie's life and feared she was somehow going to worsen Katie's condition. Although Ms. P's philosophy with her boys had been to promote self-sufficiency, Katie was clearly unable to accept this approach, as demonstrated by her intense screaming whenever her stepgrandmother left the room. Because Katie appeared uncomfortable except in her stepgrandmother's arms, Ms. P was eager to learn what she could from our visit. Her agenda appeared to be to get Katie to be less needy and to learn to manage things by herself. Yet, Ms. P often asked what she was *supposed to do* when the baby does this or that.

As the account of the children's experience in their mother's home unfolded, we began to realize Katie's behavior was largely due to severe neglect and deprivation of stimuli. It was possible she was also scared, had witnessed violence between the mother and her boyfriend, and had received harsh treatment from both of them, becoming hypervigilant.

Recognizing the importance of Katie's stepgrandmother as the primary caregiver at this point, we worked to help Ms. P understand Katie's need for increased social interaction. We interpreted Katie's behavior as an attempt to gain more input and become more attached to caregivers because she often signaled her anxiety about being left alone and wanted the reassurance of a consistent and reliable attachment figure. Rather than discouraging Ms. P from responding to Katie's neediness, we recommended just the opposite. Ms. P began to realize that to help facilitate the child's development, it was necessary to become more attached to the child. Ms. P seemed relieved to understand that Katie's ability to attach socially was more important at this time than self-reliance and self-soothing.

We began to explain and model for the stepgrandmother several ways she could promote Katie's social relatedness. First we explained the possible effects of neglect on Katie's ability to focus her gaze on other people or to engage in visual exchanges or "conversations." Also, the lack of touch and of contingent responses possibly had led to Katie's hypertonicity and difficulty in modulating her own emotions and behavior. It was also possible Katie's exposure to drugs in utero could have contributed to these features. During an office visit, we practiced a massage technique that seemed to soothe Katie; her hypertonicity diminished, and she was able to manage a brief smile when sung to. This technique could be used to calm Katie when she appeared uncomfortable, overstimulated, or upset.

Regarding feeding, we suggested to Ms. P that she hold Katie in her arms as if to mold, protect, and physically soothe her during this usually agitating and disorganized time. We also encouraged Ms. P to engage in playing animated social games, "reading" (showing pictures), and singing as a way to connect with Katie both visually and auditorily. Ms. P admitted with some embarrassment that she had forgotten songs to sing to babies, so we practiced some together: doing so seemed to give her "permission" to soothe the baby and respond to her, as she quickly remembered and felt comfortable singing to Katie. It was important to stimulate, encourage, and validate the reemerging natural mothering abilities of Katie's step-grandmother. We were relieved to see a reduction of Ms. P's level of anxiety regarding whether she could adequately care for Katie. After several days, Ms. P noted Katie cried less and appeared less scared.

Grandparents' Home

The next step in the intervention process involved leaving the office—that is, meeting Katie and her grandparents in their home environment. It seemed necessary to observe and assess Katie's behavior in her usual surroundings and to see how comfortable Katie felt without the new stimuli that were present in the office. For this home visit to Mr. and Ms. P, we traveled north of town to a neighborhood perhaps best described as being in the middle- to low-socioeconomic level. While traveling, we discussed our concerns about racial issues that might arise with other members of Katie's family, or even in the surrounding neighborhood, because one of the therapists was not Caucasian. We were aware of Ms. P's mild apprehension about the reception we would receive from her husband. (We later learned he was involved in a white supremacist group.)

As we entered the grandparents' home on a cold January day, we noticed it seemed modest but comfortable, clean, and adequately heated. Katie's older brother, Tommy, was obviously excited by our arrival, as demonstrated by his energetic overactivity. Ms. P continued to be receptive and had many questions about how to accomplish certain changes in Katie. Mr. P was cordial. (We later found out from Katie's mother that the grandparents were particularly willing to cooperate because this was their only female grandchild and their first opportunity to raise a baby girl.) During the visit, we learned from Ms. P that Katie was doing better and had fewer and less intense outbursts. She was becoming much more interested in people around her and was showing a greater range of affect and some initial verbal overtures. Her improved behavior was clearly evident as we sat on the floor and played with her and her family.

This home visit had a calming effect on the therapists, who began to think that Katie's situation was less urgently in need of remedy and that some adaptive processes and tendencies had been set in motion for both the child and her caregivers. At that time, we became more acutely aware of Katie's older brother, Tommy, who seemed to require an inordinate amount of energy to contain. Tommy was 2½ years old and seemed able to express his need for inclusion only through physical overactivity and intrusiveness rather than through verbal exchanges or reciprocal interactions. One of the family's central concerns was his rough play with

Katie. He had practically no language skills and seemed to focus on others for only seconds at a time. Thus, he seemed unable to maintain two-way interactions or to close circles of communication. His stepgrandmother described him as a "wild child" who bounced from toy to toy and seemed unable to focus on anything. Whenever anyone tried to engage him by holding him, he resisted by screaming, pushing, hitting, and trying to bite. His stepgrandmother complained that she could not do "anything" with Tommy and that he was developmentally delayed in many ways and was unable to do what many children his age could do.

The children's grandfather sat in his chair throughout our visit and spoke little. He did not appear discouraging of our efforts, but he was minimally involved with the children.

The grandparents frequently issued commands and admonitions to Tommy, with asides to us to explain he "knew better" than to climb on furniture or run around the house and he was just "showing off" by throwing things all over the place. We started to see a dichotomy of the grandparents' feelings toward her brother vis-à-vis Katie, whom they were starting to call "Miss Sunshine." In a moment of anger, the stepgrandmother said that when she was a child, she'd had her own "butt spanked" and that's how she had learned the difference between right and wrong. The grandparents expressed concern about spoiling their grandchildren if they did not use sterner measures to correct the kinds of behavior that Tommy was displaying.

This home visit also provided us with some insight into Katie's biological mother, Carla, who was the daughter of Mr. P and his first wife but had not been raised by Mr. and Ms. P. They recognized that Carla's biological mother was an "irresponsible mess" and expressed their own feelings of guilt for not having had more contact with Carla while she was growing up. This distance—emotional and geographic—and the associated feelings of guilt seemed to be their rationale for enduring the stress of raising Katie and Tommy, which was especially evident in the boy's disruptive attitude that day. In addition, the home visit helped us gain an appreciation for other stresses faced by the caregivers; to address Tommy's troubles, we worked with the grandparents to encourage methods similar to those used with Katie. Later, more individualized treatment was arranged for Tommy, who was clearly struggling with his own history of neglect and maltreatment.

Day Care Facility

Our next request was to observe the children in the day care facility where Katie and Tommy spent most of their weekdays. The day care was a home where children are looked after for 8–10 hours at a time while the stepgrandmother worked. The day care provider, Sandy, greeted us at the door. A busy, serious woman in her late 30s, Sandy usually provides day care for an average of 10 children. She immediately highlighted her permission to allow us to wear our shoes in her home; it was generally the custom for everyone to remove their shoes after entering. She quickly showed us around the first floor of her home where Katie and seven or eight other children occupied two rooms primarily. Sandy did not introduce us to the other children but instead left us to return to cooking. One of the children was very wary and anxious, crying in fear and trying to get Sandy to hold him. He signaled he wanted to be held in her arms, and she responded by telling him "It's all right" and he should not be scared.

Katie was in a walker, playing with some toys on the tray of the walker. She appeared to be trying to follow Sandy around but was not allowed to enter the kitchen. It was difficult for Katie to move the walker because of her hypertonicity and the thick shag carpeting. At this point, Katie started to cry and shake physically. She seemed completely desolate, alone, and without any internal resources to help her try to feel better. Her crying escalated to the point of screaming until she was able to see Sandy again. Katie did not seem afraid of us but, instead, seemed more bothered by Sandy going away from her into another room. Sandy finally returned to Katie, trying to soothe her by talking to her and offering her toys. Sandy did not pick up Katie because she did not want Katie to think she would be held whenever she cried. She voiced her relief about our seeing what she had to deal with all day long. Perhaps because of Katie's continued cries and requests for her arms, Sandy eventually picked up the child, who then became calmer. We told Sandy that Katie seemed to feel more secure in her arms, and we speculated aloud about how lonely Katie may have felt just previously. We suggested that Katie would not continue in the long run to be as needy once she felt more reassured and safe, and we told her this change would more likely occur with increased soothing interactions and contact from Sandy. With Sandy, we examined Katie's tendency to become tremulous, disorganized, and inconsolable. Sandy was intrigued with the idea of monitoring the level of stimulation (e.g., auditory, visual, tactile) that Katie was being exposed to and holding her to help her cope with overstimulation. She showed curiosity about all these ideas and said she would give them a try.

Tommy then became the center of attention as his overactivity and impulsivity led to combativeness with another child. He seemed unaware of how his behavior affected others and the fact that Sandy did not tolerate certain actions. Just moments earlier, he had shown a prosocial gesture toward his sister, who was upset and crying vigorously: he had brought her a toy in an effort to soothe her. We realized Tommy was reminding us of our need not to forget him in the midst of all the attention we were giving his sister.

We sat on the floor and continued to practice with the day care provider several ways to promote social exchanges, pleasurable sequences, and play between Katie and her brother. We noticed some improvements in Katie's range of affect and interest in others. She was now more likely to grab at toys with curiosity, put them in her mouth, and make social noises. She exhibited modestly improved motor coordination. Gentle massage, singing, and animated social interaction had moved Katie into a space where she was calmer and moving toward more age-appropriate developmental skills. Tommy also benefited from this sort of interaction because he no longer seemed so combative.

Biological Mother

It seemed important to try to get a firsthand version of what had happened to Katie that had previously resulted in the fractured femur and also her care prior to that incident. Thus, to complete Katie's evaluation, we needed to speak with Katie's biological mother, Carla. We also wanted to meet with Carla because she had expressed hope of getting her children back at some time. However, Carla was already having fewer scheduled and supervised visits as the process of reintegrating her into the lives of her children began. Ms. P, who was then caring for Katie and Tommy, still directed a significant amount of animosity toward Carla. Because of this difficulty, maternal visits were supervised and usually took place at various agencies. During those visits, it was clear Carla behaved in a naïve, cautious, and withdrawn manner in her interactions with her children. Nineteen-year-old Carla, who had Tommy when she was 16 and Katie when she was 18, was now 3 months pregnant with her third child. She had a different partner for each pregnancy. None of the fathers were present, and all had multiple legal and delinquent problems. When Tommy and Katie were still living with her, Carla would often sit in her chair and observe them on the floor while her stepmother and others redirected Tommy and held or played with both children.

Carla seemed interested in her children but overwhelmed with a multitude of problems, including an upcoming court appearance for beating a cousin unconscious, which resulted in a "head concussion" when she fell on a rock. Carla stated, "I'm a straightforward person, and people can't stand me." She further said, "People follow me around like dogs and stuff."

Carla said she had not planned to become pregnant a third time and explained that the contraceptive implant (Depo-Provera) in her arm had apparently failed. She admitted smoking marijuana once every 1 or 2 weeks for the first 3 months of her previous pregnancy to reduce her anxiety and insomnia. She said she also had used "crank" (methamphetamine) daily for the first 4 months of her pregnancy with Katie. In fact, she said 1 month into that pregnancy, she had overdosed on crank. But she denied using alcohol then. Carla said when she realized she was pregnant with Katie, she stopped using drugs of abuse about 3 or 4 months into the pregnancy.

We spent time discussing Katie's fractured leg. Carla denied knowing how the break had occurred. She implied that possibly Tommy—her 2-year-old son—had picked up Katie and then dropped her. She also wondered whether her boyfriend might have injured Katie out of frustration. Finally, she presented the possibility that Katie's femur was broken in the emergency room during her physical examination. Carla said, "When they started messin' around with her and stuff . . . that's when she [Katie] started screamin' and cryin' the most. They [the emergency room clinicians] could have done it."

Carla was able to acknowledge her overwhelming problems with substance abuse and limited parenting abilities. She also recognized her less-than-ideal living arrangements, which were overcrowded and chaotic. At this point, we had gained important information about Katie's exposure to drugs in utero and that similar circumstances were likely present for her brother, Tommy.

After this visit with Carla at the clinic, we decided to visit her at home. We were particularly interested in Carla's mental health and that of her developing fetus, and we wanted to suggest some interventions she might use.

Carla's home was a decrepit house in a rough part of town; the front stoop of the house lacked steps. When we were invited in, we immediately noticed a foul odor and the home's damp and desolate atmosphere. A number of people were living in this house. One man, barely clothed, was lying on the couch, with no seeming appreciation that visitors had entered his home. We asked if we could speak to Carla privately, and he left without saying much. Despite the unkempt surroundings, Carla seemed at ease. We voiced our concern about possible symptoms of depression and posttraumatic stress disorder that she evidenced, which she agreed with. We encouraged her to seek supportive services, including psychotherapy (we told her we could find her a therapist if she consented), so she could learn to cope without drugs. We mentioned medication might be an option, particularly later on, when she was able to be free of drugs.

We also suggested she needed collaborative help with her family reintegration plan. She had several excuses about why she had missed appointments with her children. We could see she was struggling to make it to numerous appointments designed for her well-being.

While getting to know Carla, we learned of her own history of trauma and neglect. She described her stepfather as a man who severely abused her physically from 5 to 12 years of age, when he died of a heart attack. She said her stepfather was a Vietnam veteran (a man with apparent symptoms consistent with posttraumatic stress disorder) who broke numerous bones in her body. She and her younger sister were repeatedly abandoned by their biological mother, who would leave for weeks at a time on drinking binges. As a result of their chaotic home, she and her sister took on the responsibility of raising themselves with some assistance from their neighbors. By age 13, Carla was abusing alcohol heavily, drinking up to two pints of tequila a day. She became involved in gang activities and eventually was placed in a locked girls' home for about a year. She dropped out of high school and became pregnant for the first time with Tommy. She mentioned that she had had multiple fractures, many of which she did not remember but which had been discovered when she had a CT scan and numerous healed fractures were discovered in her limbs.

Carla was clearly a survivor of many severe adversities. We encouraged further visits for treatment, and she continued to be a marginal participant.

FORMULATION AND OUTCOME OF TREATMENT

The primary concerns for Katie at presentation were her developmental delays and questions about how trauma and neglect had affected her short life and what could be done to help her heal from such adversities. From a biological standpoint, strong heritable factors most likely put Katie at risk for developing a mental disorder. The substance abuse tendency and alcoholism that ran deeply through her maternal side of the family may have predisposed her to other mental disorders. Unfortunately, no paternal history was available during the course of this evaluation. In addition, there were concerns about the reported severe substance abuse of Katie's mother, Carla, while she was pregnant with the child. Carla's heaviest use had occurred during the first trimester, with the overdose of methamphetamine just 1 month into the pregnancy. Clinicians will need to keep this substance use in mind when measuring the possible longitudinal effects of Katie's in utero drug exposure. This history partially explained Katie's difficulties. There were also questions about the adequacy of nutrition in the patient's mother as well as Carla's own depressed state and high level of stress and their effects on Katie in utero. Finally, Katie suffered considerable physical pain, not only from the fractured femur but also from long-standing skin irritations and rashes.

In terms of Katie's emotional life, there was evidence that her mother had much difficulty engaging with Katie in any pleasurable exchanges. The baby was also exposed to frequent quarrels and confrontations between her mother and her mother's boyfriend. It is very likely Katie was handled roughly and unempathically, thus leading to the fracture.

Given the suffering that Katie has endured, her frozen watchfulness is consistent with that of other infants who have faced this kind of life experience. The chronic trauma and neglect significantly affected her motor coordination, as well as her social, emotional, language, and cognitive developmental abilities. She has demonstrated immense anticipatory anxiety triggered by various reminders of previous neglectful and traumatizing caregivers. Nevertheless, Katie might be seen superficially as a child who was "all right" in the sense that she looked chubby and was able to eat, sleep, and gaze into people's faces for brief periods of time. Thus, the effects of trauma can be overlooked by someone unaccustomed to seeing them in small infants. Despite her significant setbacks, Katie has demonstrated a capacity to move forward in her development, aided primarily by the marked change to a more sensitive and healthful human environment.

Much of the work beyond our initial assessment was focused on educating—in the broadest sense (sensitizing, empathizing, speaking for the baby, giving permission to nurture the child)—the caregivers about Katie's needs and how to address them. This process involved meeting in Katie's environment with those who provided her care. The developing treatment alliance with Katie and her caregivers was essentially a rewarding experience as we all observed Katie's rebound from her early life adversities.

CONSULTANTS' OBSERVATIONS AND SUGGESTIONS

Dr. Kathryn Barnard

This infant's resilience and struggle to thrive and communicate are remarkable despite the obvious challenges she faces. Yet the baby has a frozen look and lacks spontaneous and relaxed activity (e.g., she rushes to suck from the bottle in a single burst). Katie's attempts to manage to hold the bottle and support it with both hands midline are impressive, as is her ability to listen to her stepgrandmother, perhaps the most important person in her life. It will be critical to see what happens over the next 6–12 months, which will be crucial in terms of supplementing her development or creating further difficulties if her needs go unmet. The essential question here might be, What can be done regarding Carla, the biological mother, and her capacity to step up emotionally to the task of mothering? After all, she is expecting a third baby, and she has started to articulate her own need for intervention. The possibility of forming a treatment alliance with her seems extremely fragile. Of particular concern are Carla's many chronic past difficulties, which may render her mistrustful as well as unable to see others as potentially helpful. She may also have difficulty developing alternative coping abilities, that is, a life without drugs.

There is also a need to continue focusing on the stepgrandmother's ability to parent Katie and Tommy by providing them with as much support as possible. In our society, grandparents who have reared their own children are frequently enlisted to rear their grandchildren. However, rearing a grandchild is an "out of step" challenge developmentally. Grandparents, who have their own personal needs and interests, must postpone many of their own activities and pursuits to devote time and energy to a small baby. This issue needs to be addressed and explored with these grandparents to facilitate their feeling of being understood and supported.

Ms. Alice Eberhart-Wright

Many questions about this highly complex family structure remain unanswered. It may be necessary to spend more time exploring the family history of these children and their parents; to this end, a detailed genogram might be useful. Obtaining a better idea of the multigenerational patterns that exist would add a perspective on Carla and her situation—beyond that of individual psychopathology—placing Carla in the wider context of a system in which themes and dramas repeat from one generation to the next. The question is whether this repetition can be avoided with this mother and her children or whether our only hope is to intervene with the children. It seems clear this baby's mother had never made a significant attachment in her own life. Further assessments should focus on "coaching" caregivers, including the biological mother, in their interactions with Katie. To be successful in this effort, it is important to use "naturalistic" assessment methods, not artificial methods such as office visits or standardized assessment tools. The more structured assessment methods might increase tension for Carla and her children and would also be less likely to give an accurate picture of their struggles and strengths.

The more a therapist insists on a traditional model of providing help (i.e., having the children's mother come to appointments at a specified time for a preestablished amount of time and behave like a participant patient), the less likely the approach is to succeed. The same would be true if a clinician with the best of intentions was to focus mostly on Carla's symptoms and weaknesses. She would likely feel misunderstood and demoralized. Focusing on what she does well or any other positive points would perhaps lead to a more promising response.

Dr. Elizabeth Fivaz-Depeursinge

Most clinicians would feel overwhelmed in the face of the enormous and long-standing problems presented by this young mother, especially in light of her devastating childhood circumstances. She obviously needs a great deal of help. But the question remains open: How much time can two young children afford to wait for their mother to improve enough so she is able to protect and care for them? My own experience leads me to believe the therapists should continue to use techniques in the here and now, such as placing the baby in the stepgrandmother's lap and helping her practice closeness, expressions of warmth, and responsiveness. This pattern of interaction has been therapeutic for Katie and facilitated her development since the intervention. The therapists may need to focus on what they have to work with, that is, a stepgrandmother and, to some extent, a grandfather. These relatives are the lifeline for these young children, given the uncertainty about the mother's motivation or ability to change within a certain time framework. While work with the biological mother proceeds on the side, if possible, the bulk of the therapeutic work can take place in the only family environment these children have now. The stepgrandmother needs to get all the support she can get to manage coping with a new and unexpected situation: being a mother to young children all over again.

Dr. Hisako Watanabe

Families like Katie's suffer the effects of the deprivation of the "everyday." That is, simple things other families might take for granted are missing from Katie's life; just being able to survive is a major accomplishment for this family. It is even a big step for these family members to just make it to appointments. In working with families or individual patients with these kinds of problems, therapists should be aware that their object world interacts with those of the mother, the infant, and other family members and caregivers. It is easy to dismiss the family as beyond help; to help a mother like Carla, the therapist has to be sensitive and be able to empathize with her situation and life history, as well as with the transgenerational themes that she represents. With hopefulness and sensitivity, the therapist can interact with the mother's internal world to convey hope (or despair). The presence of so many severe problems may lead a therapist to feel despair and even to ask (as the baby's mother may have asked), How can anyone make sense of this life of abuse?

Chaos is the norm in Carla's life. When the therapists enter her home environment, they feel unsettled and perceive sensations that make them uncomfortable. Surprisingly, Carla appears completely at ease and is unable to appreciate the stressful circumstances that are part and parcel of her world; it is as if a long time ago she had renounced any expectations of anything different. She lives in a state of being that might qualify in her eyes as having been "abandoned by God."

The role of the distant grandfather remains unclear. He apparently had little to do with his daughter in everyday life while she was growing up. Now, years later, he is instrumental in seeking a severance of contact between Carla and her children, Katie and Tommy. Yet day to day, the grandfather is more a passive observer of rather than an active participant in their lives.

CONCLUSION

Katie came to the clinicians' office with obvious, undeniable effects of maltreatment (e.g., a bone fracture). Unfortunately, this degree of maltreatment is frequent. In this case, the fracture facilitated the child's receiving help in the context of her relationship with her new caregivers. There are other infants, equally neglected or maltreated, who would receive no interventions because something as obvious as a fracture did not happen to them.

The effects of neglect and maltreatment at such a young age can easily be overlooked. A very young infant like Katie does not speak, is unable to be violent, and does not yet say "no." Nonetheless, she suffers the effects of deprivation and violence. Her emotional needs can easily go unmet if caregivers focus mostly on satisfying her physical needs. Children who have been maltreated have unique needs. Katie needs to be held a lot; she protests if she is left alone, and once she is with a caregiver, she appears unfocused and diffuse. She needs a great deal of supplementary care if she is to resume her emotional and interpersonal development.

The case demonstrates how the caregivers, including the day care provider, are able to adapt their caregiving practices to the needs of the child if they know what the needs are and are reassured that they are not spoiling her.

Caregiving by grandparents occurs frequently. It is often associated with the biological parents' use of drugs. Grandparents, even when experienced and well meaning, may need a lot of emotional support to be able to modify their lifestyle and satisfy the emotional needs of very young children. They must be able to get past their anger and resentment toward the biological parents and focus on the needs of the children who, after all, are not guilty of their parents' difficulties. In this case, the child's strengths and resilient qualities allowed her to respond quickly to the new way of relating to her, and she was able to start "rewarding" her stepgrandmother emotionally. This situation, in turn, reinforced the caregiver's motivation to continue providing for the infant's needs.

Katie is now 4½ years old. She and her brother, Tommy, who is now 6, have continued to live with their grandparents, who have adopted them. Their mother relinquished custody. After she had another baby girl, she felt that she could not take care of three children, and giving the grandparents custody of Katie and Tommy seemed to her the most sensible thing to do. Carla made several appointments around the period when we were seeing her older children. On two occasions she called, requesting to be seen as soon as possible, and said she would be there in 1 hour, as she felt depressed and desperate, and then she would not come. Carla now works as a waitress, and she is still using some drugs. Katie and Tommy see her occasionally.

Katie, who is still referred to as "Miss Sunshine" by her grandparents, is in a preschool. She has very good language skills. She makes little eye contact and has a short attention span, but she is easily engaged in things that are interesting. At times, she is brusque and, on occasion, aggressive with other children in the preschool, but her behavior is not a major problem. Her motor coordination is also not optimal, but she manages to do most things that her peers can do. Her stepgrandmother—now her adoptive mother—is not so concerned about her behavior or emotions.

Katie's brother, Tommy, has been followed by a child psychiatrist for 3 years now. He has been in individual play therapy and has had special education in preschool, including language and occupational therapy. He has taken small doses of psychostimulant medication since age 4. This medication helps with his concentration and ability to learn. He was a very angry little boy; gradually this anger has diminished. Now he is inattentive and hyperactive, but he is overall kind and has a sense of humor.

Index

Page numbers printed in **boldface type** *refer to tables or figures.*